T0265537

A SHAMA
HERBAL

"Wow! Matthew Wood, one of our great modern-day herbalists, integrates his knowledge and wisdom of spirit and soul into a rich medley of animal medicine, human health, and clinical experience. He is a brilliant poetic genius!"

ROBERT DALE ROGERS, RH (AHG), MYCOLOGIST
AND AUTHOR OF THE FUNGAL PHARMACY

"A unique and remarkable herbal that describes how plants work at a shamanic level. Through engaging stories and drawing on authentic experience, together with centuries-old wisdom, Matthew reveals how plants can assist us on a spiritual journey of transformation. Highly recommended for anyone interested in herbs and shamanism."

CAROLE GUYETT, AUTHOR OF SACRED PLANT INITIATIONS

"The title of this book doesn't begin to describe the range of what is covered within its pages. Along with fulfilling the title's promise, Matthew Wood looks at shamanism concerning Western traditions and religions."

EVELYN RYSDYK, AUTHOR OF THE NORSE SHAMAN

"When it comes to plant medicine, Matthew Wood is an absolute genius. With *A Shamanic Herbal*, he demonstrates how our ever-generous plant allies not only heal our bodies but also help our souls to evolve and guide us in experiencing wholeness/holiness."

JEN FREY, AUTHOR OF COMMUNICATING WITH PLANTS

"Matthew Wood explores the spiritual and cosmological patterns behind nature, people, and plants, showcasing how herbal medicines have the power to not only heal us physically but also to support our personal growth and spiritual development."

SAJAH POPHAM, AUTHOR OF EVOLUTIONARY HERBALISM

"As a formative, new, well-written, and well-researched book by master herbalist Matthew Wood, this book opens new doors for a greater understanding of the sacred tools used by shamans throughout the world. It is a comprehensive, inspiring, and practical journey."

ITZHAK BEERY,
AUTHOR OF *THE GIFT OF SHAMANISM*

"*A Shamanic Herbal* is an exploration of a myriad of traditions from the history of humanity in the quest for merging the messages of plants, animals, and the elements for a greater understanding of our place in the universe."

BRIGITTE MARS,
COAUTHOR OF *NATURAL REMEDIES FOR
MENTAL AND EMOTIONAL HEALTH*

"In this multidimensional study, Matthew Wood explores the various cross-cultural, mystical, and phenomenological paths that lead to a truly profound understanding of herbalism."

WOLF-DIETER STORL, PH.D.,
AUTHOR OF *THE HEART AND ITS HEALING PLANTS*

"As a lifelong practitioner of Plant Spirit Medicine and Animal Spirit Medicine, Matthew Wood gifts us with a truly profound volume. This is a book to turn to again and again, addressing both physical and spiritual needs."

ELLEN EVERT HOPMAN,
AUTHOR OF *SECRET MEDICINES FROM YOUR GARDEN*

"As an elder, herbalist, and adventure shaman, this is one book I could spend the rest of my life with."

THEA SUMMER DEER, D.S.P.S.,
AUTHOR OF *WISDOM OF THE PLANT DEVAS*

"Matthew Wood's story is told, and suddenly you realize that you are the seed growing to fruit within the cocoon, the circled filaments of this amazing adventure wound 'round until you have understood. You are the chrysalis, now ready to wiggle out into a new world."

MARGI FLINT, HERBALIST AND
AUTHOR OF *THE PRACTICING HERBALIST*

A SHAMANIC
HERBAL

PLANT TEACHERS AND
ANIMAL MEDICINES

A Sacred Planet Book

MATTHEW WOOD

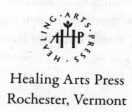

Healing Arts Press
Rochester, Vermont

Healing Arts Press
One Park Street
Rochester, Vermont 05767
www.HealingArtsPress.com

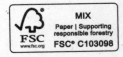

Healing Arts Press is a division of Inner Traditions International

Sacred Planet Books are curated by Richard Grossinger, Inner Traditions editorial board member and cofounder and former publisher of North Atlantic Books. The Sacred Planet collection, published under the umbrella of the Inner Traditions family of imprints, includes works on the themes of consciousness, cosmology, alternative medicine, dreams, climate, permaculture, alchemy, shamanic studies, oracles, astrology, crystals, hyperobjects, locutions, and subtle bodies.

Note to the reader: This book is intended to be an informational guide. The remedies, approaches, and techniques described herein are meant to supplement, and not to be a substitute for, professional psychological and medical care or treatment. They should not be used to treat a serious ailment without prior consultation with a qualified health care professional.

Cataloging-in-Publication Data for this title is available from the Library of Congress

ISBN 979-8-88850-020-0 (print)
ISBN 979-8-88850-021-7 (ebook)

Printed and bound in the United States by Lake Book Manufacturing, LLC

10 9 8 7 6 5 4 3 2 1

Text design by Virginia Scott Bowman and layout by Debbie Glogover
This book was typeset in Garamond Premier Pro with Angie Sans Std, Gill Sans MT Pro, ITC Legacy Sans, Optima LT Std, and Zeitung Micro Pro as display typefaces.

To send correspondence to the author of this book, mail a first-class letter to the author c/o Inner Traditions • Bear & Company, One Park Street, Rochester, VT 05767, and we will forward the communication, or contact the author directly at **www.matthewwoodinstituteofherbalism.com.**

Scan the QR code and save 25% at InnerTraditions.com. Browse over 2,000 titles on spirituality, the occult, ancient mysteries, new science, holistic health, and natural medicine.

Contents

*I dedicate this book to my late dear friend Susan Yerigan,
with whom I studied and experienced lessons on the
Medicine Path for thirty-five years.*

Journey in Unknown Lands

*None by traveling over known lands can find out the
unknown.*

WILLIAM BLAKE, *ALL RELIGIONS ARE ONE*

This is a book about spiritual growth. The primary spiritual path I
know through personal experience is the one called "shamanism." This
is based on the actualization and merger of the human self with the
animal self, resulting in the coming-to-consciousness of the dream self
or individual spirit. A shaman is anyone of any culture who experiences
their animal self as a being as complete and important as their conscious or human self. This is why the universal symbol of the shaman is
the half-animal and half-human pictograph.

From the warm-blooded animals we gain our heart—mammals take
care of their young, partner, and form communities—and the ability to
dream. Reptiles don't emotionally bond or dream; from them we gain our
raw survival and reproductive instincts. Our physical body takes after a
particular animal so that our traits resemble that animal. Our physical
appearance, instincts, and approach to life resemble our animal—Bear,
Wolf, Deer, Rabbit, Crow, Owl, Hawk. Even in rather ordinary conver-
sations we characterize people by their resemblance to animals. A lot of
people even identify with an animal, but the crucial shift occurs when
the human self recognizes its co-walker animal self in dreamtime.

In his seminal work on shamanism, cultural historian Mircea Eliade noted (1964, 94): "In a considerable number of myths and legends all over the world the hero is carried into the beyond by an animal." This can be a real event and it always does occur in alternate reality or the depths of dreamtime. In conventional society, alternate reality is looked upon as Legend; dreamtime as a weak alternative to normal reality. This book wasn't written for people with those belief systems. The animal self erupts into our world through dreamtime, from an untrodden internal wilderness.

Modern religion, East and West, does not generally address the animal self. This aspect of our psyche is largely ignored in the modern interpretation of life in the Abrahamic religions of the West and the transcendental religions of the East—with some exceptions. Ironically, the story of Abraham himself centers on the actualization of his Ram animal self on Moriah—mountain of "vision and provision." The actualization of the animal self is addressed in the authentic occult traditions of the West. This is the surviving shamanic tradition in the dominant society.

According to the testimony of the shamans, dreamtime and the Spirit World are the same—the place of "vision and provision" in the story of Abraham. The development of spiritual life requires the actualization of the animal self, which otherwise actually serves as the teeth-bared guardian of that world—waiting for the time to arrive when we are integrated and developed enough to survive the jolt into the hyperspace of the Spirit World. Sense comes from the animal world, whether it be on the physical or spiritual plane.

This is also a book about the medicinal plants that can help us in our spiritual life or shamanic journey. Because shamans work with the Forces of Nature, these plants usually are linked to such a force. "When a plant looks like an animal or is used by an animal," it is linked to that animal, which represents one of the Forces of Nature: "that is called a spirit signature and those plants are stronger than the others."* Like the

---

*Native herbalist Karyn Sanders.

warm-blooded animals themselves, these plants possess an innate link to the Spirit World.

Animism

A necessary foundation for the shamanic perspective is the experience of Nature as a living, conscious being. This is called *animism* in anthropology and is a characteristic of nearly all Indigenous and premodern societies. It was the common experience or belief in Western culture until the rise of the modern scientific paradigm in the seventeenth century and it has not completely died out among people in that culture, though their thoughts and feelings about this are not held in respect; one is "not supposed to think that way."

The word *anima* derives from the Latin, meaning "wind, air, a current of air; breath; the vital principle, life, or soul." Because of the connection to life, it also is the root of the words "animal" and "animated." The term for the "Living Nature" or "World Soul" in Latin was—still is—*anima mundi*. In *The Death of Nature* (1980), historian of science Carolyn Merchant traces the transition from a living to a dead Nature in Western culture, showing that this occurred in the seventeenth century, and was due to the rise of the scientific paradigm. It was strongly resisted by the Churches—Catholic and Protestant.

The traditional geocentric cosmology, which ruled supreme until Galileo, was innately animist because it placed the Earth at the center of a series of influential entities identified with the planets and stars. Earth was alive, receiving the influence of these celestial bodies, and we, her inhabitants, were subject to these fluctuating influences. The seven planets were identical to the seven principal gods of the ancient pagans. Their influences were not diminished, but they were no longer to be worshipped or looked upon as rivals of the Supreme Being.

The cosmology of the geocentric Earth included the four elements: earth, water, air, and fire. These are identical to the three states of chemical matter (solid, liquid, gas) and the combustible state. The word *elementum* is a Latin term referring to the four elements specifically;

only later was it identified with the elements of Mendeleev's periodic table. One wishes science would not redefine words used in a different manner in an earlier time period but introduce new terms.

In the premodern perspective, the four elements are not simply material, like the states of chemical matter, but living. According to the usual definition, the fire element corresponds to consciousness, air to intelligence (including animal intelligence), water to vitality or life itself, and earth to the mineral state, which corresponds to existence itself. The four elements in this regard also correspond to the four kingdoms of Nature: human (conscious, ensouled), animal (intelligent), plant (vital), and mineral (material).

According to another layout, fire represents the animal, characterized by movement and related to the fact that animals are personifications of the Forces of Nature. From this perspective, air represents the human, analytical principle and the self-consciousness associated with it. The *anima mundi* embraces all these attributes and consequently it is conscious, vital, ensouled, and intelligent.

The Soul World is controlled by the "laws of Nature" and even the "law of karma." All humans are bound together in that world, so that if we hurt another it comes back upon us. This extends down the evolutionary scale, so to speak. In an animist world we can disturb or hurt animals, plants, and maybe even minerals. If we have a good heart we would not want to hurt anyone and we would not want to hurt the Living Nature. If we have a nasty heart, we are going to find that the hurt is going to come back upon us and we are going to have to experience it as fully as did our victim before us—because all is continuous in that world; there are no walls of separation. This may not happen until after death, when the wall between us and the world around us will dissolve. All that is necessary to enter and live in the animist world, therefore, is an open heart and the self-responsibility to face any karma we have generated.

If Nature is alive, then how can we feel anything but love and respect for our Mother, the Living Nature? We would want to include her in our major decisions about life—individually, socially, ethically, environmentally. We would want her permission before undertaking ventures that would markedly influence the lineaments of that world. This is part of the American Indian perspective: we need to ask permission of Earth before undertaking large enterprises. I call her "Earth" because she is a being; not "the earth." The usual expression is "Mother Earth," without "the," showing that even in conventional speech she is still treated like a living being! I also capitalize the names of plants and animals because I want them to be considered "people," comparable to ourselves.

The Living Nature is also the Soul World, the natural home of the individual soul. It is a dimension of mutual feeling or empathetic connectedness. Tradition is very clear in identifying our three parts: body, soul, and spirit. The soul is not the physical body and not the individual spirit or essential self, but a being of heart and feelings. Through the body, the soul is associated with mortality; through the spirit, it touches immortality.

The existence of this world was at one time self-evident. I would maintain that it is still self-evident to the soul, but Western people train themselves not to feel or believe in it. From the research of my late friend Susan Yerigan and myself, we believe this awareness of the Soul World as a whole would normally be a natural realization that occurs as childhood draws to an end, just before puberty. This is when the individual soul is becoming self-aware—of itself and the World Soul. Both of us remember experiencing the realization that "Nature is alive" when we were about eleven.

The Snow Queen by Hans Christian Andersen is a fairy tale about this moment of challenge and change in human life. Little Kai and Gerda are fast childhood friends, but a hobgoblin makes a mirror in which everything is seen with a jaundiced and cynical eye. He and his associates take the mirror up into the sky to look at the angels, but the higher they go and the more they laugh, the more it shakes until it falls and shatters. Tiny bits and pieces blow all over the world, into people's eyes and hearts. One falls into the eye of Kai and he is taken away by the Snow Queen to the land of snow and ice. Little Gerda has to follow him there and remove the fleck before they can be returned to friendship.

The Wisdom of Nature

The Soul World touches us primarily in two ways: one through love and the other through wisdom. We have already discussed the empathic, soul, or heart connection, but not the special kind of wisdom associated with this world.

There are two kinds of wisdom. One is derived from living a good-hearted, successful life. With time we learn how to be a better person, coming from the heart—also to remove ourselves from a situation where our heart would be vulnerable or even where our soul could be damaged. We might call this the "wisdom of life."

The other kind of wisdom derives from observing and learning about the underlying patterns or archetypes of Nature in all her myriad expressions and forms, independent of the issues of soul and heart. Within the forests and fields of Nature we see the animals, who themselves represent the Forces of Nature, and the plants, representing archetypal powers and medicines. Looking up into the heavens, we see the stars and planets, which represent the primal movers and forces of the cosmos. Through the "doctrine of correspondence" there is a relationship between the above and the below, so that what happens in the heavens is reflected on earth. Others say that the celestial bodies emanate little rays, or perhaps harmonious songs, that control our lives here on Earth. I used to think the idea that there were little rays emanating from the planets was tedious and ridiculous—silly me, later I found out that this kind of relationship also exists.

We do not need to know anything about the astrological powers or the singing of the spheres to accumulate this kind of knowledge. It can be known directly through the plants, animals, and minerals. The traditional name for it in Western philosophy and theology is the "Wisdom of Nature," or *natura sophia*.

Sophia was the old Greek name for wisdom and—fortunately for Western peoples, both as Jews and Christians—she was not looked upon as a goddess but more as a type, emblem, or symbol, like the Statue of Liberty. Wisdom was highly valued in Greek, Jewish, and non-Jewish

Middle Eastern spirituality, and later in the Abrahamic religions that descended from the search for wisdom—Christianity, Judaism, and Islam. In the Septaguint, the earliest Greek translation of the Tanahk, the Hebrew Bible, the word *sophia* was used to translate the Hebrew *chokmah*, "wisdom." Chokmah/Sophia came to be personified in the Wisdom Books of the Hebrew Bible; for example, in the Book of Proverbs (9:1) it is said that her temple has seven pillars. The prophet Jeremiah complained about the worship of the Queen of Heaven before the fall of Jerusalem in 597 BCE. Sophia, the North American Star Woman, and the Queen of Heaven are variations on the same theme of archetypal wisdom or Nature Wisdom.

Sophia was therefore highly esteemed among the pagan Greeks, Jews, early Christians, and other people of the Mediterranean and Near East. Eventually, she was identified with theological wisdom as well. Finally, the Christian Roman Emperors named their central cathedral in Constantinople for her: the *Hagia Sophia*. Down through the centuries, the relationship of Sophia to the Christian Trinity remained somewhat uncertain, however, and she is still somewhat mistrusted—where she is known at all. A remarkable fictional account of Sophia—considering that the theology is closer to that of modern Evangelical Christianity—was penned by William P. Young in *The Shack* (2007). Here she represents wisdom gained from life experience.

Before this constellation of associations crystallized, there were earlier "incarnations" of Sophia, some of which had an influence on her Judeo-Christian persona. The visible representation in our world of the archetypal realm is the starry sky. This was personified as the Egyptian goddess Neith, stretched across the sky with the stars in her body. Athena was a version of Neith adopted by the Greek city, according to her early historians. Athena is certainly a goddess of wisdom. Meanwhile, some characteristics of Neith were incorporated into the emerging goddess Isis. She was associated with the hidden soul of Nature, for which reason she was shown as veiled—a characteristic later picked up by Sophia. There are also analogies between Sophia and Hathor, Queen of the Heavens, but the latter is not veiled.

Indeed, Neith is pictured as naked, stretched across the sky, her body covered with the stars.

We can see quite clearly the analogy between Sophia and the North American Star Woman. In Native America it is said that Star Woman descended from above—the birds of the air circling around her as she descended—until her foot landed on the back of Grandfather Turtle. The little water creatures were bringing up bits of mud to create the earth on the back of Turtle. When Star Woman stepped upon this inchoate surface, she impressed her stars or archetypes on it to make the individual types of the mineral, plant, animal, and human worlds.

I refer to "Grandfather Turtle" because that is how he introduced himself to me—see the account related to Gravel Root (chap. 6). My friend Sondra Boyd, a Tsalagi (Cherokee) medicine woman, preferred the term "First Turtle" or "Original Turtle," not liking to sex a primal being. However, I decided to go with the vision that was presented to me; it was powerful and engraved upon my soul.

Since Star Woman impressed her essences upon Grandfather Turtle he has been, forever afterward, associated with the Wisdom of Nature because he is the receptacle of the archetypes comprising Mother Nature. It is this knowledge that is the basis of the Language of Nature, the School of Nature, the Green Tongue, or Shamanic Speech. Turtle is the main stem from which the mammalian life-wave arose out of the reptilian, according to evolutionary biologists. Turtle is rightly be seen as the foundation of our world—in mythology, Earth is pictured supported on the back of an enormous Turtle.

Because Nature is directed by the forces of creation, following archetypal lines of expression and cosmic law, she is amenable to our understanding—especially through the intuition, the faculty that perceives patterns and wholes. Intuitive thinking was the basis for the development of the geocentric model of the four elements of Mother Earth. This is a beautiful and harmonious method of thinking and knowing that makes our sojourn in Mother Nature an even more enjoyable experience.

The Wisdom of Nature is extremely important for generating common concepts and terminology for discussion of experiences along the road of shamanism—or any spiritual path, for that matter—because there is no way to describe the spiritual world except by analogy. This is why Jesus continually spoke in parables and analogies about the "kingdom of heaven"; there was no way to describe his spiritual experience in ordinary language. Ironically, his followers don't get why this is the case and insist upon using ordinary speech to persuade themselves that they understand the alternative reality he was describing. Jesus used similes and contrasts from peasant life, because this was his milieu, rather than the animals and plants of Nature. But all of this constitutes the "Language of Nature" and the "Speech of Nature," and it is important to learn to think by analogy, inference, and contrast, instead of in rational, materialistic terms. The ability to speak this way was traditionally associated with the expression of the spirit.

Wisdom is encoded into every leaf and stone, paw and footprint. It is also found in what Eliade called "myths and legends." On this path we have many stories that inspire us, while others cannot be understood until we have experienced the inner reality conveyed by the story. Still others simply amuse us on what can so often be thought of as a long and dreary path. These are traditionally called "shaman stories." Nature is constructed to make us more complete, well-rounded individuals, both in this world and in the world to come. This Earth Wisdom, built into the fabric of the Living Nature, is an important part of the journey.

The Old, Old Path

The path of the shaman takes us beyond our "native dimension." It is not a comfortable path and it is not for everyone. It is available only to those who have the calling. If you are reading this book, you have had the calling. If you hadn't, you'd find this book unbelievable or boring.

Once I saw the shaman's path in the forest—there were leaves covering it, several years deep. It was barely discernible. A voice said, "That's the Old, Old Path that almost nobody follows today."

The shamanic path implies the existence of a world different from the one everybody is used to. It can only be described by parable, inference, and comparison. We look down and see the faint markings of the trail on the surface of Earth and from Earth we learn to see the mysteries in the heavens above. So there are actually three worlds: above, middle, and lower. J. R. R. Tolkien revived the archaic term "Middle Earth" for the world we live in, between the Heavenly and the Underworld or Netherworld. In 1648 the alchemist Thomas Vaughan wrote (1968, 52):

> Your fate is written by an unseen hand,
> But his Three Books with the Three Worlds shall stand.

The Soul World is always close to us but the Spirit World is far away. It is available to us only through dreamtime or other types of alternative reality, so it is effectively an unknown and unseen world. This is why the universal experience of the spiritual voyageur at the moment of the birth of the spirit self is the perception of total darkness, representing the sensory non-awareness we had in the Spirit World previous to that time. Don Juan called it the "black world" or "netherworld" (Castaneda 1985, 293; 1993, 45). The ancient Maya called it the "Black Dreaming Place" (Gillette 1997, 40).

When Castaneda had his first vision of the "black world," don Juan commented that this was the first time he had actually moved over from normal human perception to alternate reality (1985, 293). And that was after years of hallucinations on drugs and elaborate shamanic training. Castaneda was a sort of "Everyman of Western Culture" and a burden of disbelief weighed heavily upon him. But he opened a door.

The Whispering of the Spirit

The spirit is that which knows the truth. It is, therefore, the ground and guarantor of truth. When we know truth, our individual spirit is active. This level of experience occurs much less frequently than body and soul awareness. It is therefore something we should welcome on the rare opportunities we have to experience it.

What is spirit? Are we talking about our own individual spirit? The spirit that moves the entire universe? The divine spirit? The spirit land, where "the spirits" live? The spirit of an animal or plant? Ultimately, if we are honest with ourselves, we have to admit that spirit is a mystery we don't know. The Native American words for spirit, like *manitou* or *wakan*, mean both "mystery" and "spirit" at once. Even the Bible (John 3:8) agrees:

> The wind blows wherever it pleases. You hear its sound, but you cannot tell where it comes from or where it is going. So it is with everyone born of the Spirit.

Unlike the translators of the Bible, I don't capitalize the word "spirit" myself. It is hard to define anything that pertains to the spirit; the difference between the universal spirit and the individual is not well defined in most languages and cultures. It is traditional to capitalize Soul World but not soul, so I also capitalize "Spirit World" because it is a place—but that is the exception to my choice.

The spirit has been present with us from the moment of our birth, trying to steer our life in a positive direction. However, we are born so far from the spirit that we hardly notice or hear the little voice. It takes courage to follow what it says because it opposes the entropy of self-centered human culture. Any time we do experience and stand up for inner truth, the spirit has won a battle and we inch toward the day when we will be hardwired into the Spirit World.

The spirit has always cared for the human heart/soul. The moment we recognize the existence of the Soul World, we also become aware of the spirit. Why? Because that is a moment of truth. We have to believe in the reality of the Soul World; if we don't, we destroy our connection to soul, spirit, and truth. But that is only the beginning of the path. Until a full commitment is made, the soul is easily misled and confused, so the spirit cannot consider the soul to be a reliable partner or recipient of its message. It sends its messages, but poor little soul does not know what to make of these smoke signals and often dismisses them as mere opinions.

The spirit is always whispering to us and this whisper is like a constant IV drip telling us what would be good to do if we want to walk the good path and lead a good life. All this arrives in terms of the inner knowing of truth because that is the only language the spirit speaks. Basically, inner truth is not a language many people speak.

I use the simile of an IV drip because it is like we are stuck in triage in a spiritual hospital, virtually unconscious, on a drip line that's keeping us spiritually alive. We are just barely conscious of the spiritual voice. The IV drip is like the trail of breadcrumbs Hansel and Gretel followed in the woods. Once we are aware of it and dedicated to it, we are driven along it to survive. If we turn around or wander away, we'll end up cooked in the witch's oven.

All human beings have the opportunity to hear and respond to the whisper. Not all do, but it is with us throughout life, giving us guidance. It is not an easy job to follow that voice: we human souls are innately simple, naive, gullible, wavering, and uncertain.

Another characteristic of the spirit is freedom. It hates bondage. That's why we are so far from it. We are creatures of bondage: to falsehood, delusion, egotism, power, fear, and biological imperatives. The spirit never tries to force the soul to accept the truth or itself. That would end free will and be a form of abuse. Instead, the spirit conspires to set up situations where the person can only choose inner truth. Usually, a person's back is against the wall when he or she has to make the decision to join his or her will to the spirit.

Although the spirit respects the free will of the individual completely, it wants us to surrender that free will totally. We might think this means the spirit wants us to be its slave. Actually, that path doesn't really work. If we slavishly follow the spirit, we will suffer deprivation of our personal, soulful desires and lose the instinct to enjoy life and love. We will not want to live. Therefore, there has to be a bargaining—

and even a fighting—for personal needs, in which the individual soul justifies its personal desires and learns that the spirit will tolerate enough independence to make life enjoyable. Following this procedure, we become the partner and co-creator with the spirit, combining our funny little human foibles and desires with the most powerful force in the universe. The combination of the spiritual will with the personal will and the imagination is the origin of magic.

The whispering of the spirit is suited to life in time and space. It shows us that we are watched over, taken care of, and able to actualize our lives while we remain fully immersed in our native dimension. It leads to a unification of the personal spirit with the soul. Rudolf Steiner called this amalgamation the "soul-and-spirit," while Carl Jung named it the "Self." This combination is the basis for what is usually meant by "spirituality" and "spiritual life" in Western culture. Whether beyond us or within us, the spirit continues to roam free, unhindered by "our dimension," because the spirit is otherworldly by nature.

The Land of the Dead

The Christian West habitually confuses the Underworld with hell. In the Hebrew Bible, *Sheol* is the abode of the dead, translated into Greek as *Hades*. This is a place of life-unmaking, not necessarily of punishment. By comparison, *Gehenna* is the place of punishment in the Hebrew Bible, rabbinical literature, and the sayings of Jesus. The King James Version (KJV) of the Bible incorrectly translates both *Sheol* and *Gehenna* as "hell," showing that it is indeed a "version" and not an accurate translation. So the shaman has been tarred and feathered with the sooty pigment of the Devil.

After we die, the Lords of Death grab hold of us and we are forced to confront our deeds, fears, and accomplishments. The Underworld is therefore a place of purification for the soul, not a pit of damnation. If we don't want to cooperate with the creation and Creator, or the other inhabitants of the Soul World, we are given the opportunity to become an eternal being living in self-awareness cut off from the All-Life. Then we are exiled to the Outer Darkness. This constitutes an act of grace on the part of Creator, because otherwise the individual soul would have to be dissolved into nothingness. The grace is that the ego can continue to exist, even though it is cut off from the Soul World and the Spirit World. This is the path of the hungry ghost, always craving something it cannot have.

In the Underworld the Lords of Death hold us until we give up struggling and accept who we are and what we have done. There is no pity to be found in the process of uncovering the truth. Don Juan called this the "place of no pity." It is a hard road and the one we are on at first, as a shaman's apprentice or a dead person walking the paths of Hades. As we let go of our baggage and are attracted to a positive spiritual momentum, we spend less and less time in the place of no pity.

In his commentaries on Castaneda, Théun Mares (1998) notes that if we don't yet have true spiritual seership or awareness in dreamtime, then we can use the place of no pity to reveal truth and make fundamental changes. This is because the place of no pity is associated with dying, while vision and dream come directly from spiritual life.

There is some reason why the Underworld is mistaken for hell, and the Lord of the Underworld for the Devil. It is not just an overly zealous Christian moralism. In order to reach the Spirit World, we need to meet and pass the Guardian of the Threshold. This being is the personification of all that we fear. It is our personal Devil, forged in the depths of our unconscious, composed of all the things we fear or have been programmed to believe are bad. It takes years to save up enough energy and courage to face this entity. Then we find that it is not really the Devil after all. Jung (who had read of the Guardian in occult literature) called it the "shadow."

The shadow is the opposite of Freud's "superego," which is the projection of all that we think of as good. In our naivete, we only perceive our projections of the Devil and God and mistake them for the "real guys." If you seek Creator this side of the veil of dream and the land of legend, you will be disappointed.

The Spirit World has two faces. The first one is the dark world, presided over by the Lord of the Underworld. That is the world we see as we approach. This is because we are so filled with the darkness of the world we came from that we cannot see anything else. That darkness is the part of us that must die in the great life-unmaking in order to experience the light of the Spirit World. There is no one better suited to bring that darkness to our attention than the Lord of the Underworld. That is his job. He manifests the darkness within us, forces us to confront it, and—if it is delusory—he and his servants break the darkness down into raw, undifferentiated "soul stuff" that can be recycled. However, those parts of our soul that are conjoined with the spirit pass the great threshing floor of death and remain part of the eternal self we are building.

The Lord of the Underworld is also known as the Keeper of the Animals or the Lord of the Hunt. He is the master of the Forces of Nature, which are embodied in the animals; therefore of the ultimate spiritual genomes, totems, or species of the Animal Kingdom. Each type of animal represents a force of Nature. We have to learn to assimilate the animal power inside of us in order to be complete beings. We have to understand it, adopt it, and incarnate it without egoic attachment or rejection. We also have to assimilate the human, which is no less complicated.

In the old days, while people still felt his presence, the hunter prayed to the Lord of the Hunt for game. Right now, when the socioeconomic underpinning of the world is in disarray, in this period of transition, he is more active. All who are not doing their spiritual work, not confronting the darkness within them, have an unwilling appointment with the Lord of the Hunt.

In near-death experiences, many people report that they see their lives flash before them. That is the beginning of the "recapitulation" of life-experience that occurs after death. They also report a light, but they will eventually meet the total darkness of the Underworld and be subject to that total darkness, alone, until every fear and content comes to the surface. The path of the shaman is to recapitulate while still in the body and to meet the total darkness of the Lord of the Underworld. These pages harbor several accounts of that meeting.

The Faery Realm

The dark face of the Underworld is what we see when we approach the Spirit World. The light face is what we see on the other side of the darkness. This is the realm of the consort of the Lord of the Underworld, the Faery Queen. Now we see a new light; the faeries are sometimes called "the Shining Ones." Don Juan called them the "inorganic beings," while anthropologist Timothy Knab's shamanic mentors referred to them as "those who are not our brothers." Susan described them as the "tumblers"—the all-possible-combinations-of-existence that fall into place whenever anything in the manifest universe is created. This may be a realm of light but it is even less safe than where we were in the darkness.

Folklore points out several reasons why it is dangerous to go into the faery realm. The first one is that the tumblers are always moving. Therefore, the doorway into that world is never the same as it was the moment we came in. It is, therefore, easier to get caught in that world than to emerge from it intact. That is the basis of the ancient taboos about going to the Faery Realm. This is a danger that never goes away until we reach a kind of peace with that world. This too occurs in alternate reality or dreamtime. When we dream of the March of the Faeries or the Faery Throne Room, or some presentation of the tumblers falling into order, we are free from this spiritual tornado power sucking at us.

A second danger is that the tumblers can perceive our deepest needs and wishes because they are in fact the instruments that created them in the first place. We could call their dominion "the world where all-wishes-come-true." This is why they unashamedly cater to us, as don Juan said. By accepting gifts that cater to our weaknesses, they gain power over us and we can't leave their dominion. We want to accept the gifts that are good and appropriate for us.

From our perspective, it seems as if the faeries want to offer us a gift—this is a universal folk tale, which is reflected in sources ranging from traditional folk ballads to Carlos Castaneda. The gift is so well chosen, so suited to our personal—even our spiritual—needs that it is impossible to reject unless we have both spiritual perception of the truth and enough stamina to resist for long enough. If we can't resist this Siren's Song, we will be drawn in, defeated on our journey for spiritual wholeness.

There are some who desire the crazy ride the tumblers provide and they are fulfilled, rather than defeated—the adventure shamans. The unprepared and the weak, the accidental tourists, will be caught in confusion. It is said they will live there in the Faery Realm until the end of time. And yet others will carry on, knowing they missed the boat, but doing their best until the leveling field of death can free them from the situation. It is a risk to make any kind of agreement in that world until after we have experienced the tumblers become orderly.

One of my friends experienced a faery being connect to his heart. He found it very disturbing because of the inhuman, alien, unfamiliar vibe of the consciousness. After attaching to him it said, "Would you like to go back to the way you were before?" He answered, "Yes." The being responded by attaching itself to him permanently. In the faery realm there is no time or space, so "before" doesn't mean anything to them. He felt he had "lost his soul." He had not. It is not a sin to have "faery genes," that is, energy implantation from the tumblers. Nor is a true spiritual aspirant ever lost, because he or she will persevere no matter what.

The third problem with journeying to the Spirit World is that it is innately impersonal and nonhuman, and therefore takes us away from our heart, our humanity—the human totem, so to speak. One touch of the faeries makes it harder to love and to be human. This lesson is told to us in the lines of an old Irish ballad:

> The short cut to the Rosses
> The short cut to the Rosses
> I'll ne'er go that way again
> Because the time I went that way
> The faeries stole my heart
> And I'll never love again.

Traditional ballads are a trove of shamanic knowledge. This particular ballad is so totally true; you know that it is if you yourself have been through the same ordeal. From the short cut to the Rosses onward, you are going to have to fight to be a human. On the other hand, it is quite possible to tread the Old, Old Path and not have an experience with the faeries that has this side effect. Susan had never had this experience, but I have.

We also realize on meeting the faeries for the first time that they are omnipotent in their world and they could capture us or destroy us down to the last atom of our identity (since they are determinants of identity). This causes us to have an existential fear of them. But we also gain an existential confidence after we have met them. We now know that there is a different world, that we are spiritual beings, that there is a spiritual purpose to life. One is genetically changed (genes are a lower-octave representation of the tumblers). But one leaves the ordinary world behind and cannot explain this to anyone who has not had the experience. It is not because we have now had experiences that sound too fantastic to be believed; it is because we have had the experience of a completely nonhuman, nonorganic type of existence. Part of what reconnects us back to humanity is speech, and this is why we should have been learning and practicing, up to now, the Speech of Nature.

Because the "genes" from the faeries are nonhuman, they change the spiritual laws that govern interactions with people who have not had the faery experience. It is "against the law" to try to force people to have these experiences. Forcefulness twists the participant. It is also not kosher to give advice about human psychological situations because one does not share the same perspective. If it sounds like I am describing how a person on the autism spectrum deals with the world—well, that would be a good analogy. From the human psychiatric perspective, it may even be an explanation.

Another group are the people who have had the experience, have magical things to say, but do it in an inappropriate, forceful manner. This means some sort of doubt or egoic expression adhered to them when they tumbled in the other world. The thrashing around they engage in, trying to convince us of this or that, is a sad state of affairs. The term for this is "fallen initiate." The fact is, however, that all of us require some time for spiritual knowledge to "settle in," and we all experience this state to some degree or another. So we are all "fallen initiates."

We must remember that our natural home is the Soul World. That is the realm of the heart. We are beings of soul and anywhere else in the universe we find ourselves is going to feel onerous because it is preventing us from fulfilling our destiny as human beings.

The faeries do not identify with individuality the way we do. They have more of a hive mentality. They are the tumblers that click, not the click; we are the click, the thing, the creature.

Unfortunately, our culture has turned the tumblers into quaint fantasies. In reality, lucid dreaming can be shockingly powerful and we are on faery turf when we are there, where they are omnipotent. We, on the other hand, have no power other than that inculcated into our souls by our own spiritual discipline, or lack thereof, so that when we meet them, we are prepared as can be. We have no reference points for interaction with the Spirit World other than shaman stories that we have internalized. I chronicled the seven great shaman stories corresponding to the seven rungs on the shamanic ladder in my book *Seven Guideposts on the Spiritual Path: Shamanism in Genesis* (2021b). The old folk ballads are another set of shaman stories. So are traditional "fairy tales." If we put in our homework, these kind of stories will bubble up into dreamtime and we will have intense otherworldly experiences.

Just as the Lord of the Hunt is the ruler of the animals, the Queen is the ruler of the plants. In this regard she is called the Green Woman—and she often appears green or flowery. The English alchemist Thomas Vaughan called her "Thalia" (ever-in-bloom).

Physical plants are related to the faery folk the same way physical animals are related to the animal totems. The animals drag us to their master, the Lord of the Underworld, which requires our death and purification, but the plants (and not just the hallucinogens) can bring us directly into the Spirit World without purification. They are inherently dangerous. (Most of our modern drugs are made from venoms and plants that have been synthesized: Snake + Plant + Human; the tree of the knowledge of good and evil). Therefore, plants must be approached with care.

The closer we are to our world, the more human the faeries appear to us, but they are never fully human. On the other hand, the further we are into their world, the more nonhuman they appear. Don Juan described them as filaments of light. Since I can't move my attention as far into their world as he or Castaneda could, I have only once ever seen them this way and even then my mind anthropomorphized them—the phrase "hair of the faeries" came to my mind when I saw these filaments of light.

The consciousness of the most ancient plants is more elemental, reflecting stone, water, air, or warmth and light. With the advent of the flowering plants, we enter a new world. Until that time, the insects were minor participants in life, but all of a sudden they were needed as pollinators for the flowers. In some art, the Faery Queen is shown clothed in plant and insect parts. It is strange that these illustrations appear to depict fantasies when in fact they reflect reality. The hivelike qualities of the Faery World are reflected in the insect world.

The Lord of the Animals is the darkness of sleep while the Lady is the light of dreamtime. Blobs of unactualized psychological content deepen the unconsciousness of our sleep, while freedom from these contents allows greater consciousness in dreamtime. But sleep is a mixture of the two. The Lady is symbolically represented by Mother Nature, while the Lord is associated with the Underworld—sleep and death. Adam slept, while Eve ("Life") came into existence.

For the ancient Mayans, the Lord of the Underworld was the paramount spiritual being and ruler of the world. He was represented in their society by the shaman king, whose animal representative was—still is—the Black Jaguar. This cultural world extended north into the modern-day Four Corners region of North America. According to Martine Prechtel, there are three jaguars in the shaman stories of Central America: Black Jaguar, Flowery Jaguar, and the Tawny Panther. The latter is the one whose job it is in the outer world to trim out the sick and injured animals.

The journey beyond the Soul Realm into the Faery Spirit World is rough and hard. As I sit and write, I am not writing an advertisement for a superior or even inferior spiritual path, but merely chronicling the Old, Old Path. Also, we are transitioning into the fifth world and a lot of this shamanic stuff will be part of the culture of the new Earth.

Human Nature

It is important that we study everything we confront in the world—or worlds—if we want to gain spiritual understanding. This includes human nature itself. A lot of what we attribute to human nature is actually inherited from the Animal Kingdom, particularly the warm-blooded crowd. The cold-blooded animals do not sleep or dream and they don't have an emotional heart. They don't take care of their young; they just dump the eggs and leave. They don't form lasting relationships and they don't hunt in packs—fortunately. The warm-blooded animals, on the other hand, take care of their young. The earliest ones were the marsupials, whose pouch is a literal representation of the warmth of true parenting. The mammals often form partnerships for a season or a lifetime and often cooperate in communities and hunt in packs. Birds are also warm-blooded—this is why we see them in the wintertime—and they too take care of their young. In this case, it is the nest that is the symbol of parenting and family life. They often form partnerships, sometimes for life, and some of them have complex community lives that are not easy for us to understand. Others are solitary. So the heart came before humanity.

Just about the only thing we have that birds and animals do not is self-consciousness and the ability to separate ourselves from the rest of creation and make our own rules. That's not necessarily a good thing.

But this gives us some control over our minds, and that gives us the ability to self-analyze, to stop the images in our brain and examine them, to reflect upon our experience and even ourselves. We can even train our minds to grasp and see the images that flit through them before they get away. Carl Jung called this "active imagination." Blake differentiated between self-generated images and those that came fresh and original from the unknown. The former he called "fantasy," the latter "imagination."

The animals touch the Spirit World through dreamtime. They have never lost this connection, but they also cannot reflect back upon it or upon their own status. We, on the other hand, enter Paradise through both dreamtime and the imagination. The former is said to be the basis of the Old, Old Path; the latter of the "New Way."

There is an old Chinese expression: "On Earth, thoughts; in Heaven, images." Images are prior to words. We interpret images into words. "A face might launch a thousand ships, but a description of a face is unlikely ever to induce a single boat to raise sail" (Hedsel 1999, 12).

From the shamanic standpoint, true imagination is the "outpost" of dreamtime in the conscious world. It gives us a second route of access to the Spirit World. Animals can see images in their minds but can't control them. We can barely control them either, but through practice we can learn to watch what images enter and leave our awareness. We can learn to differentiate between fantasy (images that are not based on reality) and imagination (images that stem from some original, authentic experience of body, soul, or spirit). True imagination is spiritual seership and it is always fresh and new, like true art, coming into our mind from sources across the gardens of time and space.

We can choose what thoughts or images we wish to entertain in our minds. We can fill our time with fantasies or we can await the imagination to bring us new things from outside of ourselves. We can choose images that are beautiful or deformed, kind or mean, loving or hateful, that increase or decrease self-awareness.

For the poet William Blake (1757–1827), the Imagination, God, and Man are continuous. In *The Laocoon* he writes: "The Eternal Body of Man is The IMAGINATION. God himself, that is, The Divine Body" (Blake 1982, 273). *A Vision of The Last Judgment* (1810) is the document in which Blake gives his most extended view of Imagination, which he contrasts with allegory, or storytelling based on memory rather than Imagination. For Blake, "The Last Judgment is an

Overwhelming of Bad Art & Science" that occurs "when all those are Cast away who trouble Religion with Questions concerning Good & Evil or Eating of the Tree of those Knowledges or Reasonings which hinder the Vision of God." It is not "Fable or Allegory but Vision." Blake is aware of common criticism of Imagination. "Fable is Allegory but what Critics call The Fable is Vision itself." The distinction ought to be made "for the Sake of Eternal Life," for the "Imagination is the World of Eternity . . . into which we shall all go after the death of the Vegetated body" (Blake 1982, 565, 554–555).

Blake gives an explanation that fits the premise of our shamanic herbal (1982, 555):

> The Nature of Visionary Fancy or Imagination is very little Known & the Eternal nature & permanence of its ever Existent Images is considerd as less permanent than the things of Vegetative & Generative Nature yet the Oak dies as well as the Lettuce but Its Eternal Image & Individuality never dies.

For Blake, the Imagination is what makes us quintessentially human. To the extent that we see the humanity in others we manifest our own humanity. So, being human is a matter of "seeing human." Blake would say that we bear the human image. Going further, Blake identified the human image, the imagination, with the Divine. That led him to coin the expression that lies at the center of his theology: "Jesus the Divine Human Imagination." Jesus did a pretty good job of personifying the magnanimous potential of humanity and describing the Spirit World, the "Kingdom of Heaven," in the imagination, so for Blake he also personified the imagination. Jesus described and initiated a New Way of imagination, as compared to its more difficult predecesssssor, the Old, Old Way of dreamtime. Born to the trade of herbalism, I prefer "Nature's Open Book," inscribed almost invisibly on the floor of the great forest where our animal kin tread. But there are villages and cities, noisy, teaming in unconsciousness, so the path of the human totem is not so easy to follow either.

We have the free will to be magnanimous, expressing our humanity in the best possible way, or in the worst. We can also waste the opportunity we have in a human body, in the Earth environment we have been gifted with, consuming time and space. These are assets that could really be used to assist the evolution of human beings.

Most people are afraid to dedicate themselves irretrievably to good or evil; they just want to live unconsciously off the fat of the land. Western civilization, which was being spread across the Earth as if it were a superior form of human life, is fast destroying the Earth, and is now seemingly consuming itself. The name for white man in Dakota is *wasichu*, "eater of the fat." This won't last very much longer; we live in a time of accounting and transformation.

The path of human nature is based on empathy for others: being kind and good and thoughtful. We find this tendency to strive toward a better, higher vision of oneself and of humanity in general in all the great religions of the world. Through the imagination we see what is better and we see ourselves becoming better people. This is the New Way, as compared (not opposed) to the Old, Old Path. It is the path of humanity today, whereas shamanism is a path that is more and more rarely trod. It is more important to have a loving heart than to journey to the Spirit World.

There are at least seven traits that are essential to human nature: self-consciousness, free will, speech, the expanding heart, imagination, intuition, and inspiration. Through (1) self-consciousness we learn to reflect on our experiences and to self-examine. Through (2) free will we choose our path. In (3) speech there is a great mystery because speech weaves together disparate strands to become new arrangements of energy and character. In this it imitates or—better yet—actually manifests the character of the spirit. This is why speech is connected to magic. As we have seen, (4) the heart is crucial to our humanity (even if it comes from the animals). So is (5) imagination, as we bear the human image. Intuition (6) is crucial to the development of our wisdom and understanding of where we are in creation. All true learning is (7) inspired: we say a good teacher "inspires her students." The root of the word "inspiration" indicates that all true learning comes from the influx of the spirit and that it is as necessary as the inspiration of the breath. These seven parts of us reflect the seven mysteries that rule creation and evolution.

Individuality

In order to fulfill human nature, we need to examine and learn about ourselves and express who we really are as individuals. In addition to being Nature-based and dreamtime-based, shamanism is centered in the individual. It does not espouse a system of beliefs but advocates methods and stories for personal development. It encourages individuality through interaction with the Living Nature and the spirit. It does not inherently conflict with established religion or belief systems because it does not seek to predetermine what a person will discover on their path. Shamanism promotes personal experience, self-awareness, independence of thought, and self-responsibility. These characteristics are integral to true spiritual life, along with compassion, humility, and an uncompromising focus on the achievement of positive outcomes for all.

This brings us to the first true flaw in the shamanic system: it does not necessarily build community. The shaman very often feels— and is—isolated from society. Mircea Eliade, in the second chapter of *Shamanism*, described the characteristic profile of the shamanic neophyte: he or she is *called* as an individual, *away* from his or her society, to *wrestle* with personal spiritual matters. This often involves physical, emotional, or mental challenges, often taking the individual all the way to psychological or physical death and rebirth. Then the shaman returns to society bearing gifts from another dimension.

Individuality and community might be considered eighth and ninth characteristics of human nature, but I believe they belong to the heart, which senses individuality in itself and others yet also needs belongingness and community.

The second flaw in the shamanic system is much more serious. Shamanism is conducive to the development of the "Dark Arts," which are terribly destructive to the individual and the community. We need to be very clear about this from the beginning. The modern conceit is that there is no real good and evil, either because there is no God or ultimate reality or indelible moral code, or because God is all-forgiving, or simply because it is rude to talk about something that might embarrass somebody. Modern education has taught the people to believe that their self-generated fantasies of truth are as good as any other, as if there were no ultimate truth.

If there is no ultimate truth, then there are no ultimates—God, Mother Nature, the Soul World, the spirit. The Harvard School of Divinity recently appointed an atheist as the head of the spiritual counseling section—to the general applause of the modern, materialist, secular humanist world.

At the same time that the modern mind denies the existence of imponderables such as soul and spirit, there is a widespread indulgence in unexamined emotionalism. If there is no ultimate truth, then there is no ultimate responsibility, and if that is the case, there is no reason not to indulge our petty and vindictive feelings. This is highly visible in the socially popular ideas of our time.

Meanwhile, there has been a proliferation of the practice of "witch-craft." People like to think of themselves as "witches" because it sounds romantic or powerful. A lot of the herb books appearing nowadays have the word in their title. But self-indulgence in unexamined fantasies and power trips weakens the soul. I call these people "petty witches." But they can do a little bit of evil. They are gods who think they can determine the fate of others through psychic manipulation. I've run up against these people.

Since thoughts and feelings do have power on the psychological and spiritual planes—even when they are not acknowledged—this means that the practice of "petty witchcraft" or projecting negative thoughts on other people is widespread. In fact, we are all doing this all the time. Many of the people who say truth is relative practice "petty witchcraft," casting spells and attacking their emotional and intellectual foes. This is much more prevalent today in the dominant culture than it was when I was young. (Or maybe I am more sensitive now?)

"Petty witches" have not run across the true witches, the terrible "witches-in-dreamtime" who laugh at psychic manipulation. Their method is to alter us in our imagination and dream—on a level where most people are unconscious. It is harder to reach into the dreams of an unconscious person, so those who are in danger are those who are just becoming awake to dreamtime.

Petty manipulations of other people have to be forgivable mistakes, as far as the spirit is concerned—or God, if you will, or Mother Nature, the Soul World herself—because we all do this. But we all need to wake up and accept that we are petty, worthless individuals in the face of the eternal spirit. Many petty perpetrators do not seem ready to awaken from their "Deadly Dreams of Good & Evil," as William Blake writes in *A Vision of the Last Judgment* (1982, 563).

After the death of the body, the soul loses the leverage that kept the person from confronting their emotions, thoughts, and actions. The conglomeration that was once a living being is pulled apart by the Lords of the Dead—alligators and death-raptors. All that is left is piles of senseless rubble and undifferentiated soul material waiting to be recycled into newly minted souls. That rubble is what don Juan called the "graveyard of sorcerers."

Dark magic grows out of the opposite of individuality and community. It feeds on personality, ego, and inability to respect the value and free will of others. We cannot be so pointedly naive on the shamanic path as to ignore good and evil. On the other hand, we cannot adhere to artificial moral codes associated with our fears and projections. We have to experience good and evil. So in that respect these petty witches serve a function, although they are not "worthy opponents," as don Juan called them, but "worthless opponents" and "time-wasters."

On the path we are going to be tested by much more hideous and skillful savants of the Dark Arts, who will come at us in dreamtime, trying to twist our destinies, not just our feelings. Our instincts, our animal self, must be trained to react immediately; they must not be cluttered over with blobs of worthless, unexamined psychological energy. Other people can believe what they want, but when one becomes conscious in imagination or dreamtime, one's inner nature is nakedly exposed to the powers that be in that world, including the thoughts, feelings, and dreams of other people, living and non-incarnate. If we seek power or selfish goals, we will be corrupted and destroyed, and never become fully fledged human beings. We will become not only removed from society, but detrimental to it. We will only bear a deformed human image.

On the spiritual path, our primal individual nature bubbles up from esoteric depths and we become who we really are. Our personal moral fiber becomes clear as our responses and actions in imagination and dreamtime bring to the surface our true aims and core attributes. We feel a deep purpose and it drives us to make that purpose happen. This truth is felt by everyone regardless of their religion. A Christian author coined the phrase the "purpose-driven life." That is the root of individuality.

Shamans frequently work by themselves. They often interact with individuals in their community one by one: perhaps as physical, psychological, or spiritual healers. On the other hand, some work with whole communities. In *The Tears of the Ancestors*, the Dutch shaman Daan van Kampenhout (2008) took on the estrangement and damage caused—to the living and the dead—by the Nazi fiasco. Working with the dead is also one of the hallmarks of the shaman.

Because the path of the shaman is so individualistic, we need other protocols for community life: religious or spiritual systems that are oriented toward building and maintaining social structure. Because of the spiritual bankruptcy of the secular humanist/industrial/pharmacological complex, combined with the armchair individualism fostered by the cyber world, with the destruction of the old neighborhood-based society, we have very few institutions left that can build community naturally. Even here, where shamanism is poorly outfitted to help, perhaps it can contribute to a better social environment.

In societies in which the shamanic element is recognized as an important part of society, it enters into community events. In the Pueblo cultures of the American Southwest, there are dances and societies closely related to the shamanic impulse. This is also preserved in the Catholic festivals of Mexico and still even in some Mediterranean countries. If modern society ever becomes founded upon authentic spiritual experience, these sorts of community-encouraging events will have to spring up from the imagination. If we survive, perhaps societies of the future will enact festivals, stories, and dances that describe their interpretation of what we went through and failed to do—or perhaps did do—as we irresponsibly endangered ourselves and the whole world.

1

Shamanism from Siberia to Los Angeles

angelheaded hipsters burning for the ancient heavenly
connection to the starry dynamo in the machinery of night
ALLEN GINSBERG, *HOWL*

The word "shaman" was originally used by the Tungus people of central Siberia, adopted by a Christian priest who was having a "spiritual battle" with one of their "shamans," later adopted into the Russian language, and finally taken up by anthropologists. In *Shamans Through Time* (2001), Jeremy Narby and Francis Huxley trace the changing conception of what a shaman is in the eyes of Western culture, from witch to madman, to psychologist, to spiritual technician. It was Mircea Eliade's breakthrough book *Shamanism* (1964) that finally caught up with the spiritual dimension of the subject.

Originally, the term was applied by anthropologists to spiritual leaders in Siberian cultures involved largely in big-game hunting. Then the same constellation of practices and beliefs were found in North American cultures that were also primarily hunter-gatherer societies—although Native Americans don't apply the term themselves. The same traits were found throughout the Americas, in urban societies as well as in the jungle, forest, and tundra. The same patterns of thought, associating humans and animals, were discovered in ancient European cave paintings. They were found

30

in Australia, Africa—in fact, everywhere other than modern Western culture.

Western Shamanism: Undying but Ignored

Surely, something that is universal has to exist in Western society as well as everywhere else. Shamanism always existed and continues right under the nose of Western anthropologists. Until recently, it was termed occultism or esotericism. This is the path of Paracelsus, Jacob Boehme, Thomas Vaughan, Paschal Beverly Randolph, Helena Blavatsky, Arthur Edward Waite, Pamela Coleman Smith, Rudolf Steiner, Albert Sidney Raleigh, George Gurdjieff, and P. D. Ouspensky. All teach, in slightly different forms, the doctrine of the three selves and the transformation of consciousness in dreamtime or an alternate consciousness through *meeting the animal self.*

Let's take a look at how Steiner describes the animal self and its importance in spiritual development. In *Knowledge of the Higher Worlds and Its Attainment,* Steiner defines the "astral cloud or aura in which the being is enveloped" as "the whole range of instincts, impulses, desires and passions both of an animal and of a human being" (1947, 199). When this "aura" becomes orderly, a person begins to see animals differently. "Hitherto we had seen only a part of the animal kingdom, its external aspect"; now we begin to see the "higher forms of every creature in the animal kingdom" (Steiner 1947, 201). Steiner makes it clear that the transition to a higher form of spiritual consciousness occurs simultaneously with this change in relationship to the Animal Kingdom. Formerly, we saw a horse, now we see Horse. This surely is not Buddhism, Eastern religion, or Christianity: it is shamanism!

This realization is followed by what Steiner called "anxiety." This is exactly true—although I would have chosen the word "mortal terror" instead. The warm-blooded animal self (midbrain) brings the reptilian self (back brain) along with it when it comes into consciousness in dreamtime and then into ordinary awareness. The reptilian brain or reptilian self cannot directly perceive the Spirit World and therefore it only knows that "something terrible has happened" that could cause self-annihilation. But this is still only part of the explanation: the animal beings or "Elders" are connected to the faery beings—the "inorganic beings" of Castaneda, and they are terrifying because they are not human or animal or even earthly. They don't have genetics that we are familiar with.

The anatomical meeting place for the animal self and the human self is in the throat, just below the thyroid. This is the border between the animal (below the neck) and the human (above). Steiner identifies this point as the "throat chakra" and says that the eight upper petals of the chakra are assigned to the human, while the eight lower petals belong to the animal (1947, 135). In his plan, first the human petals are brought to awareness and then the animal petals follow. This would not be the standard method in traditional shamanism, where the animal self often comes to consciousness first. Steiner's method meets the problem, which we have in some instances, where the animal self comes to dominate over the human. On the other hand, we don't want to over-emphasize the human either.

Steiner's term for the animal self is "astral body." The actualization of this body or self is followed, according to Steiner, by the creation of what he calls the "higher self" in *How to Know Higher Worlds*:

> Now, when the gate of the senses is closed during sleep, these other impressions begin to emerge confusedly, and the dreamer becomes aware of experiences in another world. . . .
>
> When the isolated experiences during sleep begin, as described, the moment of birth is approaching for the liberated soul, for she has literally become a new being, developed by the individual within himself, from seed to fruit. . . .
>
> That this higher soul-being should be born during deep sleep will be easily grasped, for . . . the activity of the higher soul, at first so delicate and inconspicuous, can come into evidence. (Steiner 1947, 193, 210, 211)

In addition to the "astral body," Steiner also speaks of the actualization of the "etheric body." This is the part of us we feel as vitality. It is intimately connected to our physical body and in fact we can identify it with "body awareness" and "body memory." It never forgets any powerful impression made upon it, either physical or psychological. When we have an experience in any world, from normal to alternate reality, it makes an impression on the "body memory." For this reason, the etheric body is used as a repository for experiences learned in alternate reality. As Steiner says (1947, 193): "the etheric body, when developed, brings full knowledge concerning these engraved impressions derived from other worlds."

Don Juan used this method on Castaneda extensively. In fact, the whole series of books covers the same time period and experiences, but relived from a deeper and deeper awareness in this memory bank. Don Juan called this part of a person the "energy body." He often caused Castaneda to change into altered reality, where he trained him. When Castaneda later hit that speed bump, he relived the experience in full awareness.

The idea of the PC crowd that Western people, in picking up the shamanic standard, are guilty of "cultural appropriation," is not only incorrect but insulting to shamanic cultures everywhere. It implies that shamanism is not a universal path but some sort of invention of the individual culture and therefore not founded on enduring spiritual realities. Shamanism is a universal path. The old Western occultists called it the "perennial philosophy" (adopted from Leibniz) or the "Old, Old Path." It is built into the foundations of Nature, Humanity, and Animality.

From Cosimo de' Medici to Helena Blavatsky

The basic contours of the occult tradition we follow today derive from a school set up by Cosimo de' Medici (1389–1464), which still exists in Florence today (Hedsel 1999). Actually, the school would date back to the early fourteenth century, when the tarot cards were developed in northern Italy, but only the images remain to testify to this early layer of the tradition. Cosimo hired Marsilio Ficino (1433–1499) to translate the ancient *Corpus Hermeticum* and the Platonic dialogues, which were smuggled out of Constantinople shortly before its fall to the Turks in 1457. The *Corpus Hermeticum* traces back to the Roman period. One of Ficino's students was Johannes Trithemius (1462–1516), Abbot of Sponheim, the teacher of Paracelsus (Theophrastus von Hohenheim, 1493–1542) and Cornelius Agrippa von Nettesheim (1486–1535). The former penned numerous medical and occult treatises, which represent a sort of unedited flow of consciousness—according to one of his secretaries, Oporinus, he was usually drunk—while the latter wrote a carefully organized *Three Books of Occult Philosophy*. The rise of a literature of Western occultism therefore dates to these individuals. Of the two, Paracelsus is vastly more interesting and useful.

Paracelsus's insights were so important that his ideas about occult matters have not still not completely disappeared from publication. He was an advocate of *magia naturale*, or "Natural Magic," which was the use of correspondence and signatures to understand Nature and apply natural relationships to life events. This was "science" at the time—based upon the Living Nature doctrine of the Earth surrounded by nine or ten spheres—and therefore sanctioned by the Church. Paracelsus attributed knowledge to the *lumen naturae* or Light of Nature, which shone through the creation in the signatures and correspondences. He also believed in the Light of God, which illuminated things beyond Nature.

Paracelsus inspired a lot of people, including Jacob Boehme (1575–1624), who attempted to work his wild ravings into an organized corpus of Nature Wisdom (*Natura Sophia*) and Divine Wisdom (*Theosophia*). Boehme needed the Paracelsian terminology to explain his own vision: twice he saw the *Merkabah*, the Throne of God described by Ezekiel and others. The Nature Wisdom movement, founded largely on Boehme's work, was popular in German Pietism until the end of the eighteenth century. The major translations into English by William Law await the latter half of that century. One of the readers most strongly influenced by the Law translations was William Blake. Another influence upon him was Emanuel Swedenborg

(1688–1772), the "Seer of the North," who fertilized theology and esotericism with his account of journeys to other dimensions.

Swedenborg was trained as a scientist and it is said that he lived in the last generation when a single individual could master every known scientific field. When he had completed this kind of survey, he turned the scientific method upon the one subject that remained unstudied: himself. He kept a journal of his dreams: these slowly revealed an extensively detailed internal spiritual world that he described like a scientist visiting a foreign country. He called these places "heaven and hell," although Rudolf Steiner said they were visits to the "akashic records," the library of the world. I don't know. Swedenborg's anonymous writings fascinated late eighteenth-century Europe.

William Blake was one of the persons excited by Swedenborg. He also visited heaven and hell in "Vision," as he called it. Soon he developed alternative ideas and became critical of Swedenborg's scientific "voice" and attitude in describing "Vision." Blake parodied Swedenborg, especially in the book he called *The Marriage of Heaven and Hell* (1790).

The statement by Blake at the beginning this book ("None by travelling over known lands can find out the unknown") was made by a man who lived in London his whole life, save for a few years in a cottage just south of the city. He never traveled over unknown lands—except in "Vision"—but the lands he explored were indeed new.

Swedenborg and Blake are probably the greatest contributors to esoteric literature and tradition in the late Enlightenment era. Swedenborg wrote anonymously and Blake was almost entirely ignored in his own lifetime. Both were well read in Hermeticism, Platonic philosophy, the Hebrew and Greek Bible, and the esoteric worldview. Swedenborg did not attribute any of his knowledge to the Western esoteric tradition or philosophy, though it is known that he studied both. Therefore, he recounts many esoteric doctrines as if they were simply facts he had discovered. This annoyed Blake, as it is likely to annoy anyone versed in Western philosophy and Hermeticism. Despite their direct experience, the two had little influence on the occult tradition, which followed other byways.

The early nineteenth century saw an explosion of self-confidence in the American self-made man as new "liberties" encouraged free speech and thinking. This caused a deterioration in the quality of esoteric education and knowledge. This is a time period when we see the appearance of many half-baked tenets of esotericism making their way into mainstream or sectarian literature, as exampled in Mitch Horowitz's *Occult America* (2009) or D. Michael Quinn's *Early Mormonism and the Magic Worldview* (1987).

One of the most interesting and important of the American occultists was Paschal Beverly Randolph (1825–1875). Although he originated in America—a light-skinned Afro-American—he traveled the world, was friends with kings, politicians, and occultists—and was especially close with Hargrave Jennings, the prime mover in English occultism in the middle of the nineteenth century. His occultism is conveyed in his writings without a shade of protest about his humble, disadvantaged origins, without a digression on the terrifying issues ripping his nation apart.

As a free man of color traveling both north and south of the Mason-Dixon line in a time when anyone with a dark complexion could be enslaved if they couldn't present the right papers, the reader cannot help but wonder how Randolph managed to avoid trouble. He was also a black man advocating sexual freedom in the pre–Civil War period! How could he get away with this? Randolph explains how he navigated the roads of life safely: he was able to pick up on the thoughts and emotions of people around him, weaving them to suit his purposes. It is clear he possessed a familiar spirit that "went before him," protecting his way.

Obviously, such powers could easily be abused—especially if one believed in sexual freedom—but Randolph had a highly developed moral sense and differentiated carefully between self-interest and selfless service to humanity. His writings display the humility inherent in the best occult writers—Jacob Boehme, Emmanuel Swedenborg, Rudolf Steiner, and so forth. This meant that he could not use his powers to influence students to follow him and, although he was well-known in occult circles in America and Europe, he never reached too far beyond obscurity. However, Randolph deserves credit for perpetuating occult teachings in a time of horrific strife and social upheaval, before, during, and after the American Civil War. One of his students, Allan F. Odell, describes the positive and negative sides of the environment in which he taught:

> He lived and wrote in a time of mental stress and strain; in the days of the reconstruction, after the young Republic had successfully withstood the first assault upon its internal unity. Just after this struggle of brother against brother, there was an attitude of thankfulness on the part of the nation. The people breathed more easily and turned the lamps of their minds upon the ways of the spirit and the deeper things in life. Warfare, carnage, over-zealousness, mistaken devotion or forgetfulness of high ideals always seem to have been followed by a period of solemn quiet. . . . Turning away from the world, men contemplate the dim aisles of the inner self, where God is said to dwell. (Randolph 1930, xi)

Though the work of the shaman requires connection with the eternal Spirit World, one can never separate the shaman from the time period in which they live, nor from the land they frequent, where they were born, or where they choose to live. As a product of his time, Randolph demonstrates a thorough knowledge of Platonic philosophy and the traditional magical literature of the Western occult tradition. We do not know whether he also studied with Afro-American practitioners of voodoo, though he was clearly knowledgable about practitioners in New Orleans and—of all places—Long Island.

The great watershed in modern occult education occurred in 1875, when Helena Blavatsky (1831–1891), a Russian émigré, cofounded the Theosophical Society in New York City. She incorporated a lot of doctrine from Vedic philosophy and eventually moved her headquarters to India. During the late nineteenth and early twentieth century, the Theosophical Society and its offshoots literally had millions of followers around the world. Blavatsky contributed to the cultural life of the subcontinent where she lived, supporting native religion against the missionaries and education of the West.

Rudolf Steiner (1861–1925) was a citizen of Austria living in another tumultuous time, during the rise of a unified Germany, the First World War, the collapse of the Austrian Empire and the German currency, early labor movement struggles (which he supported), just before the rise of Hitler.

Steiner was a gifted clairvoyant and occultist. He predicted—to the month—the rise to power of a German dictator. He associated this individual with Lucifer, the egoic facet of evil. He also foresaw the rise to power of the second face of evil, "Ahriman," about 2012. This time, he said, the dominant power would be faceless world corporations, not egotism.

Steiner headed the German section of the Theosophical Society and never criticized Blavatsky, but he broke with her successor, Annie Besant (1847–1933) when the latter declared Jiddu Krishnamurti (1895–1966) the avatar of the age—an elevation the Indian himself later thoroughly rejected—wisely stating that each person was responsible for their own spiritual life.

By the early twentieth century, compulsory public education was pushed on the few pockets of the U.S. population that still believed in the magical worldview—the Native Americans, the Pennsylvania Dutch, and the subcultures of the American South. Today the media is heavily controlled so that subjects such as alternative medicine are seldom mentioned in the major news outlets, and shamanism or occultism even less so.

When I was young, esotericism was still much influenced by Theosophical teachings. Blavatsky, Steiner, Albert Sidney Raleigh (1881–1930), George Gurdjieff (1866–1949), Max Heindel (1865–1919), Arthur E. Waite (1857–1942), and Manley Palmer Hall (1901–1990) all maintained a fairly unified theory of occult knowledge, and when we look at their teaching, we find the same emphasis on the three basic selves, characteristic of shamanism.

Raleigh, by the way, was one of the last occultists to have been put to death for his vocation. He was charged with spreading false doctrines in Arkansas in 1936, put on a prison farm to await trail, and despite his protestations that he was sensitive to the sun, he was sent out to work and died of heat stroke on the third day of his imprisonment. He was the only premodern Western occultist whose writings show extensive knowledge of Central Mexican nagualism, in addition to Hermeticism and Vedanta.

The appearance of shamanic and Native American teachings in the late twentieth century began to change the discussion in esoteric and New Age literature. These and other forces had a fertilizing effect on the movement. A good example of an individual who was educated largely by Indigenous influences would be Max Freedom Long (1890–1971), who studied the Hawaiian Kahunas.

The Three Selves

Max Freedom Long was perhaps the first man of Western culture to discover the threefold system in the shamanism of an Indigenous, non-Western setting. He used a traditional approach to knowledge found in shamanism throughout the world: studying root words. These were the Hawaiian vocabulary relating to the magical work of the *kahunas*. He realized that the shamans or kahunas of Hawaii must have had a language to teach their students and that it had to be Hawaiian. From this insight he developed the doctrine of the "three selves": *uhane* (talking self, ego), *unihipili* (animal self), and *aumakua* (spirit self, ancestral self). He understood that it was necessary to become conscious of the animal self so that communication with the *aumakua* could occur.

Long interpreted the word *unihipili* from its roots—which is a valid approach in the study of Hawaiian, but may diverge from common usage. Since he found *nihi* (or *hini*) to mean "hidden" and *pili* designates a "servant," *unihipili* could be translated "hidden soul (*u*) that serves another." Long rightly says that this is a perfect description of Freud's "unconscious." Freud defines the id, the central guiding intelligence of the unconscious as the center of the instincts, so in this regard the id is identical to an instinctual "animal self." However, Long's translation is quite different from common Hawaiian usage. In everyday speech, *unihipili* refers to the shade or shadow that goes down into the Underworld after the death of the body.

The word *aumakua* refers to the animal totem of a clan or person. The root *u-* or *au-* means "self" or "soul" while *makua* means "benevolent ancestor" or "ancestral spirit." The word *akua* was translated by the missionaries as "god" but also means "animal totem."

Long's ideas reflect the psychiatric contributions of Freud, who also discovered "three selves" about the same time: the ego (conscious self), id (guiding intelligence of the unconscious), and superego. The latter is not actually the spirit or a spirit, but is defined by Freud as the projection of a moral code, system, or God-belief by the individual. Freud very accurately saw that all people normally are motivated by the concept of a God or morality that is a projection of their training and experience, rather than an authentic spiritual experience.

At the time Long wrote, the outlines of shamanic knowledge were so little known in Western culture that he had to make up a word to name his system. He chose *huna*, a made-up Hawaiian word, the roots of which, however, mean "secret." This makes the miracle-working *kahuna* into a "keeper" (*kahu*) of the "secret" (*huna*). However, the word *kahuna* actually seems to merely mean a practitioner of any kind of trade, art, or practice, and first appears in a Hawaiian English dictionary in 1865 as the word for a cook! By the time Long came to the islands, in 1917, the use of the word *kahuna* to signify a practitioner of occult or spiritual power was standard.

Long sussed out the character of the shamanic path and I believe he deserves credit for this accomplishment, which he dates to about 1936. He woke from a dream understanding that the Hawaiians had to have had words for their experiences and he worked out the practices from the root words. The connection between this work, however, and shamanism, was not then apparent. Nor was the connection between Western occultism and shamanism. Or Freudian psychology and shamanism!

Carlos Castaneda

It was the appearance of the writings of Carlos Castaneda (1925–1998), that brought the understanding of shamanism into both anthropology and popular Western culture. Castaneda described many important aspects of spiritual warriorship, shamanic experience, and dreamtime know-how, yet his writings are more like a travelogue without a set of directions. Castaneda did not really want to pass on the keys he had received.

In *Journey to Ixtlan*, we are informed that Castaneda's animal self is Coyote—a perfectly fine animal but a trickster through and through; don Juan notes this in his analysis of Castaneda's experience (Castaneda 1972, 250, 255). Amy Wallace's *Sorcerer's Apprentice* (2003) reveals Castaneda's character faults: he was a narcissist and womanizer who did not want to empower anyone but himself.

Luis De La Lama's *The Heart of the Serpent: Mystical Journeys to the Core of Life* (1993) gives an account of an initiation of a student by Castaneda—who, of course, did not publicly acknowledge the transfer of energy. The download was so enormous and overwhelming that De La Lama had to spend six months living in his mother's basement in Tijuana, watching Mexican soap operas, in order to learn how to be human again.

William Patrick Patterson's critique, *The Life & Teachings of Carlos Castaneda* (2008), traces the relationship between Castaneda's work and Mexican nagualism, a connection Castaneda did not make clear until late in his writings. Patterson's main effort is to demonstrate that Castaneda borrowed from George Gurdjieff's teachings. I would make this borrowing fairly minimal and attribute most of the similarity to the commonality of shamanic concepts throughout the world.

Timothy Knab's *A War of the Witches* (1995) gives the key to the shamanic model. Like Castaneda, Knab was an anthropologist trained by nagualist practitioners in central Mexico. This book shows us what Castaneda could have been: a humble, helpful, truthful spiritual student and teacher, rather than a power-hungry womanizer and trickster.

Knab was the first author I ran across who blatantly stated a simple fact: the animal self becomes the dream self.

Knab's teachers preferred to avoid contact with "those who are not our brothers"—Castaneda's "inorganic beings." Unlike Knab's teachers, Castaneda's put great emphasis on contact with the inorganic beings. While Castaneda does not empower his readers, he leaves an extensive and detailed account of many aspects of real journeying in the Spirit World. It is profoundly useful and inspiring.

In Mexico, the word *nagual* is the most common name for the animal self, the spirit self it gives birth to, the shaman who can change into an animal, and the realm in which the dream self operates. The term was defined by Daniel Brinton in the late nineteenth century (Brinton's work is reprinted in Patterson 2008). It is also used by Timothy Knab and Théun Mares (1998) in his development of Castaneda's material.

Théun Mares's analysis of Castaneda is detailed. He explains the path into the spiritual world that Castaneda took in such detail that one can actually detect the same pattern in the visionary experiences of Jacob Boehme. Many have attempted to show that Castaneda was a charlatan. He certainly was a trickster, but his accounts of another world are authentic and can experienced. It's just that nobody can prove the existence of other dimensions to an audience that has not had the experience.

We can also refer to Douglas Gillette's *The Shaman's Secret: The Lost Resurrection Teachings of the Ancient Maya* (1997). This chronicles some of the ancient lineage of nagualism. It is now well known that the monarchs of the ancient Mayans were "shaman kings"—political, religious, and spiritual leaders. The "lost resurrection teachings" of the old Mayas that Gillette describes dovetail with modern nagualism and shamanism. The "secret" in the title of Gillette's book is a reference to the awakening of the animal self (*uayob*).

The shaman kings were identified with the Black Jaguar, an animal alter ego of the Lord of the Underworld. One can only imagine the terrifying authority these shaman kings must have exercised. The chaos that ensued when these leaders were overthrown—several cultural epochs before the appearance of the Spanish—resulted in the kind of war referred to in Timothy Knab's title.

Searching for a Name

The publication of Michael Harner's *The Way of the Shaman* in 1980 brought the concept of shamanism into popular Western culture and made it into a "spiritual movement." Under the influence of Ayahuasca administered by Native practitioners in the Upper Amazon, Harner pretty much had the full shamanic experience (1990, 4):

> I became aware of my brain. I felt—physically—that it had become compartmentalized into four separate and distinct levels. At the uppermost surface was the observer and commander, which was conscious of the condition of my body, and was responsible for the attempt to keep my heart going. It perceived, but purely as a spectator, the visions emanating from what seemed to be the nether portions of my brain. Immediately below the topmost level I felt a numbed layer, which seemed to have been put out of commission by the drug—it just wasn't there. The next level down was the source of my visions, including the soul boat.
>
> Now I was virtually certain I was about to die. As I tried to accept my fate, an even lower portion of my brain began to transmit more visions and information. I was "told" that this new material was being presented to me because I was dying and therefore "safe" to receive these revelations. These were the secrets reserved for the dying and the dead, I was informed.

Harner's conscious self is largely incapacitated. He enters the Land of the Dead and here finds "giant reptilian creatures reposing sluggishly at the lowermost depths of the back of my brain, where it met the top of the spinal column" (Harner 1990, 4). The lower back brain is the reptilian brain, one evolutionary notch above the brain stem or amphibian brain. These "dragonlike creatures" claimed to be the progenitors of life on Earth:

They were the true masters of humanity and the entire planet, they told me. We humans were but the receptacles and servants of these creatures. For this reason they could speak to me from within myself. (Harner 1990, 4–5)

As we will see, the Dragons do have a claim over the human race.

This is an experience of the reptilian self and not the warm-blooded animal self. Sometimes, this is the order in which the shamanic student experiences the actualization of the animal world—as, for example, in the experience of my friend Susan, where she was visited by the King of the Alligators.

At the time when Harner was writing, most non-Indigenous people, including anthropologists and ethnobotanists, did not understand shamanism. When Carlos Castaneda began to write in 1967, neither he, his faculty advisors, nor his readers were capable of identifying the worldview of his mentor, don Juan. It eventually became clear that this was a version of the well-documented form of Mexican shamanism called nagualism. By 1980, when Harner (one of Castaneda's faculty advisors) penned *The Way of the Shaman*, the concept finally made its way into common culture. This resulted in the initiation of a popular spiritual path called shamanism or neoshamanism in New Age and alternative circles.

Popular shamanism has several different origins. The most important would be the enormously popular series of Castaneda books. A second influence came through the popularization of psychedelic drugs. Terence and Dennis McKenna and others pioneered the use of Ayahuasca, which is now widely available in North America. Another influence is the introduction of Native American spirituality and ceremony into mainstream culture. Many Indian people associate the term "shamanism" with witchcraft or dilettantism. The popular New Age movement, descended from Western occultism, was also highly influential. Finally, there is the modern pagan and witchcraft revival, closed related to the New Age. One must include the romanticism of shamanism and its paraphernalia as an additional influence. Of course, one cannot simplify mass movements down to one interpretation.

Within the Western occult tradition there must have been many others, like myself, who saw the shamanic impulse as more vivacious and alive than the rather stultified tradition that we received through our teachers and traditions. In *The UnderWorld Initiation* (1989), R. J. Stewart fondly speaks of his mentor as an "Edwardian occultist," but the path he discovered and taught is based upon interaction with the faeries and the Faery Queen. Edwardian occultism, the New Age, and shamanism are now much interconnected.

The new "imitative" shamanism has been called "neoshamanism." I don't use this term because I consider Paracelsus, Randolph, Blavatsky, Steiner, and Gurdjieff to have been representatives of an unbroken shamanic tradition that was classified as "occultism" and is still not recognized as "shamanism" by anthropologists.

Self-identification with shamanism in the popular culture has often been dismissed by many as misguided romanticism. It is also rejected by many Native Americans. Several of my Native friends begged me not to use the word "shaman" since it was associated by them with dilettantism, while another said that as a white person, I didn't have the right to use the term. I thought, on the other hand, that she had no right to determine how a Siberian term is used, or to judge another person's spiritual path. I am not referring to myself as a shamanic practitioner in some magical sense, but as a participant in a spiritual tradition found in every culture including my own. Even a person who has not merged with their animal self, but who is working with the three selves model, is working with the spiritual technology of shamanism. That includes the psychological systems of Freud and Jung.

The three selves model is not at variance with the Bible itself. Christian theologians, lacking real acquaintance with Hebrew, missed the fact that three selves are defined in the first chapters of Genesis as the human self (*neshema*), animal self (*nephesh*), and spirit (*ruach*). However, the Church Fathers derived a similar working model from Plato's doctrine of the tripartite soul, which consisted of three elements: Reason, Desire, and Will. This tripartite definition is standard Orthodox/Catholic doctrine down to the present. Even within conventional Judaism and Christianity, we find the shamanic model shining forth.

In *Seven Herbs: Plants as Teachers* (1987) and again in *Seven Guideposts on the Spiritual Path* (2021b), I outlined the extremely accurate and detailed account of the shamanic path described in the Book of Genesis.

When Harner told his experience with the reptilians to a local shaman, the man laughed and declared that these beings were not the progenitors of humanity, but only the Lords of the Outer Darkness. We'll talk about the role of the reptiles later on.

Witchcraft and Paganism

When the Articles of Incorporation of the Town of Southampton, established in 1640 on a wild, isolated shoreline in the New World, were drawn up, they included the following declaration taken from the early laws of New England:

> Witchcraft, which is a fellowship by covenant with a familiar spirit, to be punished with death. (Cotton 1641, 10)

Proclamations like this make it clear that the authorities knew exactly what witchcraft was—not herbalism or midwifery, or even psychic interference with others—but *full-fledged possession of a familiar spirit*. Unfortunately, the application of the law was very imperfect and many innocent people were put to death. In actuality, disciplined witches are virtually impossible to detect because the animal self is highly protective of the physical body and psychically protects the possessor, keeping opponents away. This is true of both good and bad shamans—if they are disciplined. J. K. Rowling had it correct when she says the real witches largely escaped the flames because the Muggle (non-magical) authorities couldn't detect them.

I have not generally worked with material from the modern witch, pagan, or neopagan movement, partly because I am not familiar with these movements and partly because it is often presented as a "belief system" rather than an experiential method. A notable exception is the aforementioned work of R. J. Stewart in *The UnderWorld Initiation*. He provides the key to unlocking the shamanic lore preserved in the Lowland Scottish ballad tradition. What I call the "animal self" he calls the "co-walker" or "companion."

The companion spirit was well known in pagan and medieval times—see Claude Lecouteux's account in *Witches, Werewolves, and Fairies: Shapeshifters and Astral Doubles in the Middle Ages* (2003). He relates a funny story about werewolfism at the end of the seventeenth century (2003, 118–20, 168–76). A homeless man was brought up for prosecution before a magistrate in Livonia for claiming to be a werewolf. The magistrate was beside himself that someone could dedicate himself to the Devil, but the man kept saying that he was fighting against the Devil. He claimed he had to change himself into a wolf in order to get the seeds for the farmers from the Devil, so that the farmers could plant them.

Actual shamans (and witches) with familiar spirits were seldom caught if they were careful and disciplined, because it is virtually impossible to sneak up on a person with an active, well-developed animal self. By its very nature, as an animal, it is highly aware, more instinctive than humans, and self-protective. It "goes before" the person, scanning the environment as only an animal can do, disarming opponents through secret negotiations with the weaker, unactualized animal selves of other people, in order to protect the shaman and those in their sphere.

The last description I can find in Europe of someone killing an adversary with their doppelganger is from a seventeenth-century account about the gentle Lutheran mystic Jacob Boehme (Okely 1780, 19–20). He was at a dinner party where a petty noble mercilessly tormented him verbally for his spiritual opinions. Before allowing any kind of rebuttal by Boehme or his friends, the man stormed off into the night. Boehme was so angered he couldn't stop himself. He told his friends he was ashamed of what was going to happen. The next morning the man was found dead with a broken neck; his horse had violently thrown him.

What finished the magical worldview in the English-speaking world was not the persecution of witches but the rise of modern science and education. This is evident in the treatment of the Pennsylvania Dutch, who still maintained a semi-medieval belief and practice of magic. Federal educational standards annihilated the magical worldview, both in Pennsylvania and in American Indian schools.

The Spirit Molecule

Recently, a slight break in the wall of orthodox scientific opposition to the shamanic worldview has occurred due to the study of the compound dimethyltryptamine (DMT). DMT occurs naturally in the brain, which even seems to crave it, but it is in short supply unless it is artificially introduced into the body via the traditional plant mixes used by shamans or by psychiatric researchers. Most famous among these traditional brews are Ayahuasca and psilocybin. So consistent are the experiences produced in the laboratory with spiritual and otherworldly descriptions from around the world, and from person to person within or outside the laboratory, that it has been called the "spirit molecule" by psychiatric researcher Rick Strassman (2001). Because this molecule reproduces characteristic experiences of a Spirit World it must now be scientifically admitted that such a world may exist—if in no other way than biochemically—within our brains. These DMT experiences are often reported as profoundly life-changing, having more "reality" than the world of science itself. Once again, we are reminded that what happens in dreamtime can determine what happens in the material world.

Those who have been "touched by the spirit" don't really care about whether science has proven or disproven the existence of the Spirit World, but for scientists it is an important development that gives them some ability to observe "spiritual" and "otherworldly" experience. It is also important to acknowledge this work because of its difficulty. Strassman had to fight against legal and professional barriers (which are now receding more and more) to conduct research with individuals taking DMT. We should also thank the scores of volunteers in these studies.

There is an important difference between the characteristic shamanic experience (animal/human) and this research. The experience of turning into an animal, or being torn apart or consumed by an animal, under the influence of Ayahuasca, psilocybin, refined DMT, or other related hallucinogenic substances is not commonly found in Strassman's work. In other words, these heroic explorations suggest the existence of spiritual experiences similar to those found in many religions and are seldom specific to the shamanic worldview. Hallucinogens do not necessarily induce the experience of the animal self.

2

Spirit and Medicine

The eternal position of all things, independent of time, without beginning or end, operates everywhere. It works essentially where otherwise there is no hope. It accomplishes that which is deemed impossible. What appears beyond belief or hope emerges into truth after a wonderful fashion.

PARACELSUS, *CŒLUM PHILOSOPHORUM*

The first thing that can be said about the spirit is that it can't be directly seen, but is only visible in its effects. It is for this reason that the spirit is so often likened to the wind in descriptions around the world. The language we use to describe the spirit is therefore going to be metaphorical and analogical, and that is the native tongue of the shaman: analogy, comparison, and inference. That's the second thing we can say about this Mystery. The third assertion is that on any legitimate spiritual path there is nothing more important than learning to recognize the effects of the spirit.

The Spirit

Shamanism pursues realms of perception that range from the far-fetched to the completely unknown. Within that spectrum something intelligent and powerful lurks that we do not interact with under ordinary circumstances. For lack of a better word, we can call it "the spirit." It would be best not to associate it with any particular religion or religious idea. We should really not think of something higher or lower, inside or outside, personlike or impersonal, religious or secular—but something that is completely unknowable yet upon which one's life depends. There is something out there, beyond the theater of the mind, which is unknown but always hovering nearby, beating its wings on our brain, trying to get through to us.

At the beginning of his apprenticeship, don Juan said to Carlos that the only thing "indispensable" for their activities was "the spirit" (Castaneda 1972, 9). The activity of the spirit is essential in the pursuit of spiritual transformation. Without it, there is no possibility of success.

Part of the reason the word "spirit" is so poorly defined in our society is that our culture dictates that serious people do not study or define the term, or even talk about it, except in rather pedestrian phrases such as "team spirit" or a "spirited horse."

The psychiatrist E. Grahame Howe (1897–1975) was one of the only members of his profession to advocate the study of the spirit in the mid-twentieth century. He pointed out that while the king and the media declared Britain would win the Second World War due to the "spirit" of her armies and people, no one bothered to study what that meant. Imagine basing the survival of one's country and armies on something that is undefined and unexamined? Howe was eventually ostracized for asking these kinds of questions.

Our word spirit is related to words for breathing like respiration, inspiration, and expiration. Inspiration is not limited to breathing in, but can also mean that one is inspired by something—a person, art, music, or a religious or spiritual experience; one has "breathed in the spirit." Many people feel called by an inner force to make sacrifices that go beyond the needs of body and soul. They may have to follow a path that drags them through tribulation and suffering. They may have to stand up for a truth that is greater than themselves or help others at great personal peril. They may have to "give up the spirit" (expire) to follow the calling (inspiration) of the spirit.

When we feel the ring of truth, we are required to take a stand. The elements of truth, judgment, and courage pertain to the spirit. Since it is up to us to accept our experiences as true or false, the spirit is also the great advocate of free will. Acting within us, it resonates with a calling from beyond soul and body for a higher truth, freedom, and way of living. Throughout life, all of us are attracted to higher truth and vision. We are incomplete until we know this spirit. We yearn for that mysterious part of us, about which we know nothing at the start, but which slowly "fills in the blanks."

Shamanism may be described as a conglomeration of traditional methods evolved throughout the world for seeking, experiencing, developing, and defining interaction with the spirit. Even anthropologists are willing to define the shaman as a "spiritual technician."

Unfortunately, a lot of people identify shamanism with the tools and articles associated with shamans in traditional societies. These external items are relatively unimportant because the spirit shines in all times and places, generating new language and tools as needed. If the item has been empowered by the spirit then it is very important.

When the spirit shows up in our world, it rocks our boat. It can't stand slavery and that's why it is rarely seen in our world. But it will send smoke signals from its abode in a faraway land. Most of the time we don't even notice the signals—the "whispering of the spirit"—and even when we do, the whispers are so inconvenient that we ignore them.

When there is a strong need for it, or when a person is imbued "with spirit," the power of the spirit can manifest in such a way that it seems like a miracle; every miracle is a salute from the spirit to a dedicated and favored son or daughter.

As we progress along the sacred path and grow increasingly in harmony with the spirit there is less and less need for suffering or mind-boggling miracles. The best relationship is one of peaceful coexistence. As Hermes says in the *Hermetica*:

> To be able to know and to will and to hope is the straight and easy
> way, appropriate to each, that will lead to the Supreme Good. When

you take that road, this Good will meet you everywhere and will be experienced everywhere, even where and when you do not expect it; when awake, asleep, in a ship, on a rock, by night, by day, when speaking and when silent. (Salaman et al. 2000, 58)

Speech and Spirit

An interesting thing about the spirit is that it generates language. When the perspective stands somewhat outside the bounds of ordinary conversation, new terms are needed to express the experience. But it seems that there is a special connection between the spirit and language.

The repackaging of old concepts and experiences for new generations is a constant refrain in spiritual tradition. Jesus remarked on this when he said, "You can't put new wine in old wineskins." In keeping with this, he seldom quoted old, worn-out passages of the Hebrew Bible but exploited literary devices that were associated with Aramaic folk culture: parables, similitudes, contrasts, parallels, and inferences. Ever since, of course, his followers have been trying to stuff the new wine of human experience into the "same old wineskins," making Christianity boring.

A similar observation was made by Rudolf Steiner (1995, 125): we cannot allow "our cognitive growth in certain areas to be held in chains by linguistic custom." Unfortunately, I would not consider Steiner to be a good representative of the creative use of language. I once complained to a German-speaker that the translations of Steiner rendered him almost unreadable and she replied, "Oh, you have to understand, he's even worse in the original—the translators try to make him more comprehensible than he is in German!" On the other hand, Steiner generated many new ideas of benefit to society, from agriculture to medicine. The gifts of the spirit come in many forms.

Another spiritual voyageur who understood the importance of language was Terence McKenna, one of the early spokespersons of shamanism and hallucinogenic consciousness-expansion, who remarked (2016): "The way you stretch the envelope of culture is by creating language." In another lecture, he stated:

You are an explorer, and you represent our species, and the greatest good you can do is to bring back a new idea, because our world
is endangered by the absence of good ideas. Our world is in crisis
because of the absence of consciousness. (McKenna 2010a)

We are the animal with the most highly sophisticated speaking
ability. This gives us the opportunity to express aspects of the spirit
that would otherwise not come into existence. The creativity therefore
runs two ways: from the spirit to the human and from the human to
the spirit.

Innovation and borrowing are as old as human culture. They are an
innate part of every society and are required in order for humanity to
grow and change. The "cultural appropriation" crowd seem to believe
that everything worth knowing is already a part of their culture so that it
need not appropriate ideas from other cultures. This shows how conceited
and biased they are: they are too good to acknowledge the importance of
another culture.

Intolerance is built into the very bones of Western culture. Logic, a
dominant feature of Western speech and thought is innately judgmen-
tal. It forces the listener to agree or not with "what is logical," with
"what is right." That creates an "us versus them" situation in which
argued "truths" determine who is right and who is wrong—and often,
down through the centuries, who lives and who dies. It is "colonizing"
in the sense that other societies have to be brought into the belief system. The argument by the anti-appropriators is innately destructive to
the cultures they pretend to protect because it is based on a Western
paradigm.

Indigenous speech does not possess the syllogism ("If . . . , then . . .").
Aristotle says that Plato was the first to use it to obtain knowledge. The
Greeks contrasted the new logic with the old form of speech, which
they called *phasis*, "describing the appearance of the phenomena."* A

---

*This is the translation by my late friend Robert Schmidt. He gave the usual translations
as "appearance," "description," and "phenomena."

person simply described what they saw, without making a conclusion. If they wanted to expand on an idea, they made a comparison between two observations through inference, analogy, contrast, or wordplays—in other words, intuition, imagination, and new experience. The great representative of the phasic method in Greek philosophy was Herakleitos the Dark. He said: "the road up is the same as the road down"; this is an observation that contains an inference. What does it mean? Empires rise and fall. Childhood gives way to adulthood and then old age. Life experiences repeat themselves. There is no "right answer," only an observation to ponder.

Real Spiritual Experience

Due to this dry gulch of a culture, we live in a time when it is hard to find spiritually experienced people. Or maybe it just seems that way. There are always people who get clobbered over the head by the spirit whether they are interested in it or not. Fortunately, a lot of teachers are available in Nature—in the fields and forests (stones, plants, animals). Rudolf Steiner said that if one could not find a human teacher, one could start with plants. George Gurdjieff said that if we were having trouble loving our fellow mankind, we should start with plants, then animals, then people.

The principle "when the student is ready, the teacher will appear" holds true, but it is hard to "get ready" in a society with so few signposts. Real spiritual experience is difficult to obtain. We don't realize that we are missing important connecting links between the human soul and the animal self and we are missing virtually all the hardwiring for perception of the Spirit World.

At first we see the world through the physical senses. That innately distorts spiritual experience, reinterpreting it into pictures of things we are familiar with in the material world. We may have a "chance seeing," as don Juan called it—an unexpected profound spiritual experience where we are touched by the authentic spirit . . . "That may be rare, but hard to miss it when it happens," commented a friend.

Because of our innate inborn limitations, it is important for us to develop the skills mentioned above—starting with observation of experience, going on to intuitive evaluation, comparison, and inference, and not overlooking imagination. Steiner maintains that some of the "petals" of the "throat chakra" are conditioned by speech and require our attention in order for that center to open up. That is an essential center, since it unifies the human, the animal, and the spirit.

As seekers we were like blindfolded people searching for something we dimly sensed but never experienced before and cannot accurately imagine. The only reason we sense the existence of the spirit is because we feel that we are incomplete in some way—but we don't know how. Even incompleteness has its purpose.

Spiritual Seership

There is a great difference between psychism, or perception of psychic phenomena, and true spiritual seership. The latter comes from an over-shadowing of the spirit. The person sees the truth, and when that per-son speaks, you know it is true. Susan was one of these people. Whether it was about God or the waitress, it was true. Fortunately, she didn't talk that way all the time. Humans need to rest. Ordinary conversation, and even psychic perception, does not give one the "sensation of truth." Psychics—even the good ones—are guessing and probing.

Medicine

Nineteenth-century white authors spoke of "medicine men" and "medi-cine women" among the American Indian people. Their practice of medicine was similar to that of the white man. It utilized medicines, purges, diets, and fasts. The Indian people therefore adopted the word "medicine" from their conquerors. However, in picking up the word, they changed the definition to fit their experience. After a long incuba-tion in the Native world, the word re-entered the now-dominant culture with new connotations.

It took a long time for the invaders to understand the term in its new, Indigenous incarnation. Awareness is not understanding. In 1950, anthropologist Jaime de Angulo (a friend of Carl Jung) described the concepts of *dinihowi* and *damaagome* held by the Pit River Indians of northern California. He did not attempt to define the concept himself but left it to his Native friends, or informants. "Some Indians translate it into English as 'medicine,' or 'power,' sometimes 'dog,'" wrote de Angulo (1950, 340–41). It was also translated as "luck."

> It was Robert Spring who first made me understand about the dinihowi. "That's what we Indians call *luck*. A man has got to have luck, no matter for what, whether it's for gambling, or for hunting, for making love, for anything." (de Angulo 1950, 345)

De Angulo couldn't understand the difference between the *dinihowi* obtained by an ordinary person and the *damaagome* obtained by a medicine person. Spring replies:

> "There is no difference. It's all the same. Only the *damaagome* that's for doctors." "How does the doctor get his *damaagones*?" "Just like you and me get a *dinihowi*. He goes to the mountain. He cries. Then someone comes and says, this is my song, I'll help you." (de Angulo 1950, 346)

Spring went on to explain how a *dinihowi* or *damaagome* is obtained. A young man might lose interest in regular life, go up in the mountains, and wander for a while until he could "catch a *dinihowi*," a blessing or a power from a helpful animal or spirit in the wilderness (de Angulo 1950, 345).

Originally, I thought de Angulo allowed his informants to give their own definition out of deference to their opinions, but I was shocked to read that he simply did not understand what they were talking about. His biographer, Andrew Schelling, explains (2017, 225):

Religion he discussed in many pages, throughout his writings on the Achumawi (Pit Rivers) and others. He said he never found among the Pit Rivers anything that corresponds with characteristics that most people associate with religion. He found no belief in a supreme being, no creation out of nothing, no priesthood, hierarchical societies, rituals, or other elements of religion. Only the constant interest in "power, power, power."

What de Angulo did not understand is that this "power" comes from the Spirit World and is in fact the basis of a sophisticated religion that is totally experiential and not abstract, theoretical, philosophical, or theological. It was totally unlike the religion he was familiar with in his own culture. If an anthropologist like Jaime de Angulo couldn't understand the meaning of the word "medicine," then who did?

In *American Indian Medicine*, ethnobotanist Virgil Vogel dodged the bullet by quoting from an older anthropologist, George Bird Grinnell (1849–1938): "All these things which we speak of as medicine the Indian calls mysterious, and when he calls them mysterious, this only means that they are beyond his power to account for" (1970, 25). This is a pathetic definition: the Indian people could not explain "medicine" because of the limited vocabulary, experience, and preconceptions of white anthropologists like Grinnell, who treated them like children. Medicine meant something very concrete and experiential to the Native population. At the same time, it also meant something mysterious. The Indigenous word for "spirit" in many Native languages means "mystery." This includes the Algonquin *manitu* or *manido* and the Dakota *wakan*. There is both a Great Mystery (*Gitchi Manito* or *Wakan Tonka*) and little mysteries, or what we would call "spirits." Medicine is both a mystery and a concrete experience with definite rules and obligations.

I met Virgil Vogel; he stayed with my parents in the mid-1970s. He was a good man and his inventory of American Indian medicinal plants and practices is valuable. The fact that an honest, solid scholar in the field could do no better than quote the vacuous, unenlightened statement of Grinnell shows that even in 1970 the Indian concept of medicine was still generally impossible for white people to comprehend.

When the first book by Carlos Castaneda appeared in 1967 he used the word "power" to translate whatever Spanish word don Juan used to describe the invisible potency hidden in acts, perceptions, experiences, and Nature all around us. Castaneda may well have been influenced by de Angulo, whose anthropological career was also spent in California, where Castaneda did his graduate work in the field.

It is clear from the first few books by Castaneda that don Juan knew his non-Indian student did not understand the concept. He resorts to stories, analogies, and even uses the word "mysterious." Castaneda never did use the word "medicine." In 1980, anthropologist Michael Harner still used the term "power" in *The Way of the Shaman.*

In 1976, Brad Steiger, a white author of popular esoteric books, entitled a book *Medicine Power.* In this book, "medicine" is associated with what would usually be called "psychic powers" in conventional white society. This is not what "medicine" actually is, but it is moving closer and it is clear that Steiger respected the Indian people and felt there was something important they were saying with the word "medicine."

In the end it would be a Native author who finally bridged the gap. Sun Bear grew up on the White Earth rez in northern Minnesota, a fairly acculturated reservation with a large Métis population. His white wife, Wabun, was a coauthor who also deserves some of the credit. In *The Medicine Wheel: Earth Astrology* (1980) they explained that Sun Bear's people used the "medicine wheel" (a circle enclosing a cross) to arrange knowledge. Sun Bear and Wabun used Western astrology as an analogy, identifying the twelve signs of the zodiac with the twelve lunar months of the Ojibwa calendar. Sun Bear and Wabun therefore moved the definition away from the psychism of Brad Steiger toward a more archetypal foundation. The inference that a "medicine" is a spiritual power, not just an archetype, also comes across. Fairly soon afterward, the full meaning of the Native interpretation of "medicine" entered English vocabulary.

Of course, we must remember that the term "wheel" is not innate to Indigenous American culture, since the wheel did not exist in pre-Columbian times. It was, however, a good metaphor in English for the circle. The Native word for hoop would actually be the better translation; it implies a wholeness that the term "wheel" does not. For instance, the Lakota Holy Man Black Elk lamented that the "hoop" of his nation had been broken, despite his best efforts as a representative of both the white man's church and his own Lakota spirituality.

Medicine is at first unknown, unseen, and unimagined. It is a rumor. But to those who have it or have seen it operate, medicine becomes increasingly experienceable, unmistakable, and subject to reference and discussion. It is an invisible substance that possesses power and produces visible effects in the world. It bequeaths a person purpose or a path in life; a skill, talent, or power; or a tool with power to make and change the conditions of life. Or it is simple "luck" and opens doors.

Although medicine is a power and gives power, a person must acknowledge it and treat it with respect or it will abandon them. It is idiosyncratic and almost temperamental, short on tolerance for error and stupidity, yet loyal beyond what humans understand. Medicine power follows definite laws and demands the same from us in return. Sometimes it is useful and sometimes a nuisance. It can be misused but it cannot be ignored.

Medicine is artistic, creative, social, political, or medical. Or it is an object, plant, animal, or person, or a vision, empowerment, transmission, or dream. It does not arise from ordinary learning or information, but comes from the spirit and therefore is essentially mysterious. At the same time, it is quite familiar to the person who holds it or upon whom it acts. The more one becomes acquainted with medicine, the more definite and identifiable it becomes.

A medicine power cannot be refused. A person can put off the "appointment" for a long time, but it will always be hanging over their head. When that alignment occurs, the spirit asks the person to do something concrete in the world. A simple offering is seldom enough; medicine is often a vocation or calling that changes the direction of life. It doesn't matter if the person delays accepting the medicine, but if they reject the calling, it kinks them up—messes up their energy; changes to bad luck. Without medicine, a person has no power, fate, or destiny, but if suppressed, it is even worse, and if misused, it is a bane to the community.

Some people feel the absence of medicine in their lives: the absence of purpose, meaning, talent, skill, or ability. And they don't know what to do about it, don't know a name for what they are missing, and don't know how to seek it. Western society is set up to cater to existence without internal purpose. If people aren't happy in the boring, superficial society they are surrounded by, they are given drugs so that they can "function." The idea of self-fulfillment through inner exploration and discovery is not a part of ordinary society. If people can't get drugs from the doctor, they buy it on the street.

Most modern Western people don't want to commit themselves to any kind of spiritual power, good or bad. It takes courage to commit oneself, even to evil. People prefer to live off the resources of the planet without paying back. They do not realize that the situation we live in was set up with a very careful balance that allows us to experience and choose between the good path and the downward spiral. They are wasting time, resources, opportunity, and the lives of other people. This type of oblivious self-centeredness starts in neutral territory, but if it is persisted in over a length of time, it creates a momentum that slowly pulls the person down.

Robert Spring uses a term that is often found in association with medicine. A person "cries" for the spirits to have pity on them and give them a medicine. Have pity upon me, so I can have a life worth living.

Internal emptiness heralds the search for medicine, as Robert Spring says. Yearning, dedication, and exploration are often necessary, though medicine can also arrive for no particular reason and can be carried down through the bloodline, too. It may go to a child or grandchild, or even skip multiple generations. However, the gift can lead to complications if the following generation does not want it. Rejection of the spirit creates troubles. Fortunately, there are several medicines that help us understand and work out these kinds of problems.

A person can also lose a medicine. If it is not treated with respect and integrity, it can abandon the man or woman, or be taken away by more responsible medicine-carriers in the person's culture. One of my friends was abusing drugs and alcohol and living on the street. One day he woke up to find a patch cut out of his jeans jacket, where he had stored a medicine that was important to his people.

A plant can be a medicine. The ability to correctly apply a plant to a situation and heal is medicine. Medicine power may arise from worldly study or experience or the teachings of an elder, but it is only real medicine if the spirit shines in and through it, empowering it into a spiritual gift and not just a low-level occupational skill. A healer with medicine can cure just by being present or thinking about a case or recommending the right remedy or doctor.

In 2008 I was visited by the daughter of an old friend who had grown up with me in the Quaker Meeting in Minneapolis. There was nothing apparently wrong with her or her husband, but they had been infertile for over seven years. I took a case history and recommended an herb. It took them time to find the herb and before it arrived, the wife was pregnant and nine months later delivered a healthy daughter. It may have been a matter of mentioning or recognizing the right herb, but the situation changed and I was given credit for the change. I appreciated that.

It turned out the new daughter had a special medicine herself. People commented on her "perspicacity"—the ability to have special insight into things and choice of words. Her given name was Cassidy.

A sort of "luck" follows a person with medicine, but this English term is not an appropriate translation. English "luck" refers to a random benefit dished out by the Wheel of Fortune, which is arbitrary in its distribution of good and bad luck.

A person can be born with medicine or acquire it on the death of an older relative. This includes bad medicine. Even the reception of good medicine can be trying and difficult. I have many times noticed people encountering very bad to even overwhelming problems after the death of a parent or relative. It can turn out that the parent was holding back energies that were detrimental to the children, not allowing them to influence the next generation, but not able to deal with them during life. The year following such a death is a time to be very observant and careful about the inner life of surviving relatives.

A friend in her twenties was sitting with her father at his death-bed. He had been an initiate of several different medicine societies in a pueblo nearby, though he was not a member of the tribe. "Do you want my initiations?" he asked his daughter. She innocently replied, "Yes." After his death she received a massive download of silent knowledge. "I almost died," she said, and her "life was torn to pieces" over the next several years, as she slowly integrated those lessons. She didn't even join the societies, only receiving the initiations on the inner level. "I'm a blabbermouth and can't keep secrets," she explained, "so I just translate the information using published mythology."

The pueblo still considered her an esteemed elder. I was there when a call from the pueblo came in, and did they hop when she gave them some advice! And her advice was tragically justified by subsequent events.

In the old days, a young person who was particularly compatible with an older teacher might go and study with him or her and marry into the family. In ensuing generations the medicine is increasingly built into the family genes. This was fine in the days when medicine power was respected, but in modern society it is rejected. This can become destructive to family life.

A strange thing about medicine is that it travels from person to person, even when one of the parties is dedicated to good while the other is dedicated to evil. This is because the essential requirement for receiving medicine is similarity of soul and spirit. The spirit does want good to prevail, but because it guarantees free will it will not interfere, even when medicine is being abused. But it sneaks up on a person and one day it levels the playing field.

A person can "buy medicine" from another. I don't know whether this is good or bad. For Christians it constitutes a sin called "simony," described in the Book of Acts in the Greek Bible. This is not necessarily a sin in Native American society but I am too programmed by Western culture to be a fair judge here.

I was once offered the opportunity to "buy medicine" from one of my deceased teachers in dreamtime, but my dream self automatically rejected the offer. He was dedicated to evil—though I saw exceptions to this in his work—and I didn't trust his intentions while he was alive—so my dream self did not trust him either. Also, medicines are suited to certain temperaments and it is best to have medicine that is perfectly matched to one's disposition, not to that of another. And finally, I didn't want to have to go around putting food out for his energy body all the time because this would keep him from processing his stuff in the afterlife.

Medicine by its very nature can never be taken for granted. It's actions can never be fully predicated in advance and not always understood after the event. It is mysterious and if we attempt to control it with our minds or expectations it will either disappear or cause us unpleasantness until we can learn. It is a delicate thing, yet powerful enough to make perceptual, dimensional, and even social shifts. The world is full of Mysteries and wonders and if we attempt to explain it all or think we can, it will become boring and there will be no medicine, spirit, or spiritual life. Mystery must be part of even ordinary life. Susan once spoke about this in a pipe ceremony.

> *There is a sacred turtle graveyard at the bottom of the ocean. Nobody knows why it is there: why they go there to die. It is a Mystery. There will be Mysteries that will unfold as the world changes. They will penetrate to the marrow of our bones. If we are not ready, our bones will be shattered.*

We are a Mystery People. We are an Eternal Truth/Beauty/Mystery People—when we let the spirit have its way with us. It will meet us everywhere: on land, in the boat, speaking or staying silent, but more than anything else, it likes impossibility and Mystery and here it will meet us most graciously.

Don Juan told Carlos that when one has accepted one's destiny without recrimination, one gains "power"—in other words, medicine.

When we stop resisting who we are, medicine will start to walk by our side, like a faithful dog. One of Castaneda's students, Florinda Donner, wrote a book called *The Witch's Dream* (1985) about the bizarre contortions of destiny that are possible. A true spiritual vocation is demanding: there is power in such a life, as well as fulfillment, but there can also be tremendous suffering. Donner's book is a bit terrifying.

Drawing on these different sources, we can say that medicine arises from the ability to walk the path with beauty and heart in certainty, satisfaction, humility, and wonder, fulfilling the design that spirit has for each one of us.

Medicine is still being misunderstood. One of the best commentators on Carlos Castaneda stated that "personal power" develops as a result of the actualization of the dream self. While it is true that medicine arises out of the Spirit World, it is not true that one needs to develop a full-fledged dream self to receive it. This is too narrow a definition and a misrepresentation of a widespread Native American concept/experience found almost everywhere in the Western Hemisphere. One of my Native friends thanked me for pointing out the misinterpretation so I pass have to pass it on; the commentator was not an inhabitant of the Western Hemisphere.

Here is a bizarre story about medicine. There were some old storefronts in South Minneapolis that had been condemned in order to make way for the building of the American Indian Center. They were usually closed but I noticed an old man inside one of them and presumed it was open for business. Yes, he waved his hand across the room full of debris, everything was for sale. His hand was heavy and he looked tired. I was interested in some architectural drawing tools. "Oh, those aren't for sale," he said.

Some little Indian boys pounded on the front door and ran away. "I hate Indians," he said. He had just come out of heart surgery and I guess he had something he wanted to pass on. "Yeah, I only ever met one Indian I liked. It was back in the Depression. I was a kid. Each day I'd pick up shoes at a warehouse and peddle them from door to door. I was at a gas station when this sleek young Indian man came in with a brand new Pierce-Arrow and a girl on his shoulder like an Indian princess. He challenged everyone in the garage to play dice with him. In five minutes he had every penny in that place. Yeah, that was a good Indian."

I was shocked to hear such a blatantly racist story told to a stranger (me) but even more shocked to hear an account of medicine from the old man. It was like it was pressed out of him just for me and I have never forgotten it.

Here's an example of a medicine I acquired myself. The spirit can be present in the little, humble objects of creation as well as in beautiful, spectacular, or large matters. Also, one need not go on vision quests or even look for a medicine. When it comes, however, one *must recognize it and take action to keep it.* One definitely also has the right to reject a medicine gift. It might seem too onerous to take on. However, this was a nice gift.

Early one morning I drove a friend to the dental surgeon so she could have a ride back after the anesthesia. Who wants to sit around in an oral surgery clinic? Instead I stood outside in the cool Minnesota air, pushing some little landscaping pebbles around on the sidewalk with my foot. It gave me something to do to push them back onto the place where they were supposed to be.

"Wow," I exclaimed to myself as my foot connected with a little pebble that was clearly a conscious being. Did I kick it across the lawn? No, it was a conscious being and it would have been cruel to consign it to anonymity, so I picked it up and put it in my pocket. I still have it today.

It turned out there was more to this Mystery than I knew at the time. Several years later I ran across a Dakota teaching about the *witai* stone. This is a stone that is alive and conscious. When a person finds one, it gives them the right to set up an altar. We can see why this would be the case: the *witai* stone indicates that one can respond to the life inside the natural world, and that means one can act as a mediator between the Living Nature and exiled humanity.

One day I was walking down the street with a friend in a large West Coast city. Both of us noticed that the enormous shade tree on the boulevard was conscious. It was truly shocking. Neither one of us had ever experienced anything like that before, but that is the way it is with medicine: it is here and not there, there and not here. The gifts of the body, soul, and spirit are not equally dispensed across Nature. Some things have medicine while others do not. Some awake, some asleep. Just like people.

3

The Shaman's Explanation

In esoteric tradition there is no such thing as unconsciousness.
R. J. STEWART, THE UNDERWORLD INITIATION

Experiences that the soul has during sleep are in a sense illuminated by the power acquired by the perceiving human soul if it develops. . . Imagination, Inspiration and Intuition.
RUDOLF STEINER, THE WORLD OF THE SENSES
AND THE WORLD OF THE SPIRIT

Mircea Eliade (1964) described the psychological profile of the shaman and this work has been largely accepted by mainstream anthropology. Very often a person becomes disenchanted with society. He or she withdraws from friends, family, society, and normal activities. The dissatisfaction is often so profound that the person may even feel a deep disaffection with the human condition itself. Sometimes the problem manifests as an organic disease. Sometimes solace is found in lonely or wild places. (Conversely, some people throw themselves into consciousness-reducing experiences—sex, drugs, and rock 'n' roll—to try to blunt the calling.) Eventually, a crisis develops that brings the disenchantment to a head: the person feels suicidal or doomed, or health problems threaten life, or avoidance causes too much pain to be ignored.

A near-death experience is a frequent precipitating factor, making a person look at mortality and whatever lies beyond the body. This can lead to the alienation or inspiration necessary to go beyond accepted social norms to confront life's deeper questions.

Some people fail to deal with their problems constructively. However, those who do come back from the brink of hopelessness, insanity, alienation, destruction, or death are changed, renewed, and strengthened. Often they feel they have been "touched by the spirit" or have gained a new "vision" or guidance arising from outside the ordinary social order. Frequently, they want to work with this vision to bring it into social awareness—though some separate themselves from society. Some are socially constructive and some are socially withdrawn. Some are viewed as special in some way—whether good or bad often depends on the society.

The shamanic predisposition exists everywhere. There is no boundary of place, people, or time that prevents it. The discontent, disease, disorder, or "bad luck" that leads to the deep alienation so typical of the calling can happen to anyone, anywhere. Even those with good health, luck, wealth, and social standing are not immune from the calling; though generally social and financial success are going to cover up the whisper of the spirit. If those who feel this calling are able to persist on their path—and not all of them can—they are not necessarily going to find happiness, success, recognition, or acceptance within modern society, nor satisfy the demands of most of their family, friends, and neighbors. They are not going to be a "success" in a conventional sense. Society does not support them. In biomedicine, there is a psychiatric category for every manifestation of the shamanic crisis—and drugs to suppress the symptoms.

The shamanic calling represents a real existential crisis. Some people work out a solution to their predicament. They plumb the depths of the human condition, free themselves from whatever it is they distrust or dislike in society or humanity itself, find whatever it is they need to lead a self-fulfilling life, and overcome this "disorder." It doesn't matter whether Western culture has declared that these people are not shamans and that shamanism doesn't exist, or it has labeled them with a psychiatric illness. These people, in every culture, have died, gone to another world, gained a renewing vision, and returned to enrich society—or be scorned by it.

Because it is a disorder that is an expected part of the path, the chaos out of which a new order arises, I call this not a "personality disorder" but the "shamanic personality order/disorder." It is a condition native to the human species and therefore to every culture in the world.

The tools and practices of traditional shamanism—drums, rattles, rock paintings, and various objects—are not the defining characteristics of the shaman. This is not a book about totems, drums, rattles, astrology, or the tarot. It is a book about the inner life of the shaman, the purpose of which is the actualization of our threefold Frankensteinian psyche: animal, human, and unfathomable.

It takes inner power and confidence to reject the narcotic pull of societal normality. Where does this come from? To what does the social outlier adhere that gives him or her the ability to believe in and practice something that is so different? Is it merely a matter of ignorance? Are we only people adhering stubbornly to a naive and foolish worldview because we are mentally ill, deluded, or "primitive"?

No. It is the power of a genuine calling and its ultimate source is something that comes from beyond society altogether and has more power than society. To resist consensus opinion, one must not only believe in an alternative truth, one needs to be commanded by it. One has to develop oneself in the direction pointed out by the spirit.

Although each person's path is different, there is only one shamanic method. Instead of transcending earth and body (which is the idea in many religious and spiritual traditions), on the shamanic path body, Nature, and Animal are the route to the spirit.

This will sound antithetical to conventional religionists, who, for thousands of years, have been fighting against body, Nature, the Wild, and the Animal within. There really is no satisfying answer to this conflict: the Wild is innately inconvenient and scary. Nature is ever-changing; not eternal or infinite. The animal world hardly seems like a source for God-knowledge. Nature and body are rejected as detrimental to the spiritual quest. But not in shamanism.

Treading the path of inner development requires a death in one's relationship to society and the social delusions we carry within us—but also a rebirth to a personhood not based on social approval or acceptance. We will not be in control when we are swept into the abyss of the unknown, where alone we will be tried and renewed as a spirit by the spirit.

Here is a story from one of my herb clients. He was a total psychological mess, on benzodiazepines and several other psychiatric medications when he was arrested for a warrant he had already paid and thrown in jail. He was cold-turkeyed off the drugs—many people die from sudden withdrawal from "benzos" and he was having up to ten seizures a day while suffering severe mental illness. When he got out of prison he was put back on meds, but a relative reported to the psychiatrist (incorrectly) that he was abusing them, so he was cold-turkeyed again. He decided never to take another psychiatric drug: if "the system" could wrench him around like this, he wasn't safe. Instead, he started "self-medicating" on a bottle of brandy a day. Finally, he decided on to end his life and said goodbye to his support system—an aunt and his mother. Two days later he was arrested on another warrant and thrown in jail.

"I prayed to Creator for help," he said. "What else could I do? I'd prayed before but I was never answered by an actual voice saying words." This time there were very precise words. The first thing Creator asked was: "Do you want to live?" "No," he answered honestly, "I don't want to." Creator continued in a clear voice: "Well, how about if I were to help you? Would that make a difference?" He thought about that—decided it would be okay. He and Creator came to an agreement. "It was like an actual contract; I'd do my part and Creator would do his."

The man was sentenced to three years in prison. Most of the time he stayed in his cell, meditating and processing his personal baggage. He didn't go out in the yard much, to avoid getting stabbed. "I liked being in prison," he said. "It was a cakewalk compared to my life before." Other prisoners would exclaim, "Hey, how come you're smiling?" He couldn't help it. "I was happy. And let me tell ya—everyone in prison is miserable."

Another story was related to me many years ago by a woman who operated under the designation "herbalist" but was also a shaman. Her Jewish family had been forced to leave Russia by violence but her grandmother had remained behind because she was the village shamaness—the Baba Yaga—and felt a duty not to abandon her people, though they were not necessarily Jews. Finally, she left and emigrated to New Jersey. The woman telling the story got very sick when she was twelve years old. The doctors gave up. This was in the late 1950s, when there was less that doctors could do. Her grandmother said to her parents, "Give her to me and I will cure her, but she must live with me until her adulthood and you will have no claim over her." So she went to live with her gramma and was trained in shamanism and herbalism.

Don Juan speaks of the "sorcerer's explanation." Here we'll study the "shaman's explanation"—the theory of the three selves. We see this in religion (spirit, soul, and body) and psychology (ego, id, superego).

Freud

Freud famously named them the ego, id, and superego. The most ancient of these is the id, which "above all," he says, is identified with the instincts. These "originate from the somatic organization," which is to say, from the body. "The sole prevailing quality of the *id* is that of being *unconscious*. *Id* and *unconscious* are as intimately linked as *ego* and *preconscious*" (Freud 1969, 2). In other words, the id is the self of the unconscious in the same way the ego is the self of the conscious world. This center of "instincts," the id, is what we identify as the animal self in shamanism.

For Freud, the superego is a projection created by our programming about good and bad, right and wrong: God, moral codes, political correctness, and so on. It influences us "from above," so to speak, as if it were a superior being, with superior knowledge of right and wrong. Freud did not teach the actual existence of any kind of higher being, because this would not have been "scientific." But also, frankly, he was correct: until we meet the spirit, we have only an idealization of higher knowledge or the higher self.

Freud's model correlates with the age-old mythos of the three "worlds" or "selves": lower, middle, and higher. Jung, the leading psychiatric voice of the following generation, advocated a fourfold layout of the psyche based on the universal mythos of four directions. Sadly, the two had a falling-out and could not get along with each other or see the importance of the other's model. At one point, Jung commented that he did not even bother to familiarize himself with Freud's theory of the id, ego, and superego. He interpreted any threefold system as a fourfold system that was incomplete!

When these two viewpoints are brought together, the underlying model of psychiatry and psychology can be seen to be complete and in line with the mythic structure of the world as seen in almost all traditional societies. There are seven primal directions: lower, middle, and higher, and at the same time we live in a world of four "directions" or "elements." Our middle self, our conscious self, is comprised of a body (sensation), emotions (feelings), intelligence (thinking), and intuition/inspiration. These are Jung's four "functions"; when they are actualized, a person is well-rounded.

This inner landscape exactly reflects the outer landscape. When Freud and Jung are integrated, even Western culture can claim a connection to mythological wholeness.

Jung dealt with the three levels by describing some psychological experiences as "autochthonous" (of the earth) and "numinous" (of the divine or spirit) but he didn't reference the mythology of three levels or worlds the way he did the four functions. It is a bit disconcerting.

Where Freud emphasized the psychology of mental illness, Jung put psychology to work on behalf of self-actualization. One of the first and most necessary aspects of self-development, according to Jung, is confronting one's "shadow," a projection of everything that we fear and hate. The superego is a projection of everything we think of as good, while the shadow is the projection of what we think of as bad. Here is a good example of a shadow experience from my own life:

> I first contracted coronavirus in March 2020. One night it hung over me while I lay in bed in the dark, like a black ectoplasm beaming hatred at me. After half an hour I spontaneously asked a question: "How come you hate me so much?" The answer was instantaneous: "I'm everything that you hate."
>
> At first I thought, I'd better be careful not to hate anyone. After a few months I thought, But there are a lot of things people do that I think I am right to hate. Within a year, society was full of hatred: vaxxers versus nonvaxxers, Left versus Right, and Right versus Left. Then there was war. . . and more war. It was like an evil genie had been let out of a bottle—and the bottle was us.

This is an eruption of what Jung called the "collective shadow." Before the beginning of the Second World War, he sensed a spreading hatred and fear projected onto "the Other," engulfing the continent.

Both superego and shadow need to be passed in order for the shamanic student to step over the threshold, on the journey of self-actualization. They are the flipsides of the same entity.

The shadow is described in occult literature as the "Guardian of the Threshold." It was named by Edward Bulwer-Lytton in *Zanoni* (1842) and the term was then used by Helena Blavatsky, Arthur Edward Waite, Rudolf Steiner, and George Gurdjieff. Another term is "Dweller on the Threshold."

Rudolf Steiner says that there are two Guardians. The first one is the animal self while the second one, if we get that far, is a nonhuman entity from the Spirit World. Castaneda reports that when he saw his own animal self, Coyote, he also saw an inorganic being—and don Juan made it clear that he had an appointment with this entity.

We need to actualize our animal part. We think so highly of

ourselves, but our best traits—heart-love, family life, and dreaming—all originated in the mammalian life-wave. Dreamtime is accessible to us only because we are part animal, not because we are part human. An evolutionary biologist, Elisabet Sahtouris, explains (2000, 156):

> We are still not sure why warm-blooded animals dream during sleep. Sleeping and dreaming are special behaviors that evolved in mammals and were passed on to their descendants, yet no one knows why.

We see, hear, taste, smell, and touch due to our animal senses, not because we are humans. It is the same way in the spiritual world. We have senses there only because we acquire them from the animal part of us. Ironically, rather than diminishing our humanity, by conjoining with our animal self we become complete human beings. The ancient Mayan culture defined the shaman who had actualized his or her animal self (*uayob*) as:

an authentic human being (Gillette 1997, xvii).

Anatomy of the Three Selves

Components of the psyche that are competitive with each other for time and energy must to a greater or lesser extent qualify as independent entities or selves. From this perspective, not only are there three selves, but there are some sub-selves that show independence within this threefold system.

Conscious Self

The human or conscious self can be split into four components. Part of us wants to be conscious at all costs ("I don't want to go to bed"), part wants to eat, drink, and have sex all the time, diminishing consciousness if necessary. Another wants to fulfill social expectations (the persona, the mask we put on for other people), while another wants to fulfill personal values and self-development (the soul).

A fifth component unites and rules over these four fractious pieces of consciousness: the ego.

Ego (composite and ruler of):

> Conscious self
> Biological self
> Persona
> Soul

The soul is the part of us that knows we are mortal and grieves death in advance, but also celebrates the joys of life.

Animal Self

We can split the animal self into a warm-blooded component and a cold-blooded or reptilian self. The former is partly unconscious (the id) but partly conscious when we are examining our loves and relationships. The latter is normally unconscious but bursts into consciousness—almost dominating us—when we are in survival mode. Reproductive mode follows close behind. Therefore, the reptilian self shows up among the entities composing the human self—I labeled it the "biological self."

When the body is alive it is energetic, or full of vitality and energy that can be directed toward various goals. This is called the vital force in alternative medicine, the etheric body in Western occultism, and the energy body by don Juan. It is associated with vegetative existence. When a person is a "vegetable," in a coma, we are looking at a pure expression of the vital, etheric, or energy body. This is what acupuncture works on.

The cold-blooded animal self works with the energy body. Whenever there is danger, the energy shifts abruptly. Mostly, however, the energy body is in "homeostasis," trying not to shift. Therefore, the energy body, vital self, or vegetable part of us corresponds to the plant world. The perfect symbol of the symbiotic relationship between the biological self and the vegetable self is the caduceus of Asclepius: a snake (or two snakes) climbing up a green leafy branch.

The plant world is characterized by the fixation of attention on one particular setting: the expression of the genome of the plant. In addition to providing the energy for life, and its homeostatic steady state, the vital body also serves as a sensory system for "energy shifts." It reacts to any strong emotional/physical stimulus. The actual mechanism is a quantum change in the electric charge on the polymers in the extracellular matrix, which controls all cellular activity simultaneously. The polymers don't act like nerves, moving electrons along their courses; rather, they store electrons and discharge them or take them up—so their method is more like a "shift" than a nerve current. This is called the "ground regulatory system." I explained about it in *Holistic Medicine and the Extracellular Matrix* (2021a, 2–5).

Alfred Pischinger, M.D., the discoverer of this mechanism, discussed it with some anthroposophical doctors and they agreed that it explained what they called the "etheric body." Additional research showed that the ground regulatory system is what is affected by acupuncture needles. Although the existence of meridians could not be proven, the points are consistent with deformations in the matrix polymers (see Pischinger 2007).

The energy body remembers anything that caused an energy shift and therefore constitutes the "body memory." There is no way to heal without reliving the body memory. The caduceus is therefore the perfect symbol for the medical craft. The green leafy stem relating to the vegetable world, including nutrition and herbal medicine; the snake to the nervous system and the survival and sexual instincts that provide the big imprints on the body memory (while also personifying spinal manipulation, massage, and therapies that address the nervous system).

The energy body is not a self or self-conscious or it would interfere with the fixation of consciousness in all the selves. The plants are entities because they have fixed self-awareness of who they are within their world, and they can share that awareness with us. Their awareness is fixated on their basic identity; they can't change focus from one thing to another, like an animal or a human.

The mineral body—the molecules—did not originally possess consciousness, but when we descended into matter, our conscious self was overwhelmed by the physical senses, so that we identify ourselves with the things we experience through the senses. Some people even think that there is no consciousness after the death of the body. After the "incident in Eden," when the frontal brain and the reptilian brain merged, our survival and reproductive instincts became highly dominant within us and plunged our awareness into a nearly complete existence in the mineral realm. This is where the reptile beings seen by Michael Harner were correct. They did create us in a sense—by changing the course of our evolution—and they have dominated us ever since. Because there was now consciousness in and through the mineral level, the beings responsible for this shift had to descend with us down into the dust. Also, because they ruled over us—we took our "prime directive" from them—they were attracted down into matter with us. They became the conscious beings in the mineral realm. I'll try to explain this when we get to the part about Dragons.

Freudian Id (composite and ruler of):

> Animal self (warm-blooded)
> Biological self (reptilian, cold-blooded)
> Energy body
> Mineral body

Spirit Self

According to esoteric teachings, the spirit of an individual is split into three parts: the *atma* (primal particle of differentiation), the archetype (individuality), and the spirit body or dream self. As I understand the teachings, the *atma* is unchangeable, while the archetype can slightly change under the influence of life experience in the physical realm. The dream self is the sensory body of the spirit self.

Spirit Self (consists of):

> Atma
> Archetype
> Dream Self

The Assemblage Point, Egoic Will, or Fetch

What we have not addressed is the capacity of humans and other beings to change the focus of their awareness. This is with us in waking and in dreamtime, so it cannot be identified with any one of the selves, but brings them to attention without having an innate identity of its own. It is simply the mechanism of focus. It shifts from one focus to another, although we are not aware of any break in the continuity of our perception in the ordinary world. In dreamtime its true nature is brought forward: we shift from image to image, or situation to situation.

This ability to "shift" suggests a connection to the energy body and the vegetable world, where identity is extremely fixed, yet possible of movement. Under normal circumstances it takes a couple hundred thousand years to create a new species.* This gives us some idea of how difficult it is to change focus and why we don't voluntarily change that easily.

Don Juan called this mechanism the "assemblage point." When it is focused, the "tumblers click," as Susan said. The ability to move the assemblage point from one click to another is defined as "intent" by don Juan, while the ability to maintain a fixation he calls "will." In order to experience otherworldly places, we must intend the assemblage point to move to those places and then fix upon them. It is very hard for modern people, such as myself, to move very far from the established reference points of the modern focus. Susan could do this better than anyone I ever met.

The assemblage point is pretty much the same as what we call "gall" or "egoic will" in English. In Chinese folklore and medicine it is called the *hun* and is located in the gallbladder. Because we are self-conscious through and in our I-self or ego, we think of the assemblage point as the "egoic will." The *hun* and the *po* (the mortal self, the awareness of mortality) are considered two "soul parts" in Chinese culture that unify

---

*I was in a class where we were doing a "plant attunement" with Hawthorn. It said to me, "I'm taking lessons from the Oak on how to be a tree." *Oh . . .* , I thought, *I'll check in with you in two hundred thousand years.* That gave me food for thought: *What would I be doing in two hundred thousand years?* We are a Mystery People.

to become our fully developed human self. They are roughly equivalent to the ego and the soul.

An archaic English name for the assemblage point is the *fetch*, since it "fetches" the contents of the unconscious, whether from the memory, imagination, or dream and brings the content before the screen of consciousness. In an Old English glossary from around the year 800, the word *fæcce* (presumably the antecedent of "fetch") is given as an equivalent for *mære*, "nightmare." This points to a connection with the animal self: when it is agitated it produces nightmares. After death, the fetch becomes the "shade" that exists in the Underworld, keeping a record of all the focalizations of the consciousness that occurred during the lifetime. The term "fetch" is still actively used by some pagans and witches. The Hawaiian term *unihipili* refers to the animal self and the shade.

A good word here is *doppelganger*, or "double." This refers to the complex of the etheric body and the animal (warm- and cold-blooded) self detaching from the physical body and operating as a separate entity. The reptilian is referred to as the "lower astral" in Theosophy and Anthroposophy; the warm-blooded as the "higher astral." This separation from the physical body and the human and spiritual elements is counterproductive before the actualization of the animal self. In healthy circumstances, the doppelganger "goes before a person," sensing trouble, so that the person is protected by it.

In order to be able to move the assemblage point with intention, we have to face our ingrained fear of the non-ordinary. It is pretty much impossible for the assemblage point to make a large shift without scaring the survival-based reptilian self. The old shamans were able to shapeshift and change dimensions, but these shifts of the assemblage point are so far from our habitual focus in the modern conscious world that they are difficult for modern people to experience.

Spiritual transformation itself requires a shift of the assemblage point. As long as this occurs under the control of the ego, the shift is worthless to the spirit, which demands that we go beyond our ego. When we dream of our animal self and awaken the dream self, we experience the first big shift, so this primal event that defines shamanism also involves the actualization of the assemblage point.

After the death of the physical envelope, the ego dissipates, but the fixations of attention that occurred during the life can never fade because they come from the assemblage point, which is ageless, timeless, and active in every dimension. Therefore, the egoic fixations remain as a record of the life of the individual—this is called the "shade" or "shadow" in folklore. It goes down into the Underworld after the death of the physical body and remains as a permanent record.

The Hawaiian word *unihipili* is also associated with the bones. The relationship between the bones and the lifetime of shifts of the assemblage point is mentioned by Rudolf Steiner (2014, 65):

> I do not want to overfeed you with the results of clairvoyant research, but this is truly interesting, namely that through the raying out of our bones as they disintegrate, the human being everywhere leaves behind him, as it were, images, spiritual pictures perceptible to Imagination.

The assemblage point exists on the physical level because things exist there, but it only begins to move on the vegetative level. The bones are our minerality and are therefore associated with the *shade* that goes down into the Earth, to preserve the record of our life. But they are also associated with the mineral element and as such they connect us to the Dragons. We'll save this matter for later.

Due to the "incident in Eden," or the placement of the human will over the will of Creator, our souls have ceased to be eternal creatures—these, like our bodies, are subject to death, as Genesis says. This is not just a physical death but the extinction of our human self, to the extent we did not learn to identify our souls with the eternal opportunities of the Spirit World that eclipse mortality. The purpose of shamanism as a spiritual path is to reunite the individual soul with the spirit self. This is also, of course, the goal of all genuine religious or spiritual application. To the extent this occurs, the soul is immortalized. To the extent it doesn't, the soul is mortal.

Interactions of the Three Selves

According to the shaman's explanation, we are animals with the addition of a human part that accounts for one basic thing: the ability to consciously select and fetch thoughts and images in the mind. This makes us self-aware and able to develop the imagination, or the ability to perceive, see, and study the pictures in our mind. Animals can't consciously select the contents in their minds. Indeed, we can barely do it ourselves. This ability to change our focus in the imagination marks us as human. An extraordinary, magical secret is hidden in the association of the imagination and the human: we are human because we have imagination and by changing the focus of the imagination to a new click of the tumblers, we perform "magic."

Image-seeing is an attribute of the animal life-wave and differentiates the animals, even the most primitive, from the plants. The connection between a human and the animal linked to them in the dream world is like the deepest bond of friendship one could experience. The two are independent of each other and yet inextricably connected. The animal self contributes the sensory portion of the combination while the human gives the ability to focus and change the image.

Neurologists believe that our emotions start as the simple instincts and sensations of animals—safe, unsafe, pleasure, pain—and, as they come to consciousness, they are articulated into more rational conceptions that "make sense" to our more sophisticated and complex minds. So our heart comes from Animal in addition to our senses.

Our physical body is an animal; it is equivalent to the animal self. We think of it merely as a collection of molecules and chemicals, but the body is a collection of neurological pathways and behavior patterns, which gives us an overall appearance, so that in addition to the "human look" we also have the look of an animal. This "look" is not just skin deep; it reflects the animal intelligence running the body, and the body is our own personal slice of Nature, through which we communicate with greater Nature.

The mystery is in the body and the way the body works itself into nature. (Terence McKenna)

The triad in Meso-American nagualist shamanism is the *tonal*, *yollo*, and *nagual*. These are more or less equivalent to what I have been describing as the ego, soul, and animal self. Castaneda had difficulty dealing with the human heart, so his account of don Juan's teachings usually only touch on the *tonal* and the *nagual*. However, don Juan clearly stated that there are three "riddles" we need to solve to unlock human nature. They correspond to the *tonal*, the *yollo*, and the *nagual*. Sometimes he very eloquently did talk about the importance of the heart and he did consider it coequal with the other two. We'll look at these terms in greater detail in chapter 5.

Only the actualization of all three will allow a person to become whole. The occultist Gottfried de Purucker said of the body, soul, and spirit (1932, 124): "these three bases spring from three different lines of evolution, from three different and separate Hierarchies of being. . . . This is the reason why man is composite." When the three selves are actualized, they will be found to be discrete entities, independent from each other and yet cooperative. Merilyn Tunneshende succinctly describes the situation in *Twilight Language of the Nagual* (2004, 80): "I had been three different beings or had lived three different lives as the same being, or had seen life with three eyes, each with its own identity."

A good literary illustration of the body, soul, and spirit would be the three main characters in J. K. Rowling's Harry Potter series. Hermione represents the rational mind, the more material perspective, the rule-follower, the ego, and the personality. She is literalistic about rules, rational about explanations, and down-to-earth about study and work. She doesn't hide her egotism about her accomplishments and Harry and Ron find her obnoxious when they first meet her. The discipline of education and learning, however, opens her up to a greater and greater perspective. Ron represents the soul. He is not very good with reasoning and he suffers from low self-esteem—the emotional qualities of the soul make him more vulnerable. However, he warms up life for the other two, interjecting humor and breaking up their overly serious preoccupations. He possesses a certain earthy understanding of how the world works, though he seldom possesses the confidence to stand up for these perceptions. The outer and inner selves need to learn to function in harmony. Therefore, Hermione and Ron are always drawn to each other and eventually become an item. Hermione increasingly looks to and values Ron for his heart. Harry, on the other hand, represents the spirit. He is not very often drawn into the competing interests of the ego or the personalities around him. He looks for the higher, spiritual demands of situations and helps to bring higher purpose forward in other people. His actions are magnanimous and high-minded. By following the noble path, he becomes a hero and yet, because he is innately disinterested in personality issues, Harry seldom thinks of the egoic benefits that accrue from his actions. It is primarily when what he knows to be true is not respected or believed by others that he gets angry, frustrated, hurt, or disengaged. His perception cuts to the core of the situation; knowledge comes to him in realizations and flashes of intuition. Hermione actively disapproves of this type of mentation, while Ron wavers in uncertainty but generally believes Harry and tries to be supportive. Harry always functions at his best when his two friends are with him and getting along reasonably well. In the end his sacrifices drag him out of the realm of personal comfort. Like the shaman, he embraces death but survives to bring healing to his community.

The three primary selves cannot be completely integrated into one. We would not want Ron to lose his sense of humor, Hermione to abandon her sharp-edged mind, or Harry to lose his inspiration. The three selves have to be streamlined into a single functioning triad, but the independence and talents of each must never be eradicated.

It is because the seams never disappear that rumors of shapeshifting, bilocation, and magic follow the shamans. These are not just evidence of the skills of a great shaman: they represent seams between the different selves that cannot ever be completely hidden. We are part human, part animal, part plant, part mineral, and part spirit. As Steiner remarks (1914, 43): "Occult science, therefore, represents man as a being composed of many principles."

Both traditional shamanism and occultism describe a basic set of seven worlds or planes of existence that students must experience in order to move beyond the confines of this world. These are the seven rungs on the shamanic ladder, referred to as "Jacob's ladder" in Genesis. I already wrote about the seven guideposts on the spiritual path in *Seven Herbs* (1987) and *Seven Guideposts on the Spiritual Path* (2021b).

The Gnostics taught that there were seven demons that imprisoned us in the world. According to others, there are Seven Powers or Spirits to whom the evolution of the planet was entrusted by Creator in the beginning of time. We are under their power, but they were not created to hold us prisoner. They are simply doing their job. It is we who have fallen under their imperium in an oppressive sense, due to our own actions and our misapprenhension of who they are. They don't even like to be around us; we always demonize or divinize them.

Earth by herself cannot evolve. Neither can the human race. All species attempt to remain in their fixed holding pattern—their archetypal/genomic mold. It is the impulse of the spirit into the world that makes evolution possible. On a small scale, evolution is like education and education requires inspiration or the student becomes bored. The Seven Powers or Spirits are working with the Supreme Spirit to further spiritual life inside the Turtle Shell of time and space.

Helena Blavatsky taught a system of seven different "selves." Gottfried de Purucker gives them as (1932, 167): *Âtman* (individual spirit essence), *Buddhi* (spirit substance), *Manas* (man, mind, or ego; "conditionally immortal" only), *Kâma* (astral soul or animal self), *Prâna* (life energy), *Linga-Śarîra* (soul), and *Sthûla-Śarîra* (physical body). Rudolf Steiner recognized seven or nine parts, as did E. Grahame Howe in his spiritual psychiatry.

Gurdjieff taught that mankind was essentially tripartite: one part intellectual, one part emotional, and one part connected to the motor and instinctive capacities. He further subdivided the human being into the (1) sexual/biological, (2) instinctive, (3) motor, (4) emotional, (5) intellectual, and two higher centers analogous to the (6) third eye and (7) crown chakras in Helena Blavatsky's system. These—called the higher emotional center and the higher intellectual center, respectively—must be developed and earned, says Gurdjieff; they are not hardwired into us at birth.

The Pharmacology of the Three Selves

Shamanism has long been associated with the use of plants for healing and as agents for shifts in consciousness. As a herbalist, my knowledge is constellated around plants—not because I have taken lots of hallucinogens, but because plants have communicated with me through a variety of channels. This includes the doctrine of signatures—the shape, color, growth habit, or environmental niche of a plant resembles the disease, organ, or energy pattern for which the plant is remedial. It also includes empathic links through which the plants communicate their properties in pictures, words, and feelings. The tastes and smells of plant medicines have induced physiological and psychological experiences from which herbalists learn. I have a lifetime of clinical experiences that has enriched my inner life—thank you, clients, for trusting me and teaching me over the years. Finally, I never lost the opportunity to learn from my own sicknesses. I went out intentionally to get coronavirus, taking ten flights in March 2020.

If we want, we can describe the shamanic experience in terms of the pharmacology of plants. This is not my first choice. I had no insight about this until the late, great herbalist John Redden of Toronto, Ontario, explained neurotransmitters in terms of the three selves.

John was a jolly Santa Claus–like guy with a razor-sharp mind. He had a good grounding in science and pharmacology and a Jesuit education, so he introduced the classical tripartite model of the soul as defined by Plato and still taught by the Catholic Church. This divides the human psyche into Reason (mentation), Desire (appetite), and Will (action, self-control, lack of control). These are reflections in the soul of the three selves. Desire is a reflection of the animal self and Reason of the human self. The spirit is the source of the power to do—Will.

Dopamine

John pointed out that dopamine is the compound that is in charge of pleasure, reward, and pain avoidance. When it is in balance, we can experience pleasure in life, but when there is not enough we feel like "life has not given us enough." We feel emptiness and grief. Too much leads to hallucinations that are characteristic: the person often sees specters of the dead or hears voices. It opens us to the voices and land of the dead. These are not the voices of the spirits and totems in the Spirit World, but the remnants of living souls being processed in the Underworld through pleasure, reward, and pain-avoidance. These are the activities that "train" the animal self. Dopamine is the neurotransmitter on that level.

Herbal remedies for lack of enjoyment of the body and pleasure include Wormwood (*Artemisia absinthium*), Mugwort (*Artemisia vulgaris*), and Damiana (*Turnera aphrodiasia*). Plants that cause visions of the dead, monsters, and specters are found in the nightshade family (for example, *Atropa belladonna*, *Datura* spp., and *Hyoscyamus niger*). These are labeled as "hallucinogens," but they give visions of an entirely different nature than DMT and related tryptamines. In homeopathic doses, the nightshades control these sorts of netherworldly misadventures. Opioids wreak havoc on dopamine receptors.

Adrenaline, Noradrenaline

The second major neurotransmitter is epinephrine (adrenaline), along with its sister, norepinephrine (noradrenaline); they serve to increase alertness, focus, vigilance, and consciousness. They keep us "paying attention" during the day. Too much norepinephrine leads to nervousness, anxiety, hyperconsciousness, and obsessive-compulsive disorder (OCD), while too little leads to restless mind, attention deficit disorder (ADD), and hyperactivity. Good remedies for OCD include Passionflower (*Passiflora incarnata*) and Horse Chestnut (*Aesculus hippocastanum*). Hawthorn (*Crataegus* spp.) and Schizandra (*Schizandra chinensis*) are good remedies for ADD. Lemon Balm (*Melissa officinalis*) is good for nervousness similar to ADD.

If we run into a perceived threat, adrenaline is poured out and we switch from ordinary alertness and awareness to "fight or flight." The blood rushes from the guts to the brain and limbs so that we can respond intelligently and forcefully by making the decision to run away or stand and fight. Unfortunately, our system has not developed to the point where we are able to differentiate between an actual threat (rattlesnake in the kitchen) and a perceived threat (work deadlines). Or even a picture in our mind of a threat. Therefore, we treat both actual and perceived threats in the same way. In this state, the sympathetic nervous system is overstimulated while the parasympathetic (rest, relax, rebuild) is suppressed. This leads to a state of anxiety, nervousness, and excitability, with exhaustion and inability to rebuild. This is called "adrenal fatigue" in folk medicine; a condition not understood in conventional biomedicine. We don't run out of adrenaline, so that is not the deficiency. What happens is that adrenaline suppresses the digestion and that reduces the assimilation of fats and oils essential for the health of the adrenal cortex. This means we need a combination of nerve sedation and lipid digestion. This condition responds to nervines for anxiety like Lemon Balm (*Melissa officinalis*), Motherwort (*Leonorus cardiaca*), or Borage (*Borago officinalis*), combined with lipids to rebuild the parasympathetic and the adrenal cortex. Burdock root (*Arctium lappa*) is excellent for rebuilding lipid mechanisms and reduces worry and anxiety.

Serotonin

The third neurotransmitter is serotonin. It operates differently at different levels. A modest deficiency causes rumination, negative self-dialogue, and melancholy; the person is stuck in their inner self, unable to solve problems or connect with the world. This is not really "depression" per se (from actual loss, grief, setbacks, etc.), but fits the old-fashioned term "melancholy," which is more of a creative or spiritual angst involving lack of imagination, artistic funk, and anxiety.

Herbalist Seán O'Donoghue notes that melancholia matches the crisis that the shamanic personality experiences, and that it is usually suppressed by drugs (MAO inhibitors) in conventional medicine, which artificially keep serotonin levels up without dealing with the problem. It is possible that one of the reasons our society is careening out of control is the suppression of this stage of life, which is required for psychological and spiritual problem-solving.

Serotonin in moderation helps a person to switch back and forth from the social world to the internal world, leading to a "well-adjusted" person. There is a balance between self and other. It supports the "gentle spiritual path," whereby the soul is constantly fed a small stream of inspiration and insight from the spirit, so that the soul develops in an increasingly mature direction, without losing contact with ordinary human society. Appropriate levels of serotonin are associated with gaining perspective on life and therefore with something that is very important: gaining impulse control. Without impulse control we cannot venture far into the shamanic world, which tests our desire, reason, and will in every conceivable way.

Serotonin also causes problems in excess. Modest excess pushes a person into an intensification of sensory input, which can be overwhelming in a social setting, so once again the person is pushed into isolation. Here there is a greater potential for creative and spiritual development, but with isolation from society. We can see that Eliade's shamanic personality is starting to form. It seems possible that we can have too much serotonin, leading to social isolation and introversion, conjoined with highly creative or unusual orientations. This resembles the autism spectrum. However, because self-understanding is built into introversion, high serotonin levels and neural receptor sites for serotonin can be associated with stability of character and impulse control.

Dimethyltryptamine (DMT)

Serotonin in balance (combined with reasonable decision-making) leads to a solid spiritual or meaningful life, within the social network, but it does not reach the Spirit World in the same way that dimethyltryptamine does. This is the "spirit molecule," as psychiatrist Rick Strassman named it, because DMT brings on visions and all-engulfing experiences of nonordinary reality. It also develops a more dense net of serotonin-receptor sites, leading to a more balanced presence in the social world. The reverse may also be true: higher levels of serotonin may enhance the DMT experience. Impulse control (serotonin) can enhance positive spiritual lessons (DMT), while DMT and the spiritual lessons it provokes can enhance impulse control and the "purposeful life" associated with good serotonin levels.

DMT is made in the brain and the brain craves any external DMT that comes along. However, it is broken down in the small intestine and does not easily get to the brain when taken orally. Shamans, drug fiends, and psychiatrists have their ways, however. Ayahuasca consists of a plant that contains DMT (*Banisteriopsis caapi*), with another herb that helps it pass the blood-brain barrier. When ethnobotanists asked Amazonian shamans how they figured out which plants to put together—there are over a thousand different species per hectare in the rainforest—they commonly said the plants told them what to do (see Luna 1984; Narby 1998).

It is possible to generate DMT simply through spiritual exercises. When Richard Alpert (Ram Dass), the early drug-researcher-turned-spiritual-pilgrim, went to India, he gave a massive dose to an Indian guru. The man did not change in the least; his brain was already awash with self-manufactured DMT.

The DMT innate to a person's own system is the only completely safe and healthy source since reliance on plant sources will tend to suppress the manufacture of native DMT, just as reliance on medical drugs to keep up serotonin levels will suppress the development of true self-regulation. Occasional use of DMT, on the other hand, might stimulate more production—or the visions that would call creativity forth. There is a long history of DMT use by shamans. Maria Sabina's work with psilocybin, in central Mexico, is a well-documented case.

Today we not only need to develop adequate serotonin levels through mindful living, but through mindful eating. This is because modern corporations play to our appetitive nature, encouraging it through the use of addictive levels of sugar, salt, unhealthy lipids, and synthetic foods. We also develop food and substance allergies to never-eaten-before processed food, spilling histamine and heparin into our system, causing allergic reactions, sensitive tissue, and changes in local blood supply. Today, spiritual consciousness requires good, sound food, as well as spiritual desire, discipline, and effort. And everyone should exercise, whether on a spiritual path or just trying to stay healthy. "Chop wood, carry water."

Cannabinoids

In the last several decades, the contents of *Cannabis* have become the darlings of popular culture and now even science. THC is the psychoactive component, but CBDs (cannabinoids) turn out to have an important pharmacological function that acts on the neurotransmitters. THC needs to be extracted by heat (smoked, baked), but the CBDs do not; they are available like an herbal extract or tincture.

While the dopamine, adrenaline, and serotonin travel "downstream" along the nerve with the flow of electrons that constitute the nerve impulse, CBDs actually go back the other way. They move backward across the nerve synapse to tone down overstimulation of the nerve by dopamine and adrenaline. In this way they relax, reduce anxiety and sleeplessness, and give pain relief. There is no evidence yet that they have a cumulative, character-building quality, like serotonin. They just seem to make life more manageable—sometimes a lot more manageable. They also can cure some physical ailments. A lot of people experience a slackening of will from THC, and a few people experience terrible paranoia.

Cerebrospinal Fluid

Modern medicine overlooks the mechanical side of physiology, in favor of the purely molecular or pharmacological side, so it overlooks the "delivery system" for the neurotransmitters. This is the cerebrospinal fluid (CSF). The neurotransmitters move through this semi-fluid to the synapses where they conduct neural traffic.

Chiropractors and osteopaths have not forgotten about CSF. Manipulations can help the flow of CSF and the work of the neurotransmitters. My chiropractic friend Dave Milgram calls the CFS the "secret little golden oil that makes it all run." It "looks like starlight," according to another DC friend, Ariel Rose.

Chiropractic was founded by a man who thought spiritual life required a healthy, balanced cranium resting atop a healthy spinal cord. Osteopathy is based on the manipulation of the blood supply, which ties in directly to the thermoregulatory system, a part of the immune system that controls heat and influences hydration. By enhancing immunity, osteopathy reverberates into the self/not-self issues associated with serotonin and measured self-awareness. We are, of course, speaking of the higher callings and right practice of these disciplines. And a lot of the time, we just need plain old structural repair.

The grand medicine in herbalism for the cerebrospinal fluid is Black Cohosh (*Cimicifuga racemosa*, *Actaea racemosa*). It has an affinity for whiplash, which "bunches up" the CSF, resulting in spinal and arthritic pain, stagnation of CSF in the brain, depression, and headache. This plant will be described in more detail under Snake Medicine.

4

Preparations for the Journey

Not all those who wander are lost.
J. R. R. TOLKIEN, *THE FELLOWSHIP OF THE RING*

A traveller thro Eternity . . .
keeps onwards in his wondrous journey on the earth.
WILLIAM BLAKE, *THE NATURE OF INFINITY*

The shaman's journey is a long and winding road. We imagine a goal but when we get there, we find something else. One thing we find is another goal. The path demands flexibility, yet good, old-time discipline. It stretches the boundaries of the assets we bring into the world. It subjects these to mysterious tests and heartbreaking losses. Then, as if this were not enough, it hurls us into unknown dimensions, the hardwiring for which is missing in the human race. And if there is a particle of egotism, indulgence, or greed in us, which we cannot let go, our soul will be thwarted and diminished. So, a great deal of preparation is necessary on the path: it's like packing for a mountain-climbing trip.

The mountaintop is where the Fool is standing in the first card of the tarot. It pictures a daydreaming youth holding a fancy traveling bag on a staff on his shoulder. He is prepared to climb a mountain—but he is about to walk off a cliff. Fortunately for him, his little dog is biting him on the leg to stop him. Right from the start, the animal self is trying to communicate with us even when we are caught up in a fantasy world. Right from the start, the masters of the Italian occult Renaissance who painted the first tarot card show their understanding of the importance of the animal self.

The number assigned to the Fool is "0." This represents vacuity well enough, but there are deeper lessons in this number. There was not always a zero in mathematics. The Greeks did not know of it; the Arabic mathematicians "discovered" zero. What a revolutionary, important, and unique discovery that was! And there was no preexisting "model" for zero. It was a realization. That's what is needed on the spiritual journey: realization, originality, creativity. So, "0" is the number for the Fool.

The tarot is an important tool of the Western occult/shamanic tradition. The most sophisticated study of the history and meaning of the tarot from a philosophical and occult perspective is, in my opinion, Robert Place's *The Tarot: History, Symbolism, and Divination* (2005).

The best evidence indicates that the tarot originated in northern Italy in the 1430s. At that time, a well-educated artisan would have had a Church education that emphasized Greek philosophy, as well as Christianity. Place recognized that the twenty-one cards of the Higher Arcana that follow the Fool are constructed on a tripartite organizational scheme based on the model of the three "souls" of Plato. This would explain why the Higher Arcana align with deep psychospiritual, occult, and shamanic experience: they are modeled after the three selves.

Like the Fool, we do not actually know what to even look for when we begin our journey. We don't see "0." We don't know that the animal self exists, that it is important, or that it is biting our leg. We don't know that imagination or dream count for anything. We don't realize that our intellectual environment is conditioned by ideas that are contrary to spiritual freedom.

The Way of the Spiritual Warrior

When we start at such a disadvantage, there is at least one thing that we can do to help ourselves: that is the cultivation of carefulness and strategy, in our dealings with ourselves and others. That's what is called "spiritual warriorship." The number VII card of the tarot, the completion of the first of the three sevenfold cycles, is the Chariot—a picture of a warrior. The first threefold cycle relates to the conscious self. Although we don't know much about the other world, and the other parts of ourselves, we can at least live carefully and strategically. And if nothing more happens in life—at least we have lived to the best of our ability.

The authors of the tarot, whoever they were, did not have an abstract relationship to warriors. Renaissance Italy was largely governed by mercenaries (*condottieri*) who held the fate of cities and countrysides, men, women, and children in their hands. They could only hope for a code of honor.

As spiritual warriors, we learn to save up our energy—emotional, vital, sexual—to express it appropriately and deliberately. Does this mean that every action is strategic, calculated, and insincere? Not quite. There is room at least for sincerity. This doesn't sound good, but most people are already calculating and insincere—those that are not simply out of control.

Don Juan called the calculated approach "stalking," but he did not mean it as the stalking of other people, but of oneself. The spiritual warrior lives a calculated life with regard to other people: first, so that one will not waste one's own energy; second, so that others won't waste it either; and third, so we don't waste other people's energy. That does not mean we have to be insincere to enjoy life; rather, like any busy person, we need to budget our time and energy. We have to live strategically because our starting position is one of great weakness. We are far, far from the spirit.

One of the great writers on war, Carl von Clausewitz, understood the principle of warriorship implicitly (1989, 108):

> Strength of character does not consist solely in having powerful feelings, but in maintaining one's balance in spite of them. Even with the violence of emotion, judgment and principle must still function

like a ship's compass, which records the slightest variations however rough the sea.

Warriorship is necessary in war, and spiritual warriorship is necessary in spiritual war—and we are at spiritual war all the time. The chief goal here is not to win the war but to "save energy," as don Juan says. Only in this manner will we reach the far-distant shores of anticipated and unanticipated spiritual wisdom. And we will be successful, not through our own efforts, but because something in the universe responds and carries us to the accomplishment of our true self's purpose. "When you take that road this Good will meet you everywhere," says Hermes (Salaman et al. 2000, 58). Terence McKenna notes that even Nature herself loves the warrior:

> Nature loves courage. You make the commitment and nature will respond to that commitment by removing impossible obstacles. Dream the impossible dream and the world will not grind you under, it will lift you up. This is the trick. This is what all these teachers and philosophers who really counted, who really touched the alchemical gold, this is what they understood. This is the shamanic dance in the waterfall. This is how magic is done. By hurling yourself into the abyss and discovering it's a feather bed. (McKenna 2010b)

On the path of the warrior, we have to be patient and accept some indulgences for the time being. Here is a "warrior story" I heard growing up in Quaker Meeting:

> William Penn was born a noble, and his social group was expected to wear a sword as a sign of their superiority over the common people, who served them in peace and war. When Penn became a Quaker, he asked George Fox, a simple shepherd from Drayton-in-the-Clay, whether he should continue to wear his sword. Fox said: "Wear it as long as thou canst."

The bully/clown/dictator/evil-genius ego within us cannot be defeated overnight or out of season. The warrior does not force change on him- or herself or others. The result will be a waste of energy, and on the spiritual path both illusion and energy-wasting are damaging.

The way of the warrior depends upon training and receiving knowledge from the reptilian self because war is threatening. Originally, I did not know of any method for teaching people about their animal self except through descriptions and stories. That was before I teamed up with Vanessa Chakour, a retired female fighter and boxing coach in New York City. She used boxing exercises to get students in touch with their animal self. She had a method; I had the knowledge of the animal self to help students recognize what they were feeling. Teaching together, we were able to help people make that shamanic leap into the animal self.

It is our duty to respect our fellow humanity, but not to give our own energy away, so we operate from within that paradigm and try to make our reactions appropriate, magnanimous, and generous, without giving away parts of ourselves. A fight with another person, though unavoidable in the great theater of life, is always a waste of time for both parties unless we take it as a challenge to learn and grow. Then at least one person benefits.

In the old days there were shamans that simply killed anyone who interfered with them. They did this not because they were evil, but because they couldn't restrain their doppelganger when they were threatened. As I was taught, this is the origin of the Tsalagi (Cherokee) name *Asgaya-dihi* ("Mankiller"), although online information says differently. In chapter 1 we saw how even the peaceful Lutheran mystic Jacob Boehme killed a man who attacked him verbally because he couldn't hold back his doppelganger.

The two major skills don Juan emphasized for his students were "stalking" and "dreaming." Stalking is a hunter's way of looking at things and therefore more often practiced by the male students on the path. The art of dreaming is another track for getting around the ego and women tend to be better dreamers. In the end, however, all of us need to cultivate both skills, though one may be more important to us than another. In the Genesis shaman stories, the roles are reversed: Joseph is the dreamer while Tamar is the warrior.

At first, warriorship is work. Then it is a habit. Then you stop thinking about it. After a while, the responses of the warrior come automatically and there is no instant of calculation: we respond directly and completely according to the laws of spiritual war, that is to say, life.

Those who are less disciplined can make up for it in strategy. Those who have neither discipline nor strategy can make up for it through dreaming. Those who are lost causes—who are without discipline, strategy, or dream—still have a chance: they're the ones Jesus loved best. They may be closest to the kingdom of heaven because squandering time and energy, losing control of themselves, and being humbled brings them to the place where they have no choice but to follow the footsteps of the spirit. The touch of the spirit sobers them up. This might be a more direct route than warriorship or strategy—but there will be quite a few casualties along that path.

Discipline of the mind, as well as heart and body, is also important. This usually involves meditative techniques. These are always a valuable asset, whether one is on the shamanic path or another. The ability to focus the mind, be aware of a change of focus, and be in control of the focus are all skills of value. There are, however, problems with this as well: like warriorship, we need to practice it, make it habitual, and then stop thinking about it. The trained mind is still only the mind. Dark magicians train the mind as much as sincere aspirants on the path; perhaps more so. When it comes to disciplining the mind, I'm a lazy bum. I can't stop my thoughts, but I still try to watch them. We do what we can.

A form of meditation that is quite valuable on the shamanic path is one in which a person learns to catch hold of the images; especially those that are spontaneous. The most valuable is the discipline of the mind to awake in dreamtime. Subduing subjective faculties (imagination, intuition, instinct) to the mind can be counter-productive because these are the more important faculties on the Old, Old Path. Education of the conscious self to be alert, the ego to manage time and energy, and the mind to think clearly but not dogmatically, are the platform for a sensible life, much less a spiritual life.

In addition, we must educate the soul. We need to be able to recognize and value the things the soul really cares for. We need to develop soul awareness and soul wisdom. We need to learn and value what is in the heart: love, desire, values, direction. Without love, our life will have no personal meaning or fulfillment. If we dedicate ourselves to the spirit without at the same time asking that our legitimate needs be taken care of, the spirit will rub us down to the bone, taking from us everything we have, until we learn to stand up for ourselves.

Spiritual Education

Closely akin to spiritual warriorship is the "right way to think." We have to re-educate ourselves, because the dominant culture teaches us how to indulge ourselves in thought and behavior that ignores and opposes spiritual life. This demands "spiritual education," which is not a matter of learning dogmas or ideas or arguments, but how to think in a manner that leads to increased spiritual understanding.

True education is a combination of drawing forth from within the student and inspiring them with new goals and themes. The underlying Latin word (*educare*) means "to draw forth from within," while the word that underlies *inspiration* (*insprirare*) means "to draw in from without." All teachers know this. The greatest subject of study was pointed out by the Delphic Oracle: "Human, know thyself."

Spiritual education is based on finding the real, the whole, and the true. The shamanic path requires thorough self-examination. Therefore, we cannot leave out some of our experiences—the subjective, the ambiguous, or the impossible. These may be the "best ones." We need to explore and cultivate every aspect of life that we experience, inner and outer. This means that we need to study and be aware of our sensory perceptions, thoughts, and feelings, as well as our more recondite faculties: psychic perceptions, empathic impressions, animal instincts, intuition, imagination, and dream. If something is ambiguous, we may especially want to study it. The spirit loves the impossible, so we need to accept even the impossible.

The Real

Each person begins with what they have: an inner and outer life that is flawed and incomplete, but real. Going on to other realities is not a matter of transcending our flawed or limited world, but of learning how to appreciate parts of ourselves that we ignore.

Experience belongs to a fleeting perceptual and mortal world and shamanism does not want to miss one flickering instant. The examination of experience is one of the tools used on the shamanic path, and one of the skills developed by being on the path. When we are fully invested in our experience, we can fully appreciate the fleeting moment. Only when we believe our experiences to be real can we really dig our claws into them. Those are the claws of Grandfather Turtle, the patron saint of wisdom. Or Grandmother Badger, the patroness of toughness. Whatever it is we learn, when we incorporate it into our humanity—*it will become wisdom and fortitude.*

The idea of cultivating the life of the soul first gains momentum in the twelfth and thirteenth centuries. We do not find it in the Hebrew Bible, nor the Greek: Jesus taught the existence, salvation, and immortality of the soul. That was a new message for his contemporaries, most of whom believed that the afterlife constituted nothing more than a dark, will-less, zombielike existence in the relentless shadows of Hades. The Christian Dark Ages squashed the life of the soul and the appreciation for the creation, Nature, in favor of a dark, will-less obedience to God. Islam also put the emphasis on obedience, rather than the cultivation of the soul. In the twelfth century, however, the light broke through. The beauty of the soul and the wonder of creation started to fertilize the arts and human relationships. This is found in the works of Hildegard von Bingen, the teachings of Rumi, the ballads of the troubadours, the art of the great cathedrals, and the great painters. Saint

Francis taught the worth of the creation and love for natural creatures. We take for granted our appreciation of the beauty of mountains, lakes, forests, fields, and rivers, but when Hildegard, Rumi, and Francis were born, people thought of Nature as a burden to be endured.

The appreciation for Nature and the individual eventually led to the development of science and technology as tools for exploiting the natural world. At the same time, literacy was encouraged, and in a few places plurality of opinion and individual expression were allowed. This was particularly spurred by the English Civil War. When the dust settled, so many people had been killed in sectarian warfare that the king wisely allowed sects to remain, as long as they would lay down their arms. That's when we Quakers originated.

Enter science. We have to address the false idea that science is based on reality and truth. In *The Structure of Scientific Revolutions* (1970), Thomas Kuhn showed that science is always based on belief systems and assumptions, never on pure fact. He called these beliefs "paradigms." Sometimes they are caused by lack of instrumentation: geocentrism was adequate until the invention of the telescope. In the more dogmatic sciences, like medicine, it is customary to deny the importance or even the existence of paradigms, while in others it is accepted practice to consider the choice of what paradigms a field is based upon. In modern medicine it is "evidence-based medicine" (EBM). Medicine is supposedly based on proven research, although critics, including editors of the *New England Journal of Medicine* (Marcia Angell), *The Lancet* (Richard Horton), and the *British Journal of Medicine* have all cast doubt on the legitimacy of modern research, due to the pernicious influences of Big Pharma profit on research.*

However, the problem with science goes beyond corruption. Modern science is based upon arguments about the nature of proof. The presumption that everyday experience is real is labeled "naive realism," meaning that only naive, unsophisticated, uneducated, or childlike people (read: the uneducated, Indigenous people, and subcultures whose thinking is not

---

*I give the original quotations from these authorities in *Holistic Medicine and the Extracellular Matrix* (2021a, 8–9).

based on logic) consider their direct experiences to be "real." The opposite perspective is labeled "critical idealism" because it is "critical" of the experience of "reality." It substitutes a constructed model or ideal for "the real."

If the real does not exist, then how do we obtain knowledge? We launch experiments that produce statistical results; the higher the probability, the closer we are to "reality." One advocate explains: "the more precise our statistical models, though always speculative, the closer we are to grasping the real world" (McGaughey 2016). This statement assumes that statistical models, "though always speculative," are capable of drawing closer and closer to reality. This, of course, is an assumption and itself a speculation; in fact, this method of thinking defines itself as unable to arrive at reality or truth.

McGaughey's argument is based on the syllogism: "If our statistical models are precise, and they are getting more precise, then we are getting closer to grasping reality." The same information could have been arranged in a different syllogism: "If our models of the world are based on speculation, then our model of the world can never be based upon reality."

The Whole

Human beings are born incomplete and we feel this throughout life. That is why we are seeking, wondering, curious. If we were complete, we would be boring. There is no end to the wandering of a Mystery People.

One of our goals as human beings is to attempt to become whole. But first we need to learn to perceive wholeness. Even here our culture opposes us. Science is based on reductionism—the attempt to find the explanation in the smallest bits, while ignoring the whole, the context within which the bits operate. It does not deny the existence of the whole: holism is considered to be the opposite of reductionism. Science basically uses holism as a foil against which to define reductionism. Holism therefore is a subject we have to learn on our own, without the help of conventional education.

It was not always so. The study of character, the whole person, was once quite popular. Just to cite one historical era, if one turns back to the writings of the Civil War period in America, one finds tremendous interest in the study of character. The personalities of the great generals and politicians offered scope for this kind of study and were discussed and brooded over continually in the newspapers and parlors of America. What else could people at home do? They craved knowledge of the character of the leaders who would determine the successes and failures of armies, campaigns, peoples, and nations. Did Grant's whiskey-drinking indicate a weakness, a flaw he could overcome, or even a strength? Sherman was a "nervo-sanguine type," anxious, fretful, but always on the move. Abraham Lincoln was labeled "poor white trash, born and educated in a slave state" by the leader of his own party, but he deftly moved through political and military minefields to outlast the expectations of his allies and opponents. Lee, the dark gentleman, was courtly, internal, careful, yet daring—in battle, a stealthy panther; in peace, the rallying point of the "Lost Cause." "Stonewall" lived up to his name. The white people of the era did not study the character of Natives or Afro-Americans, but we can remedy that today. Frederick Douglass was a manly, intelligent, charismatic, fearless black man. In the end he was the only person the friendless president looked to as a peer for advice and approval. Sojourner Truth traveled everywhere, living up to her name, "telling it like it is."

From the Civil War to the early twentieth century, the study of character flourished and fascinated people. This was a sophisticated era from the standpoint of character study. It was superseded by the birth of modern psychology. Jung's "archetypes" and his model for character-analysis are useful, interesting, and profound, but they aren't personalized by the public interest in the character of great and terrible generals, politicians, and dictators. And we can't blame Jung because none of the other psychiatrists were interested in this study either. The intense scrutiny of public and historical figures faded into the past.

Outside of the Jungian model, which is used in education, human resources, psychology, and sociology, the study of character according to ancient standards exists as some sub-department of occultism or traditional Chinese medicine. Nevertheless, it is important to be able to recognize the whole: the character, the constitution, physical or psychological, innate and acquired, in order to be able to assess oneself and other people accurately. But more than that, it is necessary to exercise and develop the faculty within us that experiences the whole in ourselves and the world around us. Jung called this the "intuition."

The whole unites the pieces. The pieces are observable and can be documented, but the whole can only be known by an "intuitive leap." That is why holism is largely ignored by modern science and education.

When we sense the whole, the pattern, the archetype, the understanding pops into place before our mind and we experience an "aha moment"—a feeling of completeness; a lightness of being within us, as it were, that is not our normal state of existence. Knowledge of the whole that unifies the pieces is transcendental and spiritual, uplifting us to a higher world.

I remember reading the account of a teacher who taught free classes for paroled convicts on philosophy. He described the Platonic world of archetypes. One of the men said: "Wow, they sure didn't teach us that in school!" It is important to develop the life of the mind so that we can see the greater perspective that makes life more interesting, and may even "keep us out of trouble."

Intuitive and holistic connections have been removed from our language, so that we cannot even think this way. I know this because I grew up where English was the second language, still subordinate to an ancient American Indian tongue, where the real and the whole were implicit to survival in the alligator-infested swamps of southern Florida. Later in life I had to search and search for a way to express these connections in English—I found it in astrology. I'm not an astrologer, though, but a speaker in whole patterns.

The True

In order to know anything definite, we need to be able to differentiate between true and false. I am not talking about a cultural value here—good or bad behavior and thought—but the truth we feel in our hearts or soul or body when we are confronted by something that simply is true.

If we can't tell what is true, what do we know? Therefore we must cultivate the ability to know and feel truth. This will start with simple detections of bad ideas from good ones, lies from reliable statements, safe situations from unsafe. One day we will be confronted by a spiritual truth. If we have been doing our homework, then we will know that we are hearing a truth and that it comes from the spirit. We will also know that *we have to believe*: if we do not believe the spirit, then our spiritual life will not develop.

The instinct for truth is an actual faculty but it is not acknowledged or described in modern culture to any degree. The current conceit is that "truth is relative" or "everyone can have their own truth." This is only possible if there is an underlying supposition that there really is no absolute truth. There is also the idea that there is only one truth. This is also a basic supposition in Western society. Originally it was a religious truth, now it is a scientific truth—or rather, science has become the new religion.

Truth—the real McCoy—is internally recognized and therefore cannot be externally advertised. It is doubtful that the purveyors of "one truth for everyone" really know the truth they claim to know. If they did, they would have had an internal experience of truth and realize that truth cannot be advertised or forced on people. It was largely in rebellion against these unpleasant people that the modern "truth is relative" fad arose. But this solution is no better. Sorry. Delusion. The laws of the universe were not made by short-lived, inexperienced tramps living on the surface of the planet for a few decades (namely, ourselves). Truth can only be recognized by the individual.

There are several "kinds" of truth. Conscience is the "whispering of the superego," which usually gives us good advice about how to live in a way that is beneficial for us and for society. It is good idea to get in the habit of listening to one's conscience and following that voice because it generally means well. And, when the spirit does speak, we will be better practiced at listening.

Then there are the "inalienable" truths so well stated in the American Constitution:

We hold these truths to be self-evident, that all men are created equal, that they are endowed by their Creator with certain unalienable Rights, that among these are Life, Liberty, and the pursuit of Happiness.

Because we are endowed with free will, we know that taking away another person's free will is wrong. Taking away a person's life or happiness crosses their will. This knowledge is hardwired into our souls.

Then there is the truth of the intuition: "Aah, yes! It all fits together"—the pieces make a "whole." There is a part of the mind that is not satisfied until all the pieces make sense, generating the "aha moment," just as reason is not satisfied until all the pieces stand in a logical order. Intuition sees "in a flash" how the data fit together. As one of the old occult teachers put it: "Intuition sees each truth separately and distinctly and never connects it with another, or with cause or effect, this being the work of Reason" (Raleigh 1929, 16).

Since it reflects perceptions and knowledge that seem to (or actually do) come from another world, the intuition encourages us to go beyond reasoning and ordinary consciousness. It also puts us in the good habit of pursuing and finding truth. Hopefully we will reach a level where the instinct for truth is hardwired into our system

The sources of this instinct do not come from our human self, but from a deeper animal and energetic level, which, ultimately, derives from the cold-blooded instinct for survival. It is actually a part of us that is reptilian. Falsehood can be deadly, so the reptilian brain is engaged in the search for what is real, whole, and true.

Truth detection does not involve thinking about right and wrong. It arises in a dark, primitive part of our waking awareness. Who would guess that the most wicked part of ourselves—a reptilian mind that is only interested in survival and reproduction at the cost of everything else—would be the part of us that eventually learns to detect truth? Or who would think that truth, which is so essential to the spirit, would be detectable by the inner lizard? We are a Mystery People.

How can we cultivate truth-knowing? It demands that we are always looking for truth—that we face it when it appears, in whatever form, not lying to ourselves or others. The development of the instinct for truth demands an exercise of all the faculties of perception and truth-knowing. If we suppress any of them, we will know less. Or not enough.

The spirit could be defined as the true, the whole, the real, and the free. However, until we have had the internal experience of these truths, this statement is merely a concept. Ho-hum.

Shining the Spirit

Even without intending to, those who know truth shine it out into the world—and sometimes people recognize it in them. That's the kind of person who is a "city on the hill," a touchstone for truth in human society. People want to touch that stone.

We should develop the habit of shining. Then we will not waste our fleeting time on Earth, nor the time of the people around us. When we receive spiritual truth, our own spirit is awakened and it is our duty to let our spirit shine. It happens naturally. It is not a matter of speech, but of being.

Shining the spirit is a shamanic technique. Don Juan mentioned it a single time, without explanation. He once said to Carlos, with regard to his domestic life: "The only thing you never did was shine your spirit" (Castaneda 1972, 42). We don't need to be realized beings to shine the spirit. We need to stand for something noble, true, uplifting—even just the pursuit of truth. And since truth is ultimately personal, we can only convey our truth by shining it out to the world, not by argumentation. Carlos was too conflicted between his spiritual path and his domestic path to shine his spirit when he got home. He didn't understand that there is no difference between one and the other. What a waste.

This is also a method that Jesus taught: "a city on the hill cannot be hidden" (Matthew 5:14). I never appreciated the physical reality of this observation until I traveled through Galilee at night: all the villages were on the tops of the hills. That's because of centuries of warfare. "Shining the spirit" rises to the top in the life of the spiritual warrior.

Uncertainty

The world is not perfect. What if we really don't know anything definite? Carl von Clausewitz had to confront this often in war, the most serious "business of life" (1989, 140):

> [T]he general unreliability of all information presents a special problem in war: all action takes place, so to speak, in the twilight, which, like fog or moonlight, often tends to make things seem grotesque and larger than they really are.
>
> Whatever is hidden from full view in this feeble light has to be guessed at by talent, or simply left to chance. So once again for the lack of objective knowledge, one has to trust to talent or to luck.

It is shocking to think of common soldiers living or dying by the "luck" of their superiors.

This is called the "fog of war." The coronavirus pandemic, and the years that have followed, offers a good illustration of this mindset in the "twilight" or "haze" of battle. As I write, these events are still unfolding. We, as a species, don't know what is going on.

Faith

If we don't look forward to the future then we can't enjoy life. This is called "faith." It gives us purpose, confidence, and forward propulsion on the path of life, however we visualize that path. As Hermes said:

> When you take that road, this Good will meet you everywhere and will be experienced everywhere, even where and when you do not

expect it; when awake, asleep, in a ship, on a rock, by night, by day, when speaking and when silent. (Salaman et al. 2000, 58)

To *know* that is to have faith.

I used to ignore this important element of the path because the word "faith" was so overused—it seemed to me—by the Christians. But to the extent that they meant an "inner knowing" that we can put our faith in—rather than belief in a dogma—they are correct.

When I was young and had the experience that "Nature is alive" and knew it to be true, it gave me faith in the future of my young life. No matter what happened, I would always be a part of the All-Life. But other things also gave me meaning on the path. Reading Castaneda a few years later, I felt the ring of truth in what don Juan said and his teachings were always a touchstone for me. Even the inscrutable tarot cards, which I first saw at about the same age, gave me faith in the ultimate meaning and outcome of life; they seemed to promise a life path with such meaning and outcome. And what was the last card of the Higher Arcana: the World, representing fulfillment, the end of the journey reached, but also picturing the very Living Nature that had given me faith in the beginning.

Knownism

One day I was talking to my late friend Arlo Omaha, who was born on Rosebud Reservation in South Dakota. While I kept using the word "God," he would use the word "Great Mystery." After a few minutes, I wondered why he wasn't using "Great Spirit." That is a common English translation of the Lakota *Wakan Tonka*. So, I listened carefully. Arlo wasn't forceful or unusual in his demeanor, but I could feel that he was teaching something. Then it struck me: he was pointing out that I was talking about something I really didn't know anything about. I was unconsciously conceited on the subject of God. The very term "God," so common in my culture, was a conceit. It implied a knowledge that out-stripped the possible. Even if we know something tangible about God, there is so much more that we don't know. We live in the middle of a Great Mystery.

There are two lessons here, not one. The first is called "known-ism," while the other is called "paying attention and deserving to know." Thank you, Arlo—I leave these teachings as a monument to you, a spiritual warrior gone on to the next world. Travel well.

One of the fallacies of Western culture is the assumption that we either know everything of essential value or we are going to know it when our technology has gotten sophisticated enough for us to investigate everything. This assumption even pervades our attitude toward the unseen worlds. Thousands of years of churchianity have encouraged us to presume that we can know God easily and directly. Both our science and our religion cause the deadly conceit of *known-ism* to spread throughout the entire culture, which explains in some measure the arrogance of modern Western culture. This is a kind of entitlement.

The teaching of fundamentalist Christianity is that God, Jesus, is a familiar, approachable God rather than a remote one. It is hard to see how this can be a bad idea under any circumstance. However, this leads to religious entitlement, which we see writ large all over the institution of Christianity, not to mention dogmatism. These kinds of religious and scientific fixations are found everywhere in Western culture.

Against close-minded fundamentalism of all kinds there is the terminal open-mindedness of the superficial seeker people in our culture who believe they can "choose" to make God whomever or whatever they want him or her or it to be. They are relatives of the "everyone can have their own truth" people. They presuppose that God is no more than a concept and a possession belonging to a person. This is another form of entitlement.

The problem of *knownism* goes very deep because it has been an inherent feature of Western culture for a very long time. The ego lives in a limited, self-determined universe and it wants to believe that there is nothing else out there but what it knows or can know. However, human beings innately feel that something is missing. Something is calling.

The path of the shaman is pointed in the opposite direction from the known. Although the shaman accepts the reality of the human experience in all its diversity, that path ironically questions even the validity of human nature itself. It does not take for granted that human nature is a good thing. Talk about skepticism! The shamanic journey takes us beyond self, family, friends, neighbors, and finally even the human genome. Let us call this the path of *unknownism*.

Shamanism is a path of death, not just for the ego and the social person, but our attachment to the human genome, humanity itself, and everything that we take for granted; the shaman survives that inner death and returns.

I do not mean that one literally dies physically, ceases to be human, loses connection with the known or sanity, or completely loses their self-identity, friends, and family. It is only required that our egoic attachments to these matters must pass away. Then, in the space created by the death of these attachments, we will discover something that is beyond the ego, the known, or even the human. At the same time, one may discover how precious is our life, the known, the human, one's family and friends.

The death of the ego makes room for something from beyond the personal to come into one's life. That ultimate transpersonal factor is the spirit—so transpersonal we don't really know what it is. The spirit is the ambassador of the unknown.

In the end, however, the known is not one iota inferior to the unknown. All things that pertain to the heart are part of the known. Within it we find the most delicate, temporal, and beautiful bits of life that will ever be lived. It is the preconceptions, the entitlements, the conceits, that are in the way.

Paying Attention and Deserving to Know

One evening, more than thirty years ago, I went out for dinner with an American Indian friend I had met in the herb store. She was a poised, well-educated woman of middle years, who resided in one of the wealthiest neighborhoods in the city. I was not expecting an education, but as she spoke, I began to realize she was teaching me. I learned more things about medicine that night than I learned in any other three hours. Now, thirty years later, I realize maybe I should have camped out on her doorstep and learned more, but because of stereotypes (my own *knownism*), I didn't think of her as the expert she was.

Indians who reflect traditional ways often teach by subtle suggestions; they don't want the listener to lose face or feel imposed upon. Being a teacher is a very delicate position. Also, they feel that people should have an inner sensitivity to the knowledge imparted. It should not be given away for free. It should—indeed—*must* be worked for. Much is asked of the student, as well as the teacher. The student who pays attention earns the knowledge and respects both the knowledge and the teacher.

Back in those days, when this conversation took place, politically correct people got uptight using the word "Indian" and replaced it with "Native American." That didn't fly in Canada, so they adopted the term "First Nation." Later there was a switch to "Indigenous."

All of this was done without asking the Indian people what they thought. The PC advocates of the time certainly didn't ask members of the American Indian Movement—the leading politically active group in Native America. While AIM did not speak for all Indian people, it was certainly well known in the American press, due to the seizure of Alcatraz and Wounded Knee, plus other run-ins with the FBI. A kid in my high school was on probation for hitting an FBI agent over the head with a pipe. It would have been respectful to ask AIM what they thought was a respectful term—but white people thought they knew better. They didn't know about "deserving to know" or even "listening." The white way, as they said on the Seminole rez, was "too-much-Jesus." Preach, preach, preach and don't listen.

My dinner friend kept pointedly using the expression "the Indian People." That caught my attention: it was like a speed bump in the road of the conservation. Why did she use the phrase? I wondered. I listened more carefully and became aware of the undercurrents behind her choice of words. They were a statement: *We are People, we are a People.* And finally there was even the deepest inference: *We are the People . . . of the Land.*

What did my friend call my people? In traditional Native teachings, the Indian educator is very polite and don't like to cause loss of face. My friend used the term only once, but it was shocking when she did: *invader.* She applied it to someone else, deflecting it from me because she didn't want to offend me. I've met Indian people much more militant than this woman, but she was the only one who made sure I knew who I was.

Although my friend was educated in the colleges of white society, she still spoke in the traditional fashion. Everything she told me was a story. Not one thing was presented as something derived from logic, which I had to agree or disagree with. She just told me stories; one after another. If I understood them, then I deserved to know. One of them, about the Bat People, I failed to understand for decades. It would take getting coronavirus for me to understand this most profound and powerful medicine animal.

Different Kinds of Knowing

The word "science" refers to a system of organized knowledge. Historians of science have listed a total of five "methods and procedures" for constructing systems of knowledge: "revelation, authority, reason, experience, and experimentation" (Clagett 1955, 4). To this must be added "commercial science," since knowledge is always harnessed to better oneself or others. "Authority" refers to expert opinion, peer review, history, and tradition. But it is "revelation" we want to dissect here. There are at least three different methods that fall into this category. Science can be intuitive (looking for connections and patterns), visionary (dream and imagination), and clairvoyant (Rudolf Steiner and Edgar Cayce).

Intuitive science is based on the detection of patterns in data, to establish the greater context. A good example of the intuitive approach would be Darwin's realization that all the different finches on the Galapagos Islands derived from one ancestral finch that had evolved into many species suited to the different food-gathering niches on the islands.

History includes well-known examples of "visionary science," like the chemist August Kekulé's discovery of the structure of the benzene ring in a dream:

> I was sitting writing at my textbook but the work did not progress; my thoughts were elsewhere. I turned my chair to the fire and dozed. Again the atoms were gamboling before my eyes. This time the smaller groups kept modestly in the background. My mental eye, rendered more acute by repeated visions of the kind, could now distinguish larger structures of manifold conformation: long rows, sometimes more closely fitted together all twining and twisting in snakelike motion. But look! What was that? One of the snakes had seized hold of its own tail, and the form whirled mockingly before my eyes. As if by a flash of lightning I awoke; and this time also I spent the rest of the night in working out the consequences of the hypothesis.
>
> Let us learn to dream, gentlemen, then perhaps we shall find the truth. (Benfey 1958, 22)

These images are remarkably similar to the "pharmacological" visions experienced by partakers of Ayahuasca in the Amazon: they also sometimes see molecules as snakes (Narby 1998)!

A modern biographer commented on Kekulé's approach: "There was not universal approval for this method of gaining inspiration" (Libby 1922, 270). Note that this biographer couldn't actually perceive what Kekulé described: *he used this method not to gain inspiration, but to acquire specific scientific information.* This difference is so far-fetched for this commentator that he was not able to read or report the account correctly! This is a good example of "cultural blindness," or "bad education."

It also turns out that this was not just a freak accident but that Kekulé's teacher trained his students in this method and Kekulé trained some of his own students as well:

> Kekulé's pupil Van 't Hoff, who at the age of twenty-two wrote the essentials of *La Chimie dans l'Espace*, seems to have shared the visual imagination of his master. For Kolbe the idea that the arrangement of atoms in molecules could be determined appeared almost as fantastic as a belief in witchcraft or spiritualism. Berthelot was not less disdainful concerning Wurtz, the teacher of Van 't Hoff and Le Bel. When some friend told Berthelot not to take the atomic theory too seriously, atoms having no objective reality, Berthelot growled: "Wurtz has seen them!" (Libby 1922, 270)

Visionary science is the essential basis for much of the traditional knowledge, culture, and religion of the Indian People. Historically, Native Americans considered dreaming to be the source of information about how to regulate and run their culture and learn about the world around them. Dreaming, for the Native American People, is/was not just an uncontrolled, mysterious experience—as it is for most people in the dominant culture—but serious business that can determine the direction of life for the individual and society. Of course, the pernicious effect of the dominant culture has badly damaged this scientific approach to life.

An Anishinabe Ojibwa elder speaking to a folklorist in the Upper Peninsula of Michigan described the use of dream in traditional Indian society. He likened it to the white man's idea of school. Children were asked to relate their dreams to their elders. At large yearly sociopolitical gatherings, dreamers were queried by experts in the community to see what meaning their experiences had for the individual or the community. The elder likened this to the process in white culture when "a lawyer goes before the bar" (Dorson 1952, 32).

Robert Moss describes the traditional Iroquois approach to dreamtime (2012, 4). In 1647 a Jesuit reported back to his superiors that for this people the "secret of the soul, especially as revealed in dreams" was considered the most important aspect of life. There was a word for this: *ondinnonk*, which Moss himself first heard in dreamtime and later in conversation with Iroquois people. Dreams were shared in the community, scanned for insights into the person, the community, the future, and the Spirit World. Society was built and maintained upon dream.

Knowledge based on dreaming is not just a willy-nilly, uncontrolled enterprise, but can be systematic and therefore a type of science, in the true sense of the word. The knowledge it provides can be accurate and deserved: Wurtz and Kekulé deserved to know and their knowledge is the basis of modern chemistry, physics, and medicine.

The comparison of dream analysis by elders to going before the bar is very insightful because the practice of law is based on a different paradigm from standard science: "case law" or "case histories." It is understood that law is a human endeavor and therefore legal truth is based on empirical experience and logic. Law, therefore, is built upon a series of case histories. Dream knowledge is like "case law": it slowly builds up an edifice of applicable personal and social understanding.

Truth-Knowing

The thing about truth is: when you feel it, you know it and you have to believe it. A spiritual test occurs at that moment: are you likely to accept truth or reject it? If you accept it you will henceforth have to acknowledge that truth in your life. It might be inconvenient; you're not going to make money off it either. When the spirit directly reveals a truth to a person and they reject it, the instrument of truth-knowing within them is *permanently damaged*. Wrong behavior is forgivable, disbelieving external facts is forgivable, but disbelieving truth is irreparable.

The Inner Light

What is the instrument of truth-knowing? This "detector" is personal and subjective. There was originally no name for it in our culture— *is that a statement or what*? Since it was the center of their religion, Quakers invented a term to fill the gap: the Inner or Inward Light. I learned about it in Quaker First Day School and it was explained by my father at home. I experienced it when I had my "mountain top experience," when I knew that Nature was alive and I had experienced a spiritual truth and I knew—even at age eleven—that I had to believe it or forever lose my ability to know spiritual truth.

The Inner Light is often mistaken for "conscience," but that is the "whispering of the superego." Still, like I said, listening to the superego is good practice and better direction than a lot of other voices. Most of what I heard growing up in Quaker meeting was the "whispering of the superego." But people were trying to hear something to guide their life by—and that is an endeavor worthy of us all.

The idea that each person possesses the Inward Light, without reference to anyone or anything else, is one of the two Quaker doctrines. The other is that truth reveals itself in all times and places. So there is also an Inner Truth which is knowable by the individual without regard to *any* external source, doctrine, or person. These were my spiritual "training wheels" when I was growing up.

This might sound like the "everyone has their own truth" miasma, but it is based on the naive assumption that there really is such a thing as "the truth." What the Quakers mean is that there is a real truth and everyone has to seek for it, work for it, and deduce whether it is truth or not from the feeling it gives them.

During the churchianity era, one was supposed to believe what the minister said, the church doctrine, or the Bible. During our own "scientific era," one is supposed to believe the conclusions and opinions of experts published in scientific journals and parroted (or even misrepresented) by the mainstream news industry.

Without the ability to detect truth, animals could not survive, nor their wounded kin, man, who still possesses animal instincts but not the ability to believe them. We destroyed the connection between human and spirit, but the connection between animal and spirit remained. That is why God told Adam and Eve to take off the fig leaves and put on animal skins: "You are animals. Don't forget it. That is the only path implicit in your wounded condition."

I looked up the passage in the Gospel of John that inspired the Quaker belief in the Inward Light: "In him was the life (*zōé*), and that life (*zōé*) was the Light of the World" (John 1:4). The Greek word *zōion* means "animal" while *zōé* means "animal life." When I looked up the usual translations in various Bibles I almost always found that *zōé* was translated as "eternal life." I could hardly believe it! These translators thought they were representing the Word of God, but they were changing the meaning completely. What John literally wrote was, the animal life was in Jesus and that animal life was the "Light of the World," the basis of truth-knowing. He could have put "eternal" in there himself, but he didn't, so translators should not either.

Most people don't have confidence in things spiritual. Many people resort to authority figures or creeds. Or they imagine they are divining the truth when they are just fantasizing. At least these people are trying. Most people don't even bother about spiritual life.

What the Inner Light finds is Inner Truth. It comes in discrete words or no words, in pictures or feelings. The common experience is that one just "knows it is true." Sometimes there is a background of silence when an internal truth is revealed. Blavatsky called it the "voice of silence." Don Juan called it "silent knowledge." The Hebrew prophets called it the "Word of God." The Quakers meet in silent meeting.

The opposite of truth is falsehood and the opposite of silence is noise. We live in one of the noisiest societies imaginable. Not only are we bombarded by words and images all the time but even by invisible electro-magnetic signals. Most people don't feel them, but a few people are bothered by them. So it is a good thing to withdraw into silence or meditation from time to time. Forests are a good place. Even a log cabin or a sauna is a good environment because something about wood shields us from the thought-vibrations of people in the world and the invisible electro-magnetic signals that are constantly coursing through the air.

The Instinct for Truth

One would think the ability to know truth would be a subject of study in any culture, but this is not the case in the West: logic dominates over the inner voice. Finally, I found a single psychiatrist who defined an internal instrument for truth-knowing: Marie-Louise von Franz, who was one of Jung's most trusted students. This came out in her lectures on alchemy: "One is capable of distinguishing the true from the false, [when] there arises or grows within the personality what one could call the instinct of truth" (Franz 1980, 172).

Von Franz attributes the appearance of this instinct to the approach of "the Self," the core integrative factor within the psyche—what I would interpret as the soul being led by the spirit:

> [W]hen the Self is so present and so strong . . . the instinct of truth gets through quickly, like a radio telegram, and one reacts rightly, without knowing why. It flows through one and one does the right thing. . . . That is the action of the Self becoming immediate, and only the Self can accomplish this. (Franz 1980, 172; punctuation slightly altered)

What beautiful observations and statements! And yet, we hardly ever have such discussions in our culture. When von Franz wandered onto this subject in her lecture, the students asked her to elucidate. From the transcript it is clear they hadn't heard of anything like this before.

As we develop this faculty, the spirit is able to draw closer to the soul because there is nothing in the spirit that is not true. Good Doctor von Franz is correct. We start to automatically understand truth because there is less and less space between soul and spirit.

Through the instinct of the animal self, we know what is true and what is not. The truth comes to us as a certainty, which we know in our body as a kind of body knowledge. It generally cannot be conveyed by external words, but only mind-to-mind or Nature-to-human. It also comes to the person as a realization. Before, one knew nothing; now, something true has been revealed.

There are words in many languages and traditions for revelation. The terms "silent knowledge" (don Juan), "inner truth" (Quakers), and "realization" (Paramahansa Yogananda, Max Freedom Long) are interchangeable.

Body Knowledge

The animal self and the energy body (vital force or etheric body) give rise to "body knowledge." In occultism these two, plus the physical body, are looked upon as a unit called the "lower vehicle," or the vehicle for the incarnation of the soul, which partakes of both the higher and the lower dimensions and inputs. We can feel body knowledge, sometimes like a shiver of recognition running down the spine.

The knowing that comes from the energy body is what don Juan called "seeing." He explains to Carlos that although he described it as if it were visual, it was actually something felt in the body. When it is fully developed, all the senses are activated so that one sees and touches and hears the truth. Or so I have heard. This creates a second body so that the shaman can be in two places at once. I know only two people who have seen a person who could be in two places at once.

That can be a pretty mundane experience, by the way. Susan was having breakfast when her teacher's teacher showed up from northern Canada. "Ah. . . Ah. . . Do you want some breakfast?" she asked. "No, I'm looking for Amos. I guess he's not here."

The term "lower vehicle" is not that good because it sounds like a value judgment and the animal self in particular is deeply susceptible to judgment. The way it thinks is like a dog: "lower is bad, so I'm bad!" So this is not a term we will perpetuate in this book; although it is not inaccurate to place the physical body, the animal self, and the energy body together as a comprehensive "vehicle."

Imagination and Fantasy

Human beings and animals can see images in their mind, and both can dream, but only human beings can willfully focus on an image or hold it in their mind's eye. Because we have a conscious mind, we can choose which thoughts and images to entertain. We can train our minds to grab and hold on to fleeting images we would otherwise ignore, and then we can study them meditatively. For this reason, the imagination is a characteristic of humanity, not of animality.

Aristotle taught that it was the ability to examine (rather than just have) the imagination, plus the rational faculty, that made us human. Imagination is the Tree of Life and logic is the Tree of the Knowledge of Good and Evil, to use the Biblical metaphor. The ability to examine images in the mind is possible because of self-consciousness, which we gained at the foot of the second of those Trees.

William Blake also concluded that it was the imagination that made us human. For the poet it is the root of our salvation from slavery in the world of the ego, cut off from the rest of creation. This is why Blake spoke of "Jesus the Divine Human Imagination." Theologians excuse Blake's exuberant eccentricities, but he had it right: imagination is the faculty through which we return to the spirit; it is the Spirit World itself. It is the Tree of Life that binds together all of creation. The seer Jacob Boehme, who greatly influenced Blake, traced vision to the core of existence: he saw the "eye of the abyss" looking out at him from the "eternal unground."

As we have seen, Blake differentiated between imagination and fantasy. Because it is so important, we can say it again: images that come from our memory or other people are qualitatively different from images that spring up fresh in our own mind's imagination. Blake called the "recycled images" fantasies; although we should not judge them so much as differentiate them from true imagination. The development of imagination requires careful self-examination of the contents passing before the mind. "You have to open the mind to let the image in, but snap it shut to catch it by the tail, before it gets away." That is such a perfect observation that I have to credit it; it was said by my best friend on the spiritual path when I was young: Peter Young.

This opening and closing of the mind's eye is analogous to the discipline of the spiritual warrior, who learns to let go and grab hold in the right proportion in the activities of life. As we discipline our outer lives, our inner life follows suit. This is a lifelong process. When we meet up against new challenges—like aging or a new love—we face the same challenges in a new form. Thank you, Great Mystery, for letting me grow.

One of the great teachers of "soul sight" was the American Rosicrucian Pascal Beverley Randolph. He points out an important aspect of Plato's definition of sight:

> The Platonic philosophy of vision is that it is the view of objects really existing in interior light, which assume form; not according to arbitrary laws, but according to the state of the mind. This light unites with exterior light in the eye, and is thus drawn into a sensuous or imaginative activity [Blake's "fantasy"]; but, when the outward light is separated, it reposes in its own serene atmosphere. It is, then, in this state of interior repose that all really inspired and correct visions occur. (Randolph 1930, 83)

This is what don Juan called "silent knowledge." When we hear the spirit deep inside of us, it is usually accompanied by silence. Of course, sometimes the spirit has to break through the clouds of our thoughts to get to us because there is some kind of "spiritual emergency." But a lot of the time the silence is discernible. I believe it is this ability to descend to this quiet and hear the spirit that gives rise to "spiritual seership." Psychic powers come from the psychic level, which primarily comes from the soul.

Not only is the imagination our vehicle for return to the Spirit World; it is the means by which we become co-creators in the grand theater of creation. By expanding in our imagination upon the scenery that flows by, as we cruise along in our spiritual vehicle, so to speak, we change the creation. As Jacob Boehme said, "magic" is the result of imagination, desire, and will—the ability to fixate the attention. The capacity to see images was present from the beginning of creation, according to the Book of Genesis, for it is said that God made "man in his own image." Before all else, we are an image.

Boehme observes something about vision that is remarkable. He says there is an "eye in the abyss," in the void at the source of creation. Vision was first, before all else. The English word "see" implies both vision and knowing.

When we understand that we possess the wonderful gift of imagination, we understand why it is that the plants and animals want to communicate with us. They too possess an image, but not the ability to change the focus of the internal images. When they are interacting with us they can participate in the wonderful unfolding of creation through imagination, magic, and even speech. There is so much that we owe to our animal relatives, but the creative use of the imagination belongs to the human life-wave alone.

Herbal Preparations for the Journey

The first preparation for the spiritual journey, in almost any place in the world, from the sweat lodge to St. Peter's Basilica in Rome, is burning incense or smudge. There are so many of these different kinds of incenses and smudge sticks that one could not count them all. There are also essential oils that serve the purpose.

According to the teachings of the genius Abbess Hildegard von Bingen, there is one plant that increases the power of animal within us, Angelica (*Angelica archangelica*), and one that increases the human, Galangal (*Alpinia galangal*). The former is a native of Europe, the latter a trade item from the "Spice Islands." A smudge of Angelica root opens up the imagination like no other vegetable teacher. Galangal strengthens the heart.

We can also use the cousins/analogues of this plant: Bear Root (*Lomatium dissectum*) and Oshá Root (*Ligusticum porteri*). They are members of the *Apiaceae* or Carrot family. All have brown, furry, oily roots that look like the paw of a bear, so they are all Bear Medicines and are closely related, botanically and medicinally. Many members of the Carrot family are abortifacients, some are moderately toxic, including the native North American *Angelica atropurpurea*, and a few are deadly, like *Conium maculatum* and the *Cicutas*.

Ethnobotanist Kat Harrison says that in every Indigenous culture she has ever visited, in every part of the world where Angelica or an analogue grows, she has found that people wear it as a mojo. It is not only protective against germs and bad vibes, but it is spiritually reinforcing and uplifting. It was used in Europe for pestilence (contagious diseases). It has a strong, sweet/spicy scent that makes it also an incense or smudge.

The European species (*Angelica archangelica*) is used in Sami medicine in the far north of Scandinavia. It grows over to Greenland and down to the Swiss Alps. Once upon a time, it was used as money in Iceland. The Indian People of North America use a native Angelica, or a cousin like Oshá or Lomatium "on the rocks," in the sweat lodge. The major native Angelicas of North America are the *atropurpurea* in the east, north, and south, and the *hendersonii* in the Pacific Northwest. Various cousins called Oshá or Oshalla are used in the Southwest and California, but as these are somewhat uncommon, they should not be picked.

Because it is easy to grow in the garden, *Angelica archangelica* ought to be the preferred medicine, unless we need one of the others for a specific reason. In New Mexican folk culture, Angelica is called "Angelica del Campo," or Angelica of the Garden, versus "Angelica del Montana," the wild mountain Oshá. *Angelica atropurpurea* is extremely common in the Eastern Woodland region so it can also be used as a smudge in place of the garden variety. It is easy to establish a wild population.

The interesting thing about these three plants is that they are suited to journeying in the three worlds: Upper (*Angelica*), Middle (*Lomatium*), and Lower (*Ligusticum*). According to herbalist Seán O'Donoghue—and I would agree—Angelica opens the inner eye of the imagination to the Upper World, Oshá to the Lower World. Lomatium, on the other hand, helps a person to control their own mind. That associates it with the Middle World of the conscious self.

☸ BEAR MEDICINE ☸

Because Bear goes into the cave every winter and sleeps for the duration, his medicines are considered to be fundamental for learning how to enter dreamtime. Bear Medicines are, in addition, very often brown, spicy, warming, and oily. It is said that upon leaving the cave in the spring, Bear seeks out these oily roots in order to fatten up and, at the same time—

because they are warming and stimulating—wake up the circulation. Because they are bitter, they also increase digestion and metabolism. The bitterness is combined with some acridity—the taste associated with hallucination (Peyote, Ayahuasca, psilocybin) and relaxation of the guts.

There are about a half-dozen Bear Roots in North America, including *Angelica*, *Lomatium*, *Ligusticum*, *Aralia racemosa*, *Balsamorrhiza*, and *Helianthus annuus* (Sunflower). There are at least two or three in Europe: Burdock, the Latin name for which is *Arctium*, meaning "of the bear," *Angelica archangelica*, and *Peucedanum ostruthium*. Another group of Bear Medicines are the berries, which bears like so much, especially Bearberry (*Arctostaphylos uva ursi*), native to the New and Old Worlds. Elderberry (*Sambucus nigra, S. canadensis*) is also a Bear Medicine, but it is mentioned elsewhere. There is a third group, the digestive bitters. We won't discuss them here, but Angelica is on that list too.

ꙮ Angelica ꙮ
(*Angelica archangelica*)

The name Angelica hearkens back to medieval Catholic folk religion and medicine—it is reported that a priest had a vision that the plant was for pestilence. There are two types of Angelicas in Europe, but one is superior to the other in medicinal potency—probably the reason it was named "*archangelica*."

Angelica is bitter, sweet, acrid, spicy, warming, and oily. It increases lipids but is drying to internal water. The native Angelicas are called Grizzly Bear Medicine in some areas of Indian Country—California, the Dakotas, and Minnesota. Since it is a hunting and fishing medicine, it is also assigned to Elk—the tops spread out like antlers. It is used to hide the odor of the hunter and relax him. Some of its botanical cousins are attractive to deer and elk.

Since the seed and root are gently warming and drying, Angelica is classified in astrology as a solar remedy, and its medicinal properties will be more fully described under the Sun Medicines. For now, we are just using the dried root as a smudge.

Angelica is an old and universal shaman remedy. It is used by the Sami in northern Scandinavia as a journeying plant. The signature here is the hollow-tubed stalk, which represents both the passage to another dimension and probably acted as a smoking tube. Angelica root is a great remedy for opening the imagination. For this, we burn the dried root in an open room on some charcoal. The sweet savor is extremely pleasant and one feels the "sphincter of the mind" open and relax and the imagination gently unfold. It helps one fall asleep at night and awaken refreshed in the morning.

ʚ Lomatium, Bear Root, Biscuitroot ɞ
(Lomatium dissectum)

This is a member of the family native to the northern Rocky Mountains, from Montana to the Pacific Coast. The root is warming, drying, bitter, sweet, acrid, spicy, and oily—more oily and sweet than Angelica. It contains various kinds of coumarin compounds, like *Angelica atropurpurea*, that are toxic to microbes, but can cause severe skin rashes and probably mucosal inflammation.

This is a very interesting plant because it was a specific in the flu epidemic of 1918. Ernst T. Krebs, M.D., the Bureau of Indian Affairs doctor for the Washoe Indian Reservation in Nevada, published a 1920 article, "An Indian Remedy for Influenza," in the *Bulletin of the Nevada State Board of Health*. In it, he writes:

> During the fall of 1918 when the influenza epidemic visited this section of Nevada, the Washoe Indians used a root in the treatment of their sick which was gathered along the foot-hills of this slope of the Sierra. The plant proved to be a rare species of the parsley family (*Leptotaenia dissectum*),* according to a report from the University of California.

---

*In the original article, Krebs used the Latin name *Leptotæmia dissecta*, a misspelling of *Leptotaenia dissectum*, a now-discontinued name. I have substituted the correct spelling.

Whether a coincidence or not, there was not a single death in the Washoe tribe from influenza or its complications, although Indians living in other parts of the State where the root did not grow died in numbers. It was such a remarkable coincidence that the root was investigated by a practicing physician who was apparently helping hopeless cases recover without any other medication or care of any kind. A preparation was prepared and employed in a great many cases among the whites, from the mildest to the most virulent types of influenza, and it proved, among other things, that it is the nearest approach we have today to a specific in epidemic influenza and the accompanying pneumonia. Where used early, it proved itself to be reliable agent in preventing pulmonary complications. Other physicians were induced to give it a trial, with the same results. It is beyond the experimental stage, as its therapeutic action in this direction is established and beyond any doubt. The cases in which it has been used run into the hundreds. There is probably no therapeutic agent so valuable in the treatment of influenzal pneumonia and, as far as being tried, in ordinary lobar pneumonia if started early. Its action on coughs is more certain than the opiate expectorants and its benefit is lasting. It acts as a powerful tonic to the respiratory mucous membranes. It is a bronchial, intestinal and urinary antiseptic and is excreted by these organs. It seems to stimulate the pneogastrics [i.e., the pneumogastric or vagus nerve] and causes a slow pulse with increased volume and reduced tension. It is a pronounced diaphoretic and somewhat diuretic, and it is a stimulating and sedative expectorant. In large doses it is a laxative, and in extreme doses emetic. (Krebs 1920, 7–8)

When I first came down with coronavirus, I woke with a heart rate of about 150. I took a bit of Lomatium over the next several minutes and the pulse returned to normal. I am sure I would have had those "pulmonary complications" Dr. Krebs referred to. Instead, I had a long, drawn-out case with mild heart symptoms that lasted three months. The plant said to me: "I am for things that are out of control." It didn't really help much throughout the long course of the illness. I used Holly and Nigella and finally White Pine.

The effect of Lomatium upon the mind is very useful on the shamanic or meditative path because it gives a person the ability to control the relentless chatter and constant self-dialoguing of the mind. For this purpose, it would be best to use as a smudge but some of us living outside of its range only have the tincture.

This is one of the two Native American invisibility remedies. I mentioned this in an article I once wrote and afterward I started to see this little old Indian gramma around—in the bank, on the freeway. I was always behind her and she didn't see me. After two weeks we met in dreamtime. She had been hired to kill me for mentioning this usage in public— to make me have a traffic accident. She smiled at me and I smiled at her. She knew it was an impossible assignment. Anyway, she'd been paid (that's why I was allowed to stand behind her in line at the bank) and she was warned to watch for the magic when it went back to her (that's why I saw her in her car). Neither one of us would get hurt— but someone was out some money.

Ultimately, it doesn't matter that much if we mention magical facts in public because virtually nobody in the dominant society believes us. The few who do don't have enough power to use them, and almost all Indigenous people dismiss non-Indigenous "shamans" as dilettantes. Magic always protects itself; it is invisible. But Mystery is better than magic.

☙ Oshá Root ❧
(*Ligusticum porteri, L. gregii*)

The name comes from the Spanish for "bear" (*osa*). There are more environmental and cultural issues involved with this member of the trio—it is less frequently encountered (except at high altitudes, where it is hard to pick since the roots intertwine with poplar). Some picking grounds traditionally belong to Native and New Mexican families. Therefore, I'm not going to recommend Oshá. It is difficult to grow in the garden, though not impossible. "Uncle Henry," a relative of my deceased friend Tony Seifert, grew it in his garden in central New Mexico. "So much for the report that it can't be grown in a garden!" commented Tony.

Unlike Angelica, Lomatium and Oshá are not classified—to my knowledge—as Elk Medicines. Although all are warming and stimulating to the circulation, and warming, drying, and stimulating to the digestion and respiratory tract, from the shamanic standpoint their actions are slightly different. Lomatium "controls the mind." Oshá Root is similar to Angelica, but causes the imagination to look downward, whereas Angelica causes one to look upward.

5

Don Juan's "Island of the Tonal"

All the world's a stage,
And all the men and women merely players;
They have their exits and their entrances,
And one man in his time plays many parts,
His acts being seven ages.

WILLIAM SHAKESPEARE, *As You Like It*

The only place the student can start the journey of self-transformation is with the only material available to him or her at the beginning: our ordinary waking consciousness. Even here shamanism presents us with an intrinsically different view from psychology.

Freud defined the ego as the focal point of consciousness, but there are subsidiary components of consciousness that the ego has to manage. This includes the conscious self ("I don't wanna fall asleep and become unconscious"), the biological self ("I wanna get drunk and pass out"), the social persona ("I want people to like or look up to me"), and the inner self ("I want to be emotionally and spiritually fulfilled"). The ego is the center and the regulator of this rebellious household.

All of these components are conscious and independent to one degree or another, though competition infers dominance and submission, and that means that different selves are being pushed forward to consciousness or back into unconsciousness at any given moment. For example, the conscious self is like a monk who wants to remain conscious at all times, wants to join "pure consciousness," have total control over the body, sexual system, and heart, leaving sensation and feeling behind, while the biological self wants to eat, drink, party, and get laid.

The one thing all of these components have in common is that they require consciousness in order to be developed and they communicate by talking. Therefore, they can all be lumped together as parts of what Max Freedom Long called the "talking self," translating the Hawaiian *uhane*. The social persona is constructed by talking to other people, the soul by talking to oneself; the monk reads scriptures, but the biological self asks for another drink.

The persona and conscious self prefer consciousness to rule as much of the time as possible, while the biological self and the soul need sleep in order to refresh themselves. The soul searches for its romantic counterpart and wants to be connected. It can lose itself in the unconsciousness of connection, or find spiritual fulfillment and increased consciousness through connection.

The Island of the Tonal

All of these selves are like actors on a stage, so we need a good term to describe the stage. Here, as in so many instances, don Juan crafted the term. He saw the conscious world as an "island" surrounded by the unknown and called it the *island of the tonal*. The word that comes closest to "conscious self" in nagualism is the Nahuatl word *tonal*. Specifically, this means the animal totem that guards the psychic components belonging to consciousness, while the *nagual* is the animal totem conjoined with dreamtime.

Don Juan's Native apprentices use the words "tonal" and "nagual" as they are used in Mexican nagualism, but don Juan translated the word "tonal" somewhat differently for Carlos, his Spanish-American apprentice. He defined it as the self-conscious being, and the island of the tonal as the sum total of everything it knows and experiences. The nagual is the unimaginable power lurking in the unknown beyond the island.

Don Juan would say the tonal keeps us imprisoned on its island. We know of nothing outside of it but we yearn for that unknown freedom.

There are also mysteries we have experienced on the island but not explored, and some of these are worth pursuing. The sincere attempt to search creates its own momentum for change.

Each day in the Mayan calendar has a different tonal: Mayan children still receive their names from the day on which they were born, so the tonal is similar to a person's astrological sign or chart in Western culture. We have already noted that there may be an animal for the physical body and one for the spirit body. The former gives us access to the instinct for truth, while the latter gives us the eyes and ears of the spirit self. The Mayan calendar name gives a remarkable profile for the conscious human self, including spiritual tendencies. I wish to thank Gianni Crow, a Mayan-born calendar-keeper, for the classes I was able to attend on this remarkable tradition.

The Outer Self and the Inner

In our daily lives we feel an ongoing tension between an inner and an outer self. We feel the tension between the two in our social relationships. When we say "I need to be true to myself," we are fighting for the inner self. A part of us craves the approval and love of those outer persons, but in conforming to their wishes and expectations we may sacrifice our "real self."

Jung identified the outer self as the "personality" or social person, or even the "mask" we wear in public, versus the inner self or "individuality" that we maintain and develop through meaningful experience. The external component he named the *persona*, from the Latin word for "mask." The idea is that we put a mask between ourselves and others to prevent being emotionally impacted too deeply by the scrapes of life that daily confront us in the social world. This theme percolated into the movie *The Mask* (1994), starring Jim Carrey and Cameron Diaz. As in that movie, a person can get trapped in the mask. One might think of the persona as a totally superficial entity, but within it Jung detected heroic qualities (1954, 171): "It is an act of courage flung in the face of life, the absolute affirmation of all that constitutes the individual, the most successful adaptation to the universal conditions of existence coupled with the greatest possible freedom of self-determination."

In the same passage, Jung also remarks that because it derives from our best efforts to adapt to the external pressures placed upon us by the environment, "Personality is the supreme realization of the innate idiosyncrasy of a living being." This definition reminds us of spiritual warriorship. Indeed, the persona is the part of us that develops the skills of war, because it must survive in the outer world. It is the part of ourselves that is naturally geared toward strategy. It works with the reptilian self, which is geared to survival.

We need to put this talented soul-part to work for us on the spiritual path. We do this first by constructing our social mask more consciously, so that we are not wasting energy fighting with the outer world and other people; we want to slip through the social waters smoothly, like a canoe on a still lake. Additionally, the persona is the master of strategy and therefore we can put it to work stalking or tracking our own egoic attachments, so that we understand our energy-wasting quirks and shortcomings.

Unfortunately, Jung felt that the average person in society identified with their persona as if it were their "true self," rather than with their native inner self. This occurs when one is living one's life unconsciously; not examining what is meaningful but identifying with social definitions rather than personal ones.

Jung identified the inner self with individuality. We protect it, hide it, and build it like a pearl in an oyster. We are an individual to the extent that we develop our sense of who we are, allowing the voice of the inner self to emerge and mature. Jung called this process "individuation" because we are becoming a true individual, not just a product of social influences.

The outer self is more closely related to the ego, while the inner self is essentially equivalent to what we call the soul in the English language.

The word *psyche*, from the Greek for "soul," signifies all functions, conscious and unconscious, which can be experienced or analyzed, so it includes the ego, id, and superego, and is not technically equivalent to the English word "soul." It is similar to the concept of the *island of the tonal*.

In *The Heart and Its Healing Plants* (2024) Wolf-Dieter Storl describes traditional remedies for the soul. He explains how the soul is identified with the heart in countless traditions and describes the many herbs traditionally used, especially in premodern European folk cultures, to treat conditions of the heart/soul. The pages are full of shamanic and herbal lore; I highly recommend this book as an adjunct to *A Shamanic Herbal*.

Conscious Self and Biological Self

The other major polarity within the *island of the tonal* is between consciousness and biological imperatives, or the conscious self and the biological self. The former wants us to stay conscious all the time and resents biological needs like eating, sleeping, drinking, partying, and sex. The biological self, on the other hand, likes to be immersed in biological needs. It is like an unruly teenager, the other like an overly moralistic parent.

The needs of the biological self come from the reptilian back brain, so we can use the terms reptilian self and biological self interchangeably. The *kundalini*, the "serpent power" in the spine and nerves, is described in Vedic philosophy. It descends down the spine from the back brain and throughout the nervous system.

The higher seat of the biological self is the back brain, or reptilian brain. This is the seat of our survival and reproductive instincts and drives. *This part of us can talk to the conscious self.* This is because our most basic survival needs have to be brought to consciousness and voiced in order to compete with the other elements of consciousness.

The battle between the "seed of the woman" and the "seed of the serpent" described in the Book of Genesis represents the continuous, circular enmeshment of the conscious self and the biological in an unending strife that typifies the post-Edenic situation of mankind.

Both are entrapped and tortured. The symbol in the Greek tradition is the *ouroboros*, or "serpent biting its tail." This is like the Wheel of Dharma in Vedic teachings.

The ability of the biological self to talk only comes up occasionally. When the blood sugar goes very low, the conscious self is turned down to the lowest notch because it is more important for basic life-survival processes to continue than consciousness. This is why a Sunday School teacher will swear like a sailor until she gets enough sugar to raise the blood-sugar level back up to censorship levels. Afterward, the person remembers nothing because the conscious mind was turned off during the experience.

The biological self gives us healthy animal instincts in order to survive in the world, but it also traps us in biological urges, just as the conscious self traps us in urges to maintain consciousness. Ironically, these same animal instincts are the origin of the instinct for truth, so the poison is the cure. This is another reason why the caduceus of Asclepius, the serpent climbing the green leafy staff, is a symbol for medicine.

Then there is the ego, whose job it is to control all of this—another contender for "king of the hill" on the unruly *island of the tonal*—while maintaining a smooth *persona* so that nobody suspects one is having difficulties that would undercut social position.

Gurdjieff's "Kundabuffer"

George Gurdjieff named the internal "installation" that the conscious self makes to protect itself against the upsurging biological self the *kundabuffer*. As the name suggests, it is a "buffer" between the conscious self and the kundalini.

According to Gurdjieff, the kundalini produces fantasies that convey its desires to consciousness. The conscious self is constantly fighting against them but the fantasies still rise to consciousness and promote a life based on them. This life, however, is an illusion because it is based on fantasy. The life lived in fantasy provides the energy that perpetuates the kundabuffer.

Gurdjieff says that each time a person imagines an outcome that is not actualized in the outer world, the kundabuffer is active and it is being manipulated through fantasies sent up by the kundalini. In contrast, imagination arises from what is true. If the person cannot fulfill the dream, they still fight for it constantly. If they give up, the battle for spiritual authenticity within themselves is diminished. The spirit generates images, dreams, art, creativity, literature—what we call inspiration—in order for us to fulfill its directives.

If we follow a fantasy and try to actualize it, it will lead us nowhere. The soul is able to differentiate between fantasy and imagination. Even the conscious self has this ability, since fantasies diminish consciousness. However, it is the ego that ultimately chooses which stream of consciousness to go with. The images streaming to the soul led us on "the path with heart" (don Juan), or the path that will actualize our soul during our lifetime. Fantasy life is never fulfillable.

The Medicine Wheel of the Tonal

The Mayan calendar name is laid out in the form of a cross with four equal sides. This is the tonal in the original sense, before don Juan and Carlos got ahold of it. The symbol of the equal-sided cross is the sign of wholeness, according to Jung, who found it in worldwide mythology and the dreams of his patients. His theory emerged shortly after his visit to New Mexico, where the state flag and a lot of Native art bears this symbol. Jung gave it the technical names *quaternio* (Latin) or *mandala* (Sanskrit), but this has been replaced by "medicine wheel," introduced by Sun Bear and Wabun. The British occultist Arthur Edward Waite named it the "Celtic Cross."

Native spiritual writers and teachers in the late twentieth century, such as Sun Bear and Vine Deloria, Jr., were well aware of Jung's work and appreciated having an ally within the dominant culture. It must be remembered that until 1978, when the federal American Indian Religious Freedom Act was passed, Indian spirituality and religion was illegal. Unfortunately, in the last several decades, almost all institutions of higher education in the United States have stripped Jungian programs from their psychology offerings.

From the Jungian perspective, the quaternio represents wholeness breaking through into the world where we humans skulk about in self-consciousness. It represents the whole, the truth, and healing coming into our lives. He also related the quaternio to the four "functions" of the psyche: intuition, rationality, emotion, and physical sensation. However, this symbol or "archetype" (in the Jungian sense), appears in many different settings, in all regions of the psyche. Jung considered the quaternio a psychologically charged symbol emanating from deep in the "collective unconscious" of the human race. Native Americans consider it to be alive. Here is a map of the medicine wheel of the conscious realm:

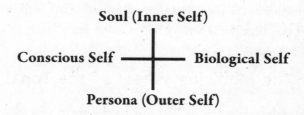

$$\textbf{Soul (Inner Self)}$$

$$\textbf{Conscious Self} \quad\rule{}{}\quad \textbf{Biological Self}$$

$$\textbf{Persona (Outer Self)}$$

The Ego

We could identify the point in the middle of the cross with the ego, the ruler of the island of consciousness. The ego is the dial that decides which of these four poles to focus on. All four competing factors function under the direction of the ego. Or at least, the ego tries to keep them under control.

Sometimes the ego identifies with one element of the *island of the tonal*, at other times with another. This fivefold constellation pulls together as a whole being, especially when threatened by danger. The biological self takes over when there is a great threat.

A lot of people have the "egoic dial" stuck on a fixed point. They are satisfied with themselves. They don't see or feel the need for substantive change. Even if they receive a message from the Spirit World, they don't do anything about it.

The Egoic Will

The ego has a strong will of its own in order to subordinate all these conflicting selves. This is called the "egoic will" or "gall." A person who pushes their own agenda forcefully is said to have "a lot of gall" in English. It definitely can be said that the ego is the most forceful component on the *island of the tonal*; that is how it manages to control the others.

In China a "spirit" or "soul" called the *hun* is said to reside in the gallbladder. A general or a politician with a strong will is said to have a "big gallbladder," while a coward has but a small one. An old-fashioned American expression for a person who lacks gall is a "yellowbelly."

Through evolution, our assemblage point has become the servant of the ego, so the egoic will is basically the assemblage point. After death it becomes the shade that records all shifts in attention a person experienced during life. It is like a blackboard with the writings of a lifetime recorded on it. "In the dissolution of a certain plane, there is nothing left but the shadow or reflection" (Raleigh, 1932, 18).

Many people just grind on and on over the same little piece of blackboard, not visiting anything new: their record would make exceedingly boring reading. On the other hand, one could ride with the assemblage point to the farthest corners of creation. To have a meaningful life, we have to scribble all over the blackboard.

In the afterlife, the *shade* has no will of its own because it no longer possesses the force of life to cause it to change positions. All that remains of our decisions are our attractions and repulsions, not actual shifts demonstrating free will. This is why people become "who they really are" after death. This is also the basis of the theory of reincarnation: the soul, purified of its dross, is no longer attracted to the processes of purification in the Land of the Dead, but is attracted to life and returns to Earth.

I was treating a young man, about twenty, who was bothered by persistent daydreams of skeletons and skulls. These would be pretty normal for some people—to judge by the prevalence of these images in our culture—but he felt them as foreign intrusions. "You're being bothered by the bone soul," I commented. I didn't consciously choose the term but it seemed the best way to say it and it just came out of my mouth. His mother, an Orthodox Jew, said: "Oh, we have the bone soul." She knew what I meant. I gave him White Oak bark tincture because it is such a hard, bonelike tree. It easily took care of the problem.

The Superego

Finally, we reach the center of the city, at the end of the Yellow Brick Road. At the center we meet the man behind the curtain pushing all the levers, the Wizard of Oz. It is Toto that tugs away the curtain to reveal the old guy, huffing and puffing. Friendly as he turns out to be, the Wizard cannot actually help Dorothy. The superego is nothing more than a false god, but he was never ill-intentioned: he wanted to direct our steps on a good path. He didn't want us to fall into the hands of the Wicked Witch.

Then the true power of Oz appears, the Good Witch of the North, with her supernatural magic wand. With it, and the deepest desire of Dorothy's soul, Glinda returns the girl and her dog home. When Dorothy wakes up, all the same people are there but now their true spirits are shining through them, revealing the wonder behind ordinary life. Dorothy's world will continue as before, but shining with spiritual light. Her desire has been empowered by her will (the magic wand) and she has learned many lessons in the Spirit World.

Losing the Human Form

Don Juan constantly stressed to Carlos the importance of "losing the human form." He never described what the "human form" was, but Castaneda himself gave an excellent description of what it felt like to lose it. The process started in his head and moved down through his body. It was as if some congestion broke up in his brain, then moved downward, giving the sensation of tension—first in the head, then down through the jaws, neck, torso, pelvis, limbs, and so on, all the way down to the feet.

This is the sensation that occurs when the hard, crystallized thoughtform a person lives within breaks up and is removed from the energy body. Until that time, the person is living inside a rigid mental thoughtform that doesn't change. The dial in the brain is stuck in one position. The blackboard is pretty boring. Afterward they become flexible and capable of "processing" and "moving energy through their system." It is easier now to be empathic.

That is not exactly an advantage, since it is quite unpleasant to have people's energy moving through oneself. However, we can now fully experience ourselves as human beings because we are conscious of our own emotions, as well as others', and can fully feel and integrate experiences from outside ourselves. Also, the animal instincts, physical sensations, and energy awareness—the doppelganger—will "go out before" the person, screening the psychic atmosphere for opposition and trouble. An empath has to have a developed animal self or he or she will get into trouble.

Some people have a rigid "human form" or rigid "mental body." Castaneda would be a good example. This kind of person has a fixed mind that makes it difficult for outside thoughts and feelings to enter into them. There is also the opposite type: people who are so porous that other people's thoughts and feelings enter them all the time, but unconsciously, so that they identify other people's emotions as their own. One of Castaneda's fellow apprentices, La Gorda, had this problem. For her, the challenge of losing the human form was to gain control over her own space. When both broke through their human form, they became much more capable of gaining spiritual insights. It was from this point on that Castaneda began to remember the teachings that don Juan had inculcated into his energy body in dreamtime—they had been unconscious up to then.

The "Soul-and-Spirit" or "Self"

Both Rudolf Steiner and Carl Jung described a process whereby the human soul or individuality became increasingly permeated by a higher "spiritual" (Steiner) or "numinous" (Jung) power. Steiner called the resulting structure within the individual the "soul-and-spirit," as if the two began to merge. Jung spoke of the appearance of "the self" as the wholeness coming from within. Even this was not tame enough for his critics, who accused him of introducing "God."

Jung called the process of becoming an individual "individuation." This leads to the "realization of the self," or identification with the "true self" at the core of a human being:

I call this centre the "self," which should be understood as the totality of the psyche. The self is not only the centre, but also the whole circumference which embraces both conscious and unconscious; it is the centre of this totality, just as the ego is the centre of consciousness. (Jung 1993, par. 44)

Several symbols represent the self for Jung. One is a circle with a dot in the middle. This is the glyph for the Sun in astrology, which has a value very much like the self. Lest we accuse Jung of taking this concept from astrology, the argument can also be reversed: modern astrology became more psychological due to the influence of Freud and Jung.

A second symbol for the self is the point at the intersection of the arms of an equal-sided cross. This is also the symbol for the ego. As a person individuates, the self gains more strength and the ego comes more under its power. This represents the integration of opposites necessary to complete the process of individuation. The actualization of all four psychic functions (thinking, feeling, sensation, intuition), rather than overreliance on one or two or three, contributes to the realization of the self.

A third symbol for the self that Jung identified is the yin and yang symbol. This shows the unification of the darkness of the unconscious with the light of consciousness. It shows that the person is willing to face the shadows of unactualized internal psychic contents.

Plants as Teachers and Medicines

Almost all plants have a specific setting of the assemblage point that is more or less permanent. Therefore, they can shift the focus of our assemblage point to theirs. Some of them are hallucinogens, but all of them have a "self" that can teach us something. "Cure" is a form of change of focus. Some plants, like Agrimony, can "change the environment" around us. Plant "doctors" are even better than human teachers in a way because they don't misunderstand, have irritating qualities, or change on us—*like every single human being.* It is very seldom that we ever have a problem with a plant—although there are a few challenging ones, like Datura.

☉ WOLF MEDICINE ☉

I always considered the signature for Wolf Medicine to be a ninety-degree angle or the equal-sided cross. This represented the extreme change between Wolf and Dog; also the Wolf remedies have to do with gallbladder energy: choice, change, even magic. Later I learned from Native herbalist Karyn Sanders that her signature for Wolf Medicine was the circle. We are both right. The circle and the square are opposites. Both are contained within the Medicine Wheel.

Nature is cyclical and circular. As it is said: "Nature abhors a square." Yet the circular year is divided into four quadrants, so the square is implied in the circle. Wolf abhors a fence because he is the great geometer of the animal kingdom, instinctually calculating the angle necessary to run down an elderly or sick animal with the least expenditure of energy.

Wolf is both circular and angular: in the unfenced wilderness the wolf pack constantly circles the caribou herd, smelling the scat, observing the plants being eaten, thinning out the elderly and the sick. Yet, when the chase is on, Wolf is an instinctive mathematician, getting just the right angle to run down the cervid. Wolf therefore incarnates both the circle and the square. One sees them in a plant like Solomon's Seal, which possesses the circular seal on the stalk but also the right angle as the vertical stem shoots up from the horizontal rhizome. The ninety-degree angle is evident in Werewolf Root as well as Agrimony.

The four angles of the Medicine Wheel imply the fifth element, the point in the middle, the *quintessence* or fifth essence, which completes, unifies, incarnates through, and constantly rejuvenates and changes the four elements. Therefore, the pentagram is also a Wolf Medicine signature. This is the signature of the human hand, which indicates the power to effect change. In practical terms we are talking about plants with five leaves—*Osmorrhiza, Potentilla, Aesculus*, and so forth.

The circle represents the unbroken wholeness of Nature, while the cross represents the fixation of the focus and the fifth essence indicates the ability to change the focus. Wolf Medicine therefore represents the wholeness and harmony of the cyclical natural world, the tension between complementary opposites (Wolf and Dog, wild and domestic), and the ability to fix or change the setting of the tumblers. Thus, Wolf Medicine is associated with magic and shapeshifting. The hand or pentangle shape is also associated with Dragon Medicine.

Wolf is the companion of the Lord of the Underworld, the Keeper of the Animals, while Dog is the companion of Man, the domesticator of animals. In the natural world, the wolves do keep the animals in balance, trimming the flocks, from the largest elks to little mice, removing the elderly and the sick in the circular dance of birth and death.

Wolf Medicines act on the tension between the wild and the domestic, the animal self and the ego, the stomach (instinct) and the gallbladder (conscious decision-making), the status quo and change, the environment and oneself, the mundane and the magical.

In modern psychotherapy and herbal counseling, most practitioners think in terms of helping a person cope with or master their situation, but the shamanic herb can change the environment. The tumblers shift under the influence of medicine plants like Agrimony, Cinquefoil, Solomon's Seal, and Werewolf Root.

℞ Agrimony ℘
(*Agrimonia eupatoria, A. grysopetela*)

Dr. Edward Bach taught us that Agrimony (*A. eupatoria*) is the remedy for those who hide their pain behind a façade. The Agrimony person is either too suave and sophisticated, or outwardly jovial and inwardly tortured, or in some way hiding his or her true inner state through the elevation of the *persona*. Sometimes also holding their breath.

I use the North American native, Sweet Agrimony (*A. grysopetela*), in place of the European *eupatoria*. It works interchangeably, although the sweetness gives the herb a more nutritive quality. I harvest the leaves from the sides of the stalk—one must not take the leader of the pack on the end—and prefer this to the flower essence. On the physical level, Agrimony is a superlative remedy for both psychological and physical tension. Since tension cuts down on the local sanguification of the tissue, atrophy will appear after a while. Sweet Agrimony is an excellent remedy when atrophy is present.

Agrimony and its cousin Cinquefoil (*Potentilla* spp.) are very powerful and easy-to-use magical plants. They have the ability to change the focus of consciousness. I wrote nearly forty pages on this subject in *The Book of Herbal Wisdom* (1997, 85–111), so I'm not going to repeat myself. However, here's a "magical case history" someone sent me after the publication of that book. The names, of course, have been changed.

When I began reading The Book of Herbal Wisdom, *I was interning at this small homestead farm with a guy named Jack. He and his wife Mary were old-fashioned vegetarians of the no-salt, no-oil, no-flavor variety, and meals would often consist solely of steamed vegetables. This was problematic for me because I was working for room and board and didn't have a kitchen of my own at my disposal. The saving grace was that they kept ten goats, whose milk was basically my sole source of protein. Some tension developed, however, because Mary wanted to sell more of the milk than was available with the three of us consuming it, and I wanted my sole source of protein. As this was going on, I read your chapter on Agrimony and Cinquefoil in* The Book of Herbal Wisdom. *I thought I'd try taking a sprig of Cinquefoil, which was growing all over the place there, and putting it in the refrigerator, which seemed like the energetic center of the tension. The next day, Mary came up to me and said: "Hey Tom, what if we bought you a gallon or two of raw cow's milk every week so that we have enough goat's milk to sell?" Up until that point everything had been silent passive aggression. Cinquefoil worked it out!*

My view of Agrimony was enlarged recently by Erica Fargione, herb teacher at Minneapolis Community Technical College. She has used Agrimony successfully more than ten times to put Tourette's syndrome in long-term remission. That's the opposite of our usual indication: instead of an prominent façade, there is no façade. The Tourette's person says what would embarrass everyone else. So we see that this is the remedy for the *persona*, whether it is too strong or too weak. Erica uses Sweet Agrimony as well.

Recently, I learned another part of the Agrimony picture. Dorothy Hall also subscribed to Dr. Bach's picture of the Agrimony temperament (1988, 77–80). She used this herb for lack of good timing in digestive function. This used to be a big problem with malaria, when the liver/gallbladder, stomach, and intestinal functions would get disturbed by the constant chills and sympathetic tension running through them. I used to see a few such cases among older Southerners, who had malaria from their youth—like our generation has Lyme disease—but this symptom has "died out" with the passage of time. Occasionally, however, it still comes up for influenzal symptoms.

One night I had a touch of the flu, with body aches, slight chills, and digestive upset. By this time the plants would sometimes talk to me and Agrimony "showed" me how my stomach and the intestine were separated: they were not timed together at all. The stomach was bloated and the food was stuck and couldn't get down to the intestine. Agrimony also showed me the difference between the "animal instincts," felt in the stomach, and the "gut-level instincts," felt in the intestines. The former are more formed and articulated, while the latter are more primitive and undeveloped. I didn't even need to take Agrimony—once I had been shown all of this, the symptoms settled down.

One client had chills and fever with tension so severe that it pulled the hips out of the hip sockets. Ouch! She was a bright, cheerful person—a constitutional Agrimony—so I suggested the remedy and within a day she was resting comfortably. But the magic happened when I hung up the phone. Agrimony said: "You can tell I'm a Wolf Medicine because of the leaflet on the end; it's the leader of the pack."

This is why we are not to pick the leaflet on the end; only the leaves on the sides.

I believe I reported the first part of the following case in *The Book of Herbal Wisdom*. A frail, middle-aged woman had a persistent high white blood count, but not enough to be diagnosed as a leukemia. She was exhausted, tense from work, slender, sallow, and atrophic. I asked her if something set off the white count. A spider bite. No façade that I could detect, but Agrimony (for the tension and atrophy) cured the case. Twenty years later, I got a call from her friends. She had been going back to her house when a snake crawled out of a woodpile. This was just a little garter snake—we don't have big snakes in Minnesota— but she was so terrified she had to leave her house and moved in with her accommodating daughter and her family. I was called over to the house and took the case history. I was going to use the Sweet Agrimony for sure, as a "constitutional." As I was zeroing in on a second remedy for her, I described how the deer don't like to be out in the center of the field, where the predators can get to them, or in the woods, where they are safer yet there is no food, but on the edges, where the food is and safety is close by. She almost jumped out of the chair: "That's me! I want to be at the edge of the field; not in the middle!" I gave her Sweet Leaf (*Monarda fistulosa*), a Deer Medicine. In a week, she was back in her house. I should have mentioned to her that although cervids are not predators, they will jump up and down on snakes to kill them; also, their hooves are sharp enough to kill an unwary dog.

☙ Cinquefoil ❧
(*Potentilla erecta*)

Cinquefoil has an ancient reputation as a magical plant in both Europe and North America. As the names indicate, this plant has five leaves (*cinquefoil*) and magical power (*potentilla*). The eighteenth- century Mohegan medicine man Samson Occom called it "Five Finger Leaf." John Goodyer, in his 1655 English translation of Dioscorides's *De Materia Medica*, noted that this plant "being poured on the hands . . . is excellent good against fears & enchantments" (Gunther 1968, 436). For this purpose, both Agrimony and Cinquefoil can be used, as well as other *Potentillas* and even some cousins in the *Geum* (Avens) clan.

The leaves of Cinquefoil are used to unblock energy interfering with one's calling or occupation, or problems between employers and employees, landlords and tenants, or other hierarchical relationships. I discussed Cinquefoil and Agrimony at length in *The Book of Herbal Wisdom*. Strangely, this is the single most reliable thing I know in herbal medicine: Cinquefoil or Agrimony will smooth out hierarchical problems in a totally fair way. If you are in the wrong, they will work against you. If you are in the right, take them to court.

In *The Earthwise Herbal* (2008–2009, 1:400), I told the story about how I used Cinquefoil for a friend who was suffering from a life-threatening asthmatic attack. When I walked into the room and saw her, I said: "My God, death is in your aura." My energy body reacted sharply, because the asthma was so dire.

My asthmatic friend was "tortured to capture her breath." That's an indication for Agrimony or Cinquefoil, a plant that looks super tense. I went out in the twilight and found some Cinquefoil; it looked even more tortured than usual and was all over the sides of the yard.

The woman's relief was almost instantaneous and she would always say for years, "That was the last terrible asthmatic attack I ever had"—though she had many lesser ones. Her husband often said to me, "Those words were so exact for her: she was 'tortured to capture the breath.' We thought she was going to die."

"Tortured to capture the breath" is what we call a "specific indication" in herbal medicine. It is so specific that it indicates only one remedy—or a small group. At the same time it points to a basic patho-logical condition that corresponds to the nature of the plant. In this case: tension. We see tension in the bristling appearance of the plant (the signature), the psychology, and the physiology.

This phrase goes back to one of Dr. Bach's friends, in the 1930s. When I included it in *The Earthwise Herbal Repertory* (2016), an overzealous copyeditor changed it to "tortured capture of the breath." I couldn't believe it. There was no need to revise the phrase and she changed the meaning entirely. It is terrible to see someone who can't capture their breath; they truly are tortured. "Tortured capture of the breath" would mean that when they finally catch their breath they are still tortured. But that makes no sense, because capturing the breath gives the ultimate relief. *In herbalism, as in medicine and shamanism, words are exact.* They can capture the essence of the energy or miss it completely. These types of phrases and specific indications arise from experience, and that is an invaluable resource. My Muskogee teacher would sometimes mention a specific symptom—enunciating it slowly—handing on specific indications that were perhaps thousands of years old. I had to go over my manuscript to make sure the copyeditor had not removed any of these entries.

When "death is in the aura" it really shakes up the energy body, as in the above case. I felt the same with Susan when death left her body: "Susan, death is leaving your body—right now!" She got mad at me for scaring her.

ৎ Solomon's Seal ৩
(*Polygonatum* spp.)

This is one of my favorite medicinal plants and one of the most widely applicable of any I know—it loosens, tightens, and nourishes tendons, so it is excellent for the joints. It appears to act on the fibroblasts, chondroblasts, osteoblasts, and tendon-generating cells, so it is wonderful for the connective tissue and has been used from time immemorial in this arena. I have already written extensively about the medicinal properties in *The Book of Herbal Wisdom* (1997, 397–406) and elsewhere. It is a Wolf Medicine par excellence, and combines well with Agrimony.

Solomon was the wise king and therefore *magical* knowledge was assigned to him. The plant Solomon's Seal or *sigillum Salomonis* was named after him because of the little circles on the roots—they look like magical "sigils" (signs) used by magicians to call spirits. The Latin name is *Polygonatum multiflorum*. We can also use the ornamental *P. odoratum* var. *variegatum*.

Solomon's Seal helps a person be in the flow of things, improves one's timing, the swing of the baseball bat, and helps us adapt to changes that were too precipitous. It is worn as a mojo. Otherwise, it is a great remedy for tendons, ligaments, bones, and joints. It adjusts them to the right tension, even structures that have been altered by surgery.

Solomon's Seal is identified as "High John the Conqueror" by Crellin and Philpott (1990) in their treatment of the old Georgia herbalist Tommie Bass. It is named after King Solomon, the king associated with wisdom, because the scars on the rhizomes look like a magical "sigil" or "seal." The rhizome, cut in half, can actually display what looks like a letter "S."

This is a very important plant in Afro-American folk medicine. High John was specifically used by enslaved people to prevent being struck. In the *Narrative of the Life of Frederick Douglass, An American Slave* (1845, 66–73), Douglass describes how he was being beaten and whipped by the "slave-breaker," so he ran away into the woods. There he met an old black root doctor named Sandy Jenkins, who told him he was going to have to go back, but he would give him a root that would make it impossible for anyone to strike him. Douglass did not identify it, but it was certainly some version of High John (more than one plant is known by that name), and probably Solomon's Seal. He went back, fought with the slave-breaker for an hour, and no one ever touched him again.

I had an email from a young woman who wanted an herb like the one Sandy Jenkins gave Frederick Douglass because her husband would strike her and she didn't have family or friends to go to. After I sent her the root she figured out how to get him to stop. Eventually, she left him.

Solomon's Seal rhizomes have another important property. Herbalist Cathy Skipper, who has worked in the U.K., France, and the U.S., explained that Solomon's Seal is for the "resonance in the bones, memories stored in the bones. It guards the resonance of the person after the person has passed on. It smells like burnt bones." Remember what I said about the shadow that goes down into the ground when a person dies. I did not know that this needed protection.

Cathy added, "It can loosen people up so that their feelings can really come out," bring realignment in family trauma, and "shift people." Here again it would combine well with Agrimony or Cinquefoil.

Swani Simon, another friend, an herbalist in Saarland, Germany, told an interesting story. "An old man had a dream about a plant. He dreamed about it again. He found out it could be Solomon's Seal. He talked to his priest about it. He was a Christian, but he wanted some of the plant." Swani sent him some at his request and he wrote back: "Now I know I am ready to pass on." She didn't hear from him again.

Swani has also used Solomon's Seal for spondylosis, which is hard to heal. This agrees with John Gerard's comment in 1633 that it is used "among the vulgar sort of people in Hampshire" for setting bones and for swellings on the bones, in themselves and their cattle Gerard (1975, 906). (My Muskogee teacher commented: "You got to watch out what those 'vulgar people' know.")

Solomon's Seal heals simple connective tissue problems, but if it is used for serious problems the person may have to change. This shows us how Solomon's Seal is a Wolf Medicine.

One day I was teaching in upstate New York about fifteen years ago, and a student had a family emergency and was forced to leave early. I said, "You need a good-luck remedy." I was inspired by Harry Potter's good-luck potion, but I didn't have that on hand so I had to make one up: Solomon's Seal, Cinquefoil (or Agrimony), and Ghostpipe. For environmental reasons, I'd prefer the reader use Rabbit Tobacco instead of Ghostpipe.

Claudia Keel, an herbalist from New York City, was sitting nearby and perked up. "Hey," she said, "Wait, wait—I want to know Matt Wood's Good-Luck Remedy!" So she wrote it down. Otherwise it would have been lost. It was a spur-of-the-moment thing. Later I forgot about it but Claudia had significant good luck and she told her story while introducing me for a class ten years later. I said: "Wait, wait—I want to know my Good-Luck Remedy!" We not only have to find the medicine, we have to grasp it before it gets away.

Claudia and her husband needed a break desparately. She saw a raffle with the winning ticket getting an all-expenses-paid vacation. She bought some, she put the formula on the tickets, they won, and got their well-deserved vacation.

Solomon's Seal helps you be in the right place at the right time. Cinquefoil or Agrimony gets rid of blockages of disbelief in yourself (so it doesn't matter whether you believe in this remedy or not) or blockages from interfering people. Rabbit Tobacco changes the dial on the other side so that we can access all the possibilities. But this is only a formula for "good luck," not for changing your destiny.

Solomon's Seal is also a magical herb in ancient Taoist medicine. There is a good report about it by Heiner Fruehauf (2016), the founder of the College of Classical Chinese Medicine. He tells us that it entered Chinese herbalism more through the Taoist magical and alchemical tradition than through the standard Chinese medical world.

One of the most relaxing combinations I know is: seven parts Agrimony, four parts Solomon's Seal. This relaxes the mind and body. Another good combination is: seven parts Hawthorn and one to four parts Solomon's Seal. This opens the rib cage and the circulation to the heart, thymus, and lungs.

Solomon's Seal is not overpicked—yet—but the person who wants to use it should grow it or spread it in the wild. This is a plant that requires payment. He Who Must Not Be Named, my Muskogee teacher, treated a friend of mine with Solomon's Seal for poisoning from red tide. He said: "You're going to have to make a payment when this plant heals you. Your destiny is going to change." After she recovered, she had to move to a different state. No return of the disease after twenty years.

☙ Werewolf Root ☙
(Apocynum androsaemifolium)

This is an extremely powerful medicine plant. It told me to call it "Werewolf Root." This is the plant used in the Grand Medicine Society to teach people how to shift their assemblage point. Movement of the assemblage point is what causes shapeshifting. Every little change of consciousness or refocusing of the mind is a shapeshift, but the little shifts are normal.

Some shamans are reputed to change into animals. If the animal rules the human, then the shaman shapeshifts into an animal. Then the person is forced to become that animal; they don't have a choice. If the human rules the animal, then he or she can appear as a human in two places at once. This is a forceful plant; you don't play with it. You don't pick it or use it unless life is in the balance. The motto of Werewolf Root is: *Change or die*. If the person has suffered a life-changing injury (like a deer-tick bite), a concussion, or stands to be destroyed spiritually or physically, the remedy is appropriate. The person who is not at this extremity may have a change brought down upon them that is life-changing.

I mentioned an asthmatic case under Cinquefoil. After that remedy, I gave Werewolf Root. It too helped. What I didn't know was that this woman had been touched by a werewolf and this had started the whole condition:

> When I was thirteen, I woke up in the night and felt compelled to go to the window and look out. On the roof of the back porch I saw a little figure that was part man and part fox, dressed in a little coat and standing on two legs. As I looked at him, his head turned and our eyes met. I went into a shock that brought on my asthma.

He Who Must Not Be Named visited a year later and commented: "He was a relative, so he didn't kill you."

The egoic will naturally conflicts with the spiritual will—which is "stored in the kidneys," according to traditional Chinese medicine. The kidneys hold the fleck of fire that is the "pilot light" for all the yang or fire in the body. It is like a fire "on loan from the spirit." Our spirit is not able to incarnate fully on Earth, but provides the basic support for our life here. The primal *jing* or essence is also stored in the reins or kidneys; it is the source of the primal yin and yang. The "*qi* of the abyss" (the primal constitutional energy) is also stored in the kidneys.

So, Werewolf Root works out problems between the egoic will and the spiritual will. That is why it is so powerful. I described this medicine in *The Book of Herbal Wisdom* (1997, 130–31). I only give drop doses, occasionally. On a mundane level, this plant is a gallbladder medicine: it is used when the stool is gray from lack of bile and an inactive gallbladder.

☉ SWALLOW MEDICINE ☉

The Celandine plant could be considered a Wolf Medicine, but European folk tradition has long tied it to the swallow. It is an excellent remedy for a too-strong ego. Richard Folkard, in *Plant Lore, Legends, and Lyrics*, writes (1884, 143):

> The ancients entertained a strong belief that birds were gifted with the knowledge of herbs. . . . Aristotle, Pliny, Dioscorides, and the old herbalists and botanical writers, all concur in stating that Swallows were in the habit of plucking Celandine (*Chelidonium*), and applying it to the eyes of their young.

The late Maurice Mességué, the famous Gascon herbalist, describes being shown by his father how the swallows rubbed the leaf on the eyes of their hatchlings to open them up when they were gummed shut (Mességué 1991, 8). His father was a country herbalist, hunter, and woodsman in the period between the World Wars. Even then, in his remote village, Mességué senior was a disappearing breed.

The word *Chelidonium* means "of the swallow" in Latin, and Celandine is sometimes known as "Swallow Wort" in English. Another old English name is "Kenning Wort." The word "kenning" refers both to seeing and knowing, as in the Scotch "I ken," much like our English "I see." So, this plant is associated both with seeing and knowing.

Because the tail of the swallow fans apart at an angle—like a Masonic compass—Swallow Medicine is similar to Wolf Medicine and is associated with the sphincter of the mind, mental focus, and egoic will. In Wolf Medicine, there is a conflict between the ego and the spirit. In Gentian, it is between the ego and the animal self. In Celandine, it is between the egoic will and "kenning." There is really no other word for it: knowledge, material, occult, or spiritual. It is one of the few remedies for abusing occult knowledge or trying to "storm the gates of heaven" with hallucinogens or egoic will. In ordinary practice, however, *Chelidonium* is usually just a remedy for gallbladder problems, migraines, or a bit of egotism.

ꙮ Celandine ꙮ
(*Chelidonium majus*)

The sap of the leaf produces a bright orange-yellow juice that is a capital signature for the bile. The leaves are lobular—a signature long associated with the liver. Chelidonium is a hot, bitter remedy that gets the gallbladder going when there is jaundice, stones, or underactivity that needs a stimulant. There may be thickening of the bile, congestion, mucus, and stones. It is also associated with people with a strong ego or egoic will. That is not, of course, a bad thing entirely. I don't get to use it much for this, but I have seen it cut down on "me-me-me-ism."

Chelidonium has a symptom that came up in the homeopathic provings of its cousin Opium: a person sees a terrifying image and can't get it out of his or her mind. I once helped an otherwise healthy three-year-old boy who had seen a scary cartoon character six months before on TV (this was in pre-computer days). Chelidonium in dilution cured him in under a month. The mother thought it was just that he got over it. She couldn't see.

Chelidonium is indicated in cases of people who abuse occult powers due to a strong ego and the belief that they can control the forces of Nature and personality. It is also for people who mess up their brain by trying to "storm the gates of heaven," as Peter Young, my friend and fellow student on the esoteric path put it; they take hallucinogens or try too hard to achieve spiritual goals through spiritual exercises or drugs. It may also be for old people who are starting to become confused after a lifetime of strong mentality—one case only. Look for a coating on the tongue that goes all the way to the tip, indicating "phlegm" obscuring thought. The tip of the tongue is the reference point for the brain.

Chelidonium is the great remedy for migraine with sensitivity to light. The symptoms were brought out in homeopathic provings in the nineteenth century. This kind of migraine is called "gallbladder head-ache" in traditional Chinese medicine because the pain ascends the gallbladder meridian: is felt at the occiput and then across the temporal bones, on one side, into the eye, and sometimes down to the cheekbone. It has cured scores of cases.

Chelidonium has an ancient reputation in cataracts that is deserved. The formula: put some fresh Celandine leaf juice into goat's milk and apply externally. I know of several instances where this has worked and I have seen it once myself. It worked in less than two weeks! It is also called the "Strabismus Herb" in Swedish, I am told. The plant is very active and should be used in small doses (1–3 drops; 10 is the maximum even in conventional dosing). The tincture is made from the leaves.

❂ HORSE MEDICINE ❂

I learned most of my Horse Medicine from Sara Annon, a "horse sha-man" (I would call her) in New Mexico; my friend Susan, who dreamed with her two or three horses; and my friend Peter Young. The horse is an extremely sensitive animal. One element of that sensitivity shows in their ability to synchronize their hearts to the same beat. In a herd they synchronize their hearts so that if one horse has an increase in heart rate from fear, the rest of the tribe knows there is danger. They can perceive a human heartbeat only feet away. Because they are so sensitive, horses can attune to people with deep neurological problems, like autism.

During the coronavirus pandemic, a considerable number of horse-owners had trouble with their horses because the vaccine caused the horses not to be able to recognize their owners. This was substantiated in many cases of which I am aware. Usually the alienation passed after several months. However, the incidence of myocarditis, pericarditis, and other cardiovascular effects among the vaccinated is widely reported. Many unvaccinated covid survivors also have suffered cardiac effects.

How was such a sensitive animal as the horse domesticated? Probably through direct mind-link or dreaming, suggested Sara. Susan always dreams with her horses; they show her things and bring her places in the Spirit World. The white horse and the black horse would always come to her. She would always take the black horse, which would go downward, while the white horse would stay in the conscious world. Peter also dreamed of being in herds of horses—hundreds of times.

Sara proposes that there was originally a group of people who specialized in knowledge of horses; how to call, train, ride, and care for them. This group would have existed as a "mystery school" or shamanic society, like the Masons and other trade guilds, passing on the secrets, dreams, spiritual wisdom, and genetic linkages associated with Horse from generation to generation. She believes they were particularly associated with what became the Spanish warhorse, which was a valuable military weapon in the premodern era. Imported to the New World, this became the "Indian pony" of the Great Plains. Unfortunately, the federal government, under both Presidents Trump and Biden, has chosen to exterminate the wild horses on public lands—over 95% of them are gone as I write—so the wild pony is facing extinction at the hands of our overdomesticated species.

The Four Horsemen of the Apocalypse

The cultus of the horse shaman has survived the ages, according to Sara. It is the source of the story of the Four Horsemen of the Apocalypse, which shows up at the end of the Christian Bible. The Lakota Holy Man Black Elk had a similar dream of Six Grandfathers and the Four Horses a few years before the Black Robes (priests) showed up. This is a vision that rises out of the horses themselves. Sadly, it is a vision which seems to occur when a society is facing annihilation—just as is pictured in the Book of Revelations. In 1875 it was the Lakota Nation; now it is the dominant culture of the world.

Horses, like many animals, come in four basic colors: white, black, red, and "yellow" or "pale." These four colors of horses usually have four basic kinds of personalities, corresponding to the four horsemen. The black horse occurs due to a dominant gene, explained Sara. The other colors are hidden within the black horse because they are carried on recessive genes.

The black horse is associated with darkness and absence of light, which is always associated with the unconscious—and therefore with the process of going within, willingly or not. In the Book of Revelations, the rider of the black horse holds a scale and represents economic tyranny and collapse, resulting in food scarcity and famine. However, the scales also represent justice. The ultimate place of justice is the Underworld, where the dead are judged and we have to face the karma of our actions.

The white horse occurs due to a withholding of pigment; it doesn't flow into the hair, so to speak, and as Sara notes, white horses usually have tumors under their skin and don't live as long as the other horses. The loss of pigment is an unhealthy characteristic. Susan agreed, "Yeah, my white horse had tumors and didn't live that long." The white horse represents the opposite or complement of the black: the realm of the conscious or egoic mind. The god of the conscious mind today is science, and the high priesthood of science is medicine (represented by white). The corruption of the medical system is characteristic of our time.

Revelation (18:23) says that in the end times the population will perish by *pharmakeia*, which more or less means "the use of potions." The usual English translation is "witchcraft," but the word speaks for itself in this era of medication run amok. I met one other person who understood this interpretation—the herbalist David Christopher, son of the legendary herbalist John Christopher.

The red horse is represented by the brown, chestnut, red-brown, and reddish colors. These horses are known for being feisty and difficult to handle. "The stereotypical red chestnut," says Sara, is known for

its "impetuous, irritable, untrainable nature." It is easy to see the connection to blood, passion, and conflict. The red horse and rider "take
peace" from the world and introduce social strife. They represent the
impulses of the blood untrained and rampant becoming dominant in
social affairs. Violence of thought and language, as well as action, represents the red horse. Looking around, as I write, we see a lot of evidence
of the red horse—social division and name-calling everywhere.

The fourth horse is the pale horse. The original Greek word in
Revelation (6:8) is *chlōros*, meaning "pale, bleached out" or "yellow." For
example, a chlorotic plant is yellow, pale, and bleached out. *Chlōros* does
not designate a complete lack of color. In equine terms, it refers to the
palominos and various shades of yellow, gray, and pink that are pale,
says Sara. Genetically, they contain all color possibilities and when two
are bred together, anything can happen.

The pale horse is associated with pestilence (epidemic disease)
and death in the Bible. The Clint Eastwood movie *Pale Rider* (1985),
features a mysterious man who comes to correct social imbalances.
His origin is unknown, but he wears a minister's collar and is named
"Preacher" by the people who take him in. He carries scars from bullets
that indicate that he should be dead. He has survived death and is, as a
consequence, melded with Death. "Preacher" has a supernatural or holy
aspect that is never fully explained.

Conscious constructs (medicine and science), economic tyranny
and famine, factionalism and war, are all visible powers, but the pale
rider is associated with something unseen and invisible—the eruption
of an overwhelming power from the unseen worlds. Like "Preacher," it
is unclear where this power comes from, what it is doing, or how things
will end. On the mundane level, one is reminded of the infiltration of
ideas into the unconscious from the news and entertainment industries. This invisible influence reinforces the tribal blood lusts of the red
horseman. Like the black and white horses, the red and pale are opposites and complements.

There is a fifth horse, the Medicine Hat or Paint, which is produced
by a very rare recessive gene. It was exterminated by European breeders

and is only found nowadays among the Indian ponies of North America—which are unfortunately being decimated by the federal government. The Paint is generally white with a red-brown forehead and ears. Sometimes there is a big spot like a shield on the chest. They can look as if they had been splashed by paint. Sometimes they have one or both eyes blue. The more distinctive the markings, the more prized the horse.

As the name Medicine Hat reveals, this horse is thought to have special powers. They are considered harder to see, so they were thought to have the ability to protect their riders from danger and protect them in battle (Fought 2020). Some people have visionary experiences just from their presence. This, suggests my mentor in Horse Medicine, Sara, is why this kind of horse may have been exterminated in Europe.

Horse Medicine Plants

Horse Medicines strengthen the heart and therefore they overlap a considerable amount with Lion and Sun Medicines. I have placed most of the direct heart remedies in the latter category.

Both St. John's Wort and Centaury are classified as herbs of the Sun in Western astrology because they are gently warming and drying. Sun remedies are like sunlight vaporizing the puddles on the sidewalk; Mars remedies are hot and fiery. However, both plants are also associated with horses or centaurs. There is a connection between the Sun and the horse; Apollo is pulled across the sky by his chariot and horses. St. John's Wort flowers on or around Midsummer Day, the sunniest day of the year.

In addition, both of these plants have alternating leaves on the stalks that produce "crosses" when looked at from above. The four-sided cross is both a symbol of the Sun (like the flag of New Mexico) and of the four colors of the Horse Nation; but it is also a Wolf Medicine signature because these animals are the "geometers" of the animal world—wolves are major predators on the horse.

Coltsfoot is named because it grows along the side of the road—in the old days, the horse path. It is perhaps another Horse Medicine. *Aesculus hippocastanum* (Horse Chestnut) is used for calming the muscles of horses when they ripple with tension.

⚘ St. John's Wort ⚘
(Hypericum perforatum)

There is a great deal of interesting lore about St. John's Wort; partly because it is so valuable in injuries and wounds, but also because it has such a long history of religious and magical connotations. It is one of the major items in the materia medica of the medieval Catholic peasantry, who associated plants with Jesus, Mary, the saints, King Solomon, and other biblical figures. It was called St. John's Wort because it blooms on or close to Midsummer Day, the feast day of St. John the Baptist. It continues blooming until late August. The leaves bear a red-pigmented oil that was likened to the blood of John, who was beheaded by King Herod at the request of Salome. Hypericum was adopted into homeopathy. It is considered a mighty remedy here, as in herbalism, and is used on similar indications.

The residence of John the Baptist, living in the wilderness, from which he obtained his clothing and food, as well as his association with midsummer, when the "green power" is at its peak, suggested an association with the "Green Man." This is not only an important figure in northern Europe, where green summer contrasts with white winter, but in the Middle East, where the lush greenery contrasts with the stark desert. It is possible the two are connected: during the Roman period, merchants, migrants, and soldiers carried ideas and cults from one end of the empire to another.

In the north the Green Man never seems to have been a god but more of a representational figure, like the Statue of Liberty. In the Middle East, however, his origins (and destination) are more complex. The ancient Canaanites recognized a God called Kothar: wherever he sat, green foliage sprang up. He appears in the Hebrew Bible as Jethro, the Priest of Midian and the father-in-law of Moses. His role as a priest is intentionally diminished: he was only allowed to give Moses advice about time management, not spiritual matters. He is also mentioned in the Qur'an. Muhammad also tamed him, but did not entirely remove his spiritual associations. He is called the "Servant of the One" and identified not by name but by his residence, which was between the "two seas," the Red and the Gulf of Aqaba. This, of course, is where Jethro lived. His name, pronounced "*Yitro*" in Hebrew, survived as Yasser in Palestine.

Neither the Hebrews, the Christians, nor the Muslims have been able to whip this religion. Today the "Servant of the One" survives as the prophet of the Druze, who are the still-surviving descendants of the Canaanites. The cult of John the Baptist also survived in the desert of western Iraq, although it may have been displaced by ISIS.

This strange history does not end here, which is testimony to the enduring importance of oral history and folklore in the region. When the Greek writings of Hermes were encountered by the followers of Muhammad, he was identified with this individual and he became Idris in Arabic. As monotheism swept the Middle East, the last citadel of paganism survived in Harran, birthplace of Abraham and mother city of the three Abrahamic religions. In 830 the Caliph of Baghdad, Al-Ma'mun, on his way to fight the Byzantine Greeks, encountered people along the road in Harran who were not dressed like Christians, Jews, or Muslims (the "allowed religions"). On inquiry, he was told they were the pagans of Harran, worshippers in the ancient Temple of the Moon. He told the leaders of the city that, by the time he returned, they must become members of one of the "allowed religions" or they would be wiped out. Al-Ma'mun never returned from the crusade, but the leaders of Harran took his threat seriously. They consulted an Islamic religious authority, who informed them that there was an additional "allowed religion" called the Sabians. Nobody knew who they were, so if they declared Saba to be their prophet and adopted some scriptures attributed to him, they would escape censure. Ironically, the Sabians were the followers of John the Baptist, a few thousand of whom still survived in the desert south of Harran. We can see how the associations interwove in such a way as to be a bit believable.

The pagans of Harran continued to exist for another two hundred years and contributed greatly to the culture of Mesopotamia but were eventually annihilated by another group of pagans, the Mongols. A thousand miles away, the Mongol generals had determined that Harran was in a strategic location where they didn't want a citadel, and the inhabitants either had to abandon the city or they would come and reduce the citadel themselves. By this point it had, in fact, been eclipsed as a city and was more of a military settlement. It was abandoned and the *Hermetic Writings* were brought to Constantinople and from there, eventually to Renaissance Italy, where they were translated by Marsilio Ficino under the care of Cosimo de' Medici, in another fabled city. Trithemius of Sponheim studied in Florence with Ficino, and his students, Paracelsus and Agrippa von Nettesheim, popularized the teachings of Hermes.

St. John's Wort is a member of the *Guttiferaceae* family. It is native to Kothar's territory—the Levant. Finding compatible ground on other hardscrabble hills and plains, it has spread throughout the world, and is now found on every continent, and is considered a noxious weed wherever cattle are raised. It causes sunburn and irritation of the skin in cattle that have been fed on large amounts of it, to the extent that they can die, and it can cause sun sensitivity in humans. It is the reason most grazing cattle today have been selected for their black coat.

The green leaves have tiny glands that sunlight shines through, like windows. Here, the photosensitive red oils are generated. They are also present in the flowers, which are the part we use. They are picked and placed in alcohol or an oil—often left in the sun. The important constituents are better extracted in oil, but the blood-red color and the constituents come out in both mediums, turning the tinctures and oils red. This is a "signature" for St. John's Wort usage in healing wounds.

Traditionally, the flowers are extracted in olive oil, letting the bottle stand for forty days in the sun. So valuable was this oil that it was taken to the Holy Land by the Crusaders—or more probably, brought back by them from the land of its nativity. St. John's Wort may also have been looked upon as a form of spiritual blessing and protection for the crusaders, since, when looked at from overhead, the alternating leaf stalks along the main stalk look like an equal-sided cross.

St. John's Wort and Wood Betony were the two most important remedies for psychiatric medicine in the Middle Ages; in other words, they were used for protection against "demons and witchcraft." Consequently, St. John's Wort fumigant was also known as *fuga demonum*, Latin for "devil take flight." One old English name for it is Devil Scare.

Fuga can mean "fleeing, escape" or simply "flight." The plant was also associated with flying off with the faeries. In Brittany it was reported that a young girl who stepped on St. John's Wort in the evening would ride on a faery horse until morning. Father Sebastian Kneipp, the great water-cure priest—who was also an herbalist—called Hypericum the "plant of the faeries."

There is more to this than mere folklore. The late Kim Dudley, of Canberra, reported that one side effect of St. John's Wort was the "sensation of levitation." I would have laughed at this but I experienced it myself. In fact, I re-enacted the sensation in front of a girlfriend and she actually grabbed me because she also felt the sensation that I was going to levitate. I put the remedy down: I didn't have enough nerve to actually levitate—opportunity missed! This was a mixture of St. John's Wort, Cat's Ears Lily, and something else. Good thing I forgot that last ingredient!

Hitching a ride to the New World, St. John's Wort was adopted by the Indian People. My Muskogee teacher passed on the observation of his teacher: "We don't know who St. John was, but we know he was an important man to the white people, so we know this is an important plant." He taught too that it protected the house against lightning.

The practitioners who really understood this plant were the late Dorothy Hall, of New South Wales, and one of her favorite students, the aforementioned Kim Dudley, of Canberra. Dorothy must be given credit for being the first to develop a constitutional profile for St. John's Wort, but this was deepened in curious and interesting directions by Kim, who was a profound thinker and philosopher of Nature. I have relied on unpublished notes taken from several lectures by Kim on St. John's Wort (Dudley 2012) and the account in *Dorothy Hall's Herbal Medicine* (1988, 266–70).

Pharmacology

Hypericum is known to contain flavonoids, phenolic acids, hypericin and pseudohypericin (and their precursors), hyperforin (and allied compounds), tannins, volatile oils, saturated fatty acids, alkanols, vitamins, sesquiterpenes, and small traces of other compounds. The hypericin, hyperforin, and similar compounds found in the red glands on the leaves, causing the beautiful red color in the tinctures, are protoporphyrins. As medicinal constituents go, they are pretty much unique; I don't think there is another plant that I use that contains them. This accounts for their unique properties; I couldn't understand St. John's Wort until I read about porphyrins, which are sensitive to sunlight. It is traditional to pick the flowers for medicine at midsummer, when the sunlight is acting on it most strongly, and to make the blood-red oil and tinctures in sunlight.

Most of the attributed properties of Hypericum in traditional and scientific literature are related to hypericin, but the effects are due to complex synergies that are still to be determined. This includes the famous mild antidepressant action and the antiviral and antibacterial capacities. Possible anti-mutagenic properties are also attributed to this herb.

Porphyrins

These square-shaped molecules are pigmented photosensitive compounds that facilitate the use of oxygen by life-forms. Chlorophyll in plants and the heme molecule in hemoglobin are both porphyrins, as are the cytochrome enzymes. Basically, porphyrins are used by all living beings to deal with the highly reactive oxygen atoms that will oxidize or tear down organic molecules wherever and whenever they can. For a detailed, well-documented account of porphyrins, see chapter 10 of Arthur Firstenberg's *The Invisible Rainbow: A History of Electricity and Life* (2020). The following list shows the properties of porphyrins and the use of St. John's Wort (*in italics*):

1. The heme in hemoglobin facilitates the exchange of oxygen and carbon dioxide in the blood. *A minor remedy in anemia and*

malnutrition. Culpeper (1652, 69) writes that it "strengthens parts that are weak & feeble." This description also fits the following.

2. Cytochrome c enzyme facilitates cellular metabolism. *Kim used it for nervous weakness, nervous breakdown, dribbling from weak bladder, and such conditions; often combined with Wood Betony. "Brings the nerves back to life." Used for detached tissue.*

3. Cytochrome oxidase facilitates oxygen uptake in the lungs. *Not used to facilitate oxygen exchange, except as a tetanus remedy, reducing respiratory spasms. This usage is documented in the old homeopathic literature.*

4. Cytochrome P450 facilitates phase I pathway in liver and cell metabolism. *Well known for facilitating the cytochrome P-450 enzyme in Phase 1 of metabolism in the liver and cells.*

5. Porphyrins facilitate nerve flow in the myelin sheaths and nerves. *Traditionally used for severed and severely injured nerves. Many herbalists—including Dorothy, Kim, and myself—have seen and collected horrible case histories of severed and severely cut limbs dramatically healed.*

6. Porphyrins facilitate the piezoelectric current on the surface of the bone. *Bone-healing, especially non-healing fractures. Kim Dudley collected many case histories.*

7. Porphyrins are active in pain receptors and promote the relief of pain. *Pain relief. There is hardly an herbalist that cannot testify to this.*

8. Porphyrins relieve mild depression (perhaps due to the pain-relieving influence). *A major remedy for moderate depression, especially seasonal adjustive disorder (SAD).*

9. Influenza season is aggravated by lack of sunshine in the winter. Contains calciferol (vitamin D). *A known antiviral, but differential symptoms are lacking.*

I have rendered detailed accounts of the medicinal properties in *The Book of Herbal Wisdom* (1997, 307–15), *The Earthwise Herbal* (2008, I: 293–96), and *Holistic Medicine and the Extracellular Matrix* (2021a, 72–73, 101, 118).

Electricity

St. John's Wort was traditionally used to prevent lightning from striking the house, by putting it on the house. This may have been suggested by the appearance of the plant from above: it looks like a cross. This fits with its use in nerve and piezoelectric tissues and suggests a relevance all the way down to the ground regulatory system in the extracellular matrix. Kim comments: "St. John's Wort can protect you from lightning or attract it." I wish I knew how he limited that to the repellent action. It does look possible that Hypericum is remedial for electromagnetic-field (EMF) problems. These are more prevalent than one would suppose. Arthur Firstenberg covers the effects of EMFs in his book *The Invisible Rainbow* (2020).

The ground regulatory system of the extracellular matrix relies on changes in fixed electrical charges in the polymers in the matrix in order to send signals to and from cells. This unifies the entire organism, on the cellular level, into a single whole being. St. John's Wort ought to have an action on this level, but it would be hard to observe and document. The next level of electrical organization involves the piezoelectric charge on the bones and connective tissue. This is facilitated by the fascia, which store the body memory.

"Baptism in the Theater of War"

Kim notes that St. John's Wort is the "treatment for baptism in the theater of war." It is "good for all injuries of war, especially in the days when horses were around." A horse bites the finger or there is a cut from a rusty metal; tetanus sets in. Horse serum is used to provide vaccination against tetanus.

Kim had a case of stuttering in a man who suffered a "machine gun wound forty years ago" that "never healed." The feet hurt badly; he had plantar fasciitis on the soles of his feet, which became tender. The feet, the stutter, and the wound all improved with St. John's Wort. Kim had another case where a Vietnam vet was suffering from cyclothymia: "unstable moods, aggressive outbursts; wild, untamed fury; huge mood swings, often seen in post-traumatic survivors." He "slowly stopped traumatizing his family." Kim also cites the homeopath Margaret Tyler (*Homoeopathic Drug Pictures*), regarding a soldier who had a bad shoulder wound, with great pain, from his service in WWI.

Constitution

Dorothy Hall describes the constitutional type in her book and unpublished lectures. She says "St. John's Wort people" have a sensitive nervous system and skin, and are therefore heir to numerous spontaneous skin problems innate to their oversensitive constitutions, including sunburn, skin rashes, eczema, and allergic reactions to plants and insect bites that would hardly bother another person.

The St. John's Wort person often has prominent white fibers in the iris. These are interpreted as evidence of nerve intensity, meaning the person has a strong and sensitive—one would say, overreactive—nervous system. They are innately irritable, not angry or overstimulated, but easily irritated and impatient. St. John's Wort people are quick in all regards: to grow, mature, go out into the world; make observations and respond to situations; think, sense, feel. Their nervous energy outstrips their muscular skill so that they have a tendency to clumsiness. Dorothy is a bit more specific: the white fibers are especially visible toward the top of the iris, which would be associated with the brain, intellectual faculties, and the five senses. These people have very acute senses. They can be acutely sensitive to sound and touch, which can irritate them. But they also can enjoy sensory input—beautiful views, music, and so forth—more than other people. This type of constitution favors hyperactivity in children.

The St. John's Wort people are sensitive to pain, not because they are crybabies (like Chamomile), but because they have so many nerve endings. They especially fear the needle of the doctor and the sharp instruments of the dentist. Do not make fun of them, comments Dorothy. They really are more sensitive to pain and they retain a body memory of needles and such that makes their next appointment terrible for them to apprehend.

The St. John's Wort person is often faster than the teacher (or the herbalist) and impatient with slow speech and progress. They choose their friends not because they are good or bad, but because they are stimulating. They will always be busy on the phone, computer, or with a book.

Dorothy wrote that they are quick to resolve personal and interpersonal problems, but on this point, Kim had a lot more to add. He found that the supersensitive Hypericum person, when profoundly injured, could not recover. It is like a part of their soul was severed from them. This pattern is pointed out by Eliot Cowan in *Plant Spirit Medicine* (2014, 150–51): the plant itself told him it would heal when a part of the soul was separated. Kim develops this theme in depth, using many stories, case histories, experiences, and well . . . opinion.

Depression

For a while, St. John's Wort was a fad herb for minor depression, until Big Pharma put their sights on it and tried to implicate it in high blood pressure and other problems that are caused by the SSRI drugs (but not by Hypericum). It was assumed that it was a selective serotonin reuptake inhibitor (SSRI) because this was the ridiculous, unproven model (not even a theory) used to account for depression in the late 1990s and early twenty-first century. Today we know that the mechanisms associated with depression are far more complex, involving the immune system, thermoregulation, and many other factors (see Maletic and Raison, *The New Mind-Body Science of Depression* [2017]).

What is worse than depression? Self-harming. St. John's Wort is a remedy for "self-harming," according to an Australian stockman who attended one of my classes in Canberra. The Russian herbalist Zevin says that too much Hypericum in the pasture (a worldwide problem) causes animals to bite their sensitive parts. Perhaps St. John's Wort would be a remedy for self-harming, or for those that seem to want to remain in a psychological funk.

Sexuality

The symptom of "injury to areas rich in nerves" includes the genitals, both physically and psychologically. Kim identified St. John's Wort with the Grail story. This revolves around the Fisher King, who is wounded in the genitals, suffering unremitting pain. His kingdom withers and all suffer. The knight Parzival wanders into his dominion and is welcomed into the Grail Castle, where he sees a complicated ceremony involving the inhabitants. A mysterious vessel is carried in, borne by the Grail maidens. He wonders what is wrong with his uncle, the Fisher King, but holds back his tongue. In the morning, Parzival awakens and the castle is gone; he and his horse are simply in a clearing in the forest. Over a long period he learns, to his great shame, that he did not ask the "right question," losing the opportunity to heal the Fisher King and become the new king. He can win any martial endeavor but he is without happiness. Finally, a hermit in the forest explains that he did not show his host empathy in asking the right question. After more adventures Parzival again finds the Grail castle, again is seated next to the Fisher King, and finally asks the question, "Uncle, what ails thee?" The king and the land and Parzival are all healed. Parzival had to become more sensitive.

Following the tradition of the Fisher King, Kim called the St. John's Wort injury the "genital wound." It is so deep that it affects the person's sexuality. As a result, there is "extreme loneliness, no fulfillment in love, no relationship is meaningful." St. John's Wort is suited to this injury. It "goes deeper than any psychologist. Suicide, insanity, schizophrenia." It is for "wounds, not just physical; also those which only time will heal; like being jilted, etc." He likens it to tetanus, "a wound to the psyche; like an 'anaerobic environment' deep in the mind. Wounded conscience, wounded spirit, wounded honor, wounded sexuality." One Australian herbalist explained it this way: "the picture of what you want to be has been destroyed."

But one must be very careful. "A lot of abuse-sufferers do well on St. John's Wort, but be very gentle," noted Kim. "If it aggravates it can be very threatening. Where their trust is wounded and too much wounding is brought to the surface too quickly, a person can be driven to madness and put on antipsychotic medicine for life." Through the cytochrome P450 pathway in the liver, hypericin will break down hormones more quickly. Therefore, St. John's Wort is not recommended for people who are taking hormone therapy—from transgender people to those on birth-control pills.

Horse Medicine

We have seen several reasons why St. John's Wort is associated with horses, warhorses, and warriors. The great sensitivity of the St. John's Wort person reminds us of the horse.

"Some herbs get people to focus on animals," observed Kim. "With St. John's Wort it is the horse. The urge may be uncontrollable: boys to mustangs, girls to stallions." Upon recovery from the use of St. John's Wort, people may "dream of horses" or of "letting go of the reins." (Giving the animal self more free rein, I would guess.) Dolphins can also occur in St. John's Wort dreams and visions, notes Kim. He had a case of chronic lower back pain in a woman. "Acupuncture caused the back to go into spasm." There was an abusive father in the background. She "got an image of a horse when she was being needled—she was terrified of horses. With increased needling and visions of horses, she got brave enough to get nose to nose with a horse."

Faery Medicine

Travel in the otherworld is often associated with horses or the winged horse. The "faery steed" is a horse that takes a person on a ride through the supernatural faery world.

Preparation

Preparations have already been described. As to dosage, Kim recommends: the more severe the physical wound, the more herb is needed, but the more severe the psychological wound, the smaller the dose, so that the person doesn't get traumatized by the sudden eruption of previous unknown or hidden contents.

Formulations

Here is a formula for oversensitivity: St. John's Wort, Skullcap, and Jewelweed or Yarrow. For nightmares, combine with Thyme, and for "processing experience," with Reishi, the "metabolizer of experience" (Matthew Becker).

Specific Indications

Moderate depression; postpartum depression (Dudley); nervous breakdown; seasonal affective disorder; depression in the winter (cf. Calendula);
fear of the dark (cf. Calendula); nightmares in children; sleeplessness; lurching awake, 2:00–4:00 a.m. (John Redden)—this symptom
is often characteristic of low blood sugar; meningitis (Hall, Dudley);
"injuries to areas rich in nerves" (homeopathic indication, excellent for
herbal use as well); CFS (Dudley); sharp, shooting pains along a nerve;
parts detached—helps regrowth; tetanus (Kent and other homeopaths);
spasms; pain relief—acute (repeat frequently), chronic (larger, long-term
doses); "stomach ailments," especially in men (Clymer); toxicity due to
low CP450-function in liver and cells; enuresis; hormonal imbalances
due to liver action; fractures; plantar fasciitis (Dudley); blood poisoning;
streak running up the arm (cured, Wood); abscess (external application);
herpes (external); basal cell carcinoma (Dudley).

℞ Centaury ℘
(*Centaurium erythraea*)

This is a member of the Gentian clan with properties that are similar but milder than Gentian. It is native to Europe and still so widely
picked that there are limitations to keep the population from decimation in Germany.

There is a legend that goes with Centaury. Prometheus stole fire
from the Gods. In punishment he was bound to a rock and given
over to an eagle that would eat a part of his liver every day. It had
been prophesied that Prometheus could never be freed from his torture until an immortal died. Chiron had been wounded in the foot
and suffered from excruciating pain so he volunteered to die for
Prometheus. However, before he passed on, Chiron taught mankind
several herbs, including this one, which Hippocrates called *Kentareion*
in his honor.

Another ancient name for this plant was given to it by the Romans:
because of its intense bitterness, the yellow color of its root, and its use

as a remedy for the liver and gallbladder, it was called *fel terrae* ("bile of the earth"). It was sometimes called "Felwort" in English. This may be related to the Roman name or to another common English name, Feverwort. There is some confusion regarding the botanical name. *Centaurium* or Centaury must be differentiated from *Centaurea*, a genus in the unrelated *Asteraceae* assigned to the Knapweeds. There is no medicinal overlap. The Latin name was interpreted in the Middle Ages to mean "hundred" (*cent*) "gold (piece)" (*aurum*), giving rise to the name "Hundred Guilder Herb" and—through inflation—"Thousand Guilder Herb."

The stamens of the flower of our Centaury are five in number. This is the symbol, again and again, of the magical hand, both interfering and protecting. It is an insignia of Wolf Medicine, as we have seen—predators of the horse. The five-finger hand is associated with change in the secret alphabet of Nature. Wolf Medicine is associated with shapeshifting and Chiron is the shapeshifter.

"The anthers have a curious way of twisting themselves round after they have shed their pollen," comments Maud Grieve (1994, 182). Twisting usually indicates something that entangles or traps, like a twisting serpent. The Saxon herbalists used it for snakebite. However, twisting also indicated to some people an ascent, like Jacob's Ladder. Centaury is sometimes called "Christ's Ladder."

It is also tempting to see the twisting aspect of Centaury as representative of the caduceus in the hand of the *medicus*—the snake twisting up the green staff. Chiron taught Asclepius, whose symbol is the caduceus.

Centaury had an almost supernatural reputation in Europe as a healing plant. The *Lesser Book of Albertus Magnus* (which was not, as a matter of fact, written by Albert) counts Centaury as one of the most important of the magical herbs of the ancients. In modern European herbalism, Centaury is used as an aromatic bitter tonic or carminative to improve appetite and digestion. The dried herb is used, so the root need not be extirpated.

The dried herb is given in infusion or powder, or made into an extract. It is used extensively in dyspepsia, for languid digestion with heartburn after food, in an infusion of 1 oz. of the dried herb to 1 pint of water. When run down and suffering from want of appetite, a wineglassful of this infusion Centaury Tea—taken three or four times daily, half an hour before meals, is found of great benefit. The same infusion may also be taken for muscular rheumatism. (Grieve 1994, 183)

Centaury has been naturalized in North America, where it does not enjoy any such popularity. There are about forty different members of the genus. The specific one in medicine is the red one—flower pink to red—but others have been used. It is an intense bitter with properties reminiscent of Gentian. Both are used as bitters for the digestion. Many species of *Gentianaceae* are used in its place.

Nicholas Culpeper proclaimed of all the Centauries (1850, 45): "They are under the dominion of the Sun"; this is because "their flowers open and shut as the Sun, either shews or hides his face."

Weak Egoic Will

Dr. Bach introduced Centaury as one of his thirty-eight flower essences. It is for people who suffer lack of self-confidence so that they are afraid to make decisions, flee from decisions, and let other people walk all over them. This is similar to its cousin, Gentian, which is good for people who don't trust their own instincts, or people who bully others so that they don't trust themselves—we will get to this herb later.

Two friends were visiting my house and one of them commented how she couldn't stop her cat from picking at her fur. The other was a flower-essence practitioner. She said: "Your cat needs Vervain, and you need Centaury so it won't walk all over you."

In this regard Centaury is the opposite and complement of Celandine. It is for a weak egoic will while the latter is for a strong ego—and both are for migraines going up the gallbladder channel. They can often be alternated, since the egoic will can switch from one extreme to the other.

Migraine, Gallbladder Meridian

Herbalist and acupuncturist Francis Bonaldo of Montreal says Centaury is for migraines coming up the gallbladder meridian into eyes, with blindness, sometimes set off by family arguments. Pain in back of the neck, below the cranium, on the right side, emanating up across the temporal regions, into the eye, sometimes down to the right scapula. The gallbladder meridian runs from the gallbladder back to under the scapula, up over the scapula to the bottom of the cranium and across the temporal bones, to the eye and down to the cheekbone. These symptoms are also found under Celandine but that remedy has the strong will.

There may also be deteriorating eyesight.

Aromatic Bitter for the Digestion

Centaury has been most famously used for bloating, dyspepsia, flatulence, and lack of appetite. Francis has confirmed these indications. As a bitter it enhances gastric secretion, stimulates the appetite, and improves the digestion. It is a long-term, slow-acting tonic to the GI tract. When the stomach is deficient, the signal to the gall ducts to open and dump bile and digestive enzymes is weak. So this is also a bitter for the liver. Returning to digestion, Centaury is an antiparasitic. Herbalist David Winston points out that the aromatic bitters are the group of herbs from which all the great vermifuges originate—Wormwood, Wormseed, Black Walnut hull, and so forth.

Liver and Gallbladder

Receiving its signal from the stomach, Centaury acts on the gallbladder to increase digestive juices. It has been used to treat jaundice, which would indicate blockage of the bile at some point between the liver and the duodenum. Returning to the psychological symptoms, Centaury is beneficial when a person has a hard time making decisions. The gallbladder, as the seat of the egoic will, is associated with decision making. The old doctors thought that it acted on the liver and kidneys to "cleanse the blood" but exact symptoms are lacking.

"Feverwort"

This is one of the old names for Centaury. It is considered to be anti-inflammatory and even sedative—said to "cool the blood." Since it is for wounds and snakebites, that suggests an antiseptic application. Bitters were often also used for the chills and fever of malaria.

Bitter Tonic

Richard Hool notes that an "excellent tonic for delicate and elderly people" is an infusion of Centaury and Raspberry Leaf in equal portions: take a "wineglassful" three times a day; "Centaury acts particularly upon the heart as a general strengthener" (1918, 11).

Contraindications

At least one online source reported that this herb should not be used when there is esophageal reflux or stomach ulcers. This is the kind of information we get from "armchair herbalists" who have no practical experience. This is a specific remedy when the reflux is due to a sluggish digestion which needs stimulation. Stomach ulcers are due to sluggish digestion as well. If anyone is afraid of the herb they should just use the Bach flower essence or drop doses of the tincture for these kind of symptoms.

⌧ Horse Chestnut ⌧
(Aesculus hippocastanum)

This is a majestic tree that came out of Turkey several hundred years ago but is now widely naturalized in Europe and to a lesser extent in North America. Because I have profiled this herb elsewhere in *The Earthwise Herbal* (2008, I:50–53), I will not cover it extensively here, except in regard to its relationship to Horse Medicine

It has a heavy, sleep-inducing quality. I remember one summer when I picked the flowers for the tincture and woke up twelve hours later. The sleep was so deep I couldn't figure out where I was, who I was, or how old I was, until I was fully awake. It truly felt like I had been out in the cosmos somewhere. (My assemblage point got shifted far away). At one time it was thought to be a narcotic, but this label was rejected.

Yagho Tahnaga explained to me why this is called "Horse Chestnut." She grew up near the racetracks in Sarasota in a small Native community and some of her first employment was on a horse farm. "They put me to work collecting the nuts from the Horse Chestnut trees. They would make it into a liniment and put on the muscles of horses—you know, like how the muscles in a horse shiver?"

Dr. Bach called this "White Chestnut" and used it for what we would today call "obsessive compulsive disorder" (OCD). It is a specific and I have used it many times with success in this dreadful affliction. It is also specific in the physical condition that reflects this mentality: tension in the blood vessels causing backup, varicosities, hemorrhoids, phlebitis, and glaucoma.

Horse Chestnut is my remedy for the quick pulse. My friend Francis Bonaldo used Passionflower (*Passiflora incarnata*) for the quick pulse. That's another remedy for obsessive thinking. The quick pulse is not rapid in beats per minute; it is rapid in the rise from the bottom of the beat to the top. That's a Greek pulse not found in Chinese medicine.

This is another plant with five leaves and a strong association with the gallbladder, so it probably has magical properties and should be associated with Wolf and Dragon Medicine.

◉ WARRIOR MEDICINE ◉

The Warrior is often associated with the Horse. The mounted rider is a picture of a harmonious relationship between the human self and the animal self, but it is also associated with warfare. In feudal societies, the rider on the horse was the landowner or overlord. The peasants weren't mounted and when the landowner had to raise an army, he went mounted, followed by foot soldiers selected from his tenants and serfs. Whatever we may think of the fairness of this system, it was the form of government from the Roman period down to early modern times.

Within this culture the need to train leaders and warriors was very important. In addition, however, it was recognized that the leaders needed to live according to an effective code of ethics, if possible. We can also see the necessity of teaching the young men to follow a code of honor to avoid brigandage and social chaos. Within this milieu, the ideal of the knight or mounted warrior as a paragon of virtue arose. This led to the appearance in the twelfth century of songs and stories of chivalry told by troubadours and storytellers. This was the milieu in which King Arthur and Parzival arose from obscurity as semi-legendary Celtic chieftains to a prominence that is still with us.

The stories less often feature the women, except as auxiliary to the men, but it is in these stories that we first find pictures of female psychology that reflect actual women. The Grail cycle by Wolfram von Eshenbach, *Parzival* (ca. 1200), is generally considered to be the first literary work in which women and children were accurately portrayed as having realistic feelings. Wolfram's account of Orgeluse, a deeply wounded woman, is an example.

Figures like Arthur and Parzival were pictured as happily married, but this changed in the later versions of the stories, which were intentionally taken over and rewritten by monks who wanted to demote sex, marriage, and women to an inferior status. The faithful husband Parzival now could only glimpse the Grail from afar, while Sir Galahad, who had renounced sex, was the only one who could actually obtain the sacred artifact.

The Grail mythos appears suddenly, fully developed, with no antecedents in the Church or Celtic legends. Sara Annon suggested that this is because the cult had already been highly developed and maintained in secrecy. She traces the association of the warrior, the horse, and the cup back to the Beaker People who lived on the shores of the Atlantic in the time period after the building of the stone monuments, before the rise of Celtic identity and culture. These people probably traded by horse and ship—their remains are scattered along the coasts and the big rivers, and they were probably associated with what became the Spanish warhorse (which we know in North America as the "Indian pony"). This horse has an angular structure in the hips and shoulders that makes it a stronger weight bearer, and it is the only kind of horse that is not afraid to enter a ship.

Sara suggests that the people who raised and took care of horses comprised a kind of trade guild or shamanic school whose teachings burst into the public eye in the late Middle Ages when the Grail mythos was merged with folk Christianity. The Spanish-born Pope Callixtus III (1455–1458) issued a papal bull enjoining people from carrying out ceremonies in a cave decorated with images of horses and a horse statue (Bahn 2007).

After the colonization of the New World began, Queen Isabella forbade the exportation of Spanish warhorses to the new colonies, knowing that they would be used against her operations. They were nonetheless smuggled to the New World and became the "Indian pony" of the Southwest and Great Plains. Since the killings of the wild American horses under Trump and Biden, there are only a couple hundred left in North America. They no longer exist in Spain; are endangered in North Africa; and the rarest among them, the "Paint," is extinct in the Old World.

The major Warrior Medicines are Yarrow and St. John's Wort, both of which are for wounds. As a general class, the astringents belong here because they toughen up the exterior boundaries of the body against loss of fluids and in this way increase stamina. This fits Schizandra, which I also include here. The most powerful astringent is the "mighty Oak"—as the remedy for integrity issues it also seems to fit with the Warrior Medicines. We have already discussed St. John's Wort.

๛ Yarrow ๏
(Achillea millefolium)

I dedicated twenty pages to this herb in *The Book of Herbal Wisdom* (1997, 65–83) and I wrote about it again in *The Earthwise Herbal*

(2008–2009, 2:51–57). Yet, I still have more to say about it from a shamanic standpoint and even in terms of its ordinary action. This is in part due to my own expanding knowledge, but especially due to accounts from the late Kim Dudley of Canberra, Canadian herbalist Christine Dennis, and Irish herbalist Rosari Kingston. So we can call this an international herbal rock star.

This powerful wound medicine was another of the herbs taught by the centaur Chiron to Achilles, Hercules, and Jason. The name Chiron means "hand" (*chiro*), and he was considered to be the master of all arts and crafts. He had been taught by his adoptive father, Apollo, and his sister, Artemis, the arts of healing and herbalism, music, and many other skills.

The Latin name *Achillea* comes from Achilles, in testimony to his use of it to staunch bleeding, as reported by Homer (ca. 700 BCE). According to the *Iliad*, Achilles bemoans the fact that he does not have his herb with him when he is wounded and dying. There are several accounts of the successful use of Yarrow in the *Iliad*, including a case where Achilles treats Telephus for a severe spear injury with Yarrow and the rust gathered from the spear. *Achillea* would long be known in European folk medicine as the remedy for injuries with iron. However, it was also known in Native America for hemorrhage before the appearance of iron—so, in reality, that is not an essential characteristic of the Yarrow wound. Anyway, the rust off an army spear might be contaminated with tetanus, which is endemic (and non-fatal) in horses.

The name *millefolium* means "Thousand Leaf," referring to the leaves that look, as Mattioli says, like "the wispy feathers of young birds" (1590, 401).

My friend Rosari Kingston, an Irish herbalist, says that the most common Gaelic name for Yarrow is *Athair thalún* ("Father of the Earth"). She asked linguists and botanists what that meant and none of them had an answer. However, she observed that the tangle of feather-like leaves at the bottom of the plant collect dust and after a few years in gravelly soil, the plant will enrich the ground. This could account for the fact that Yarrow is said to have an enriching effect on plants growing nearby. The same property is attributed to its cousin Chamomile, which also has lacy, featherlike leaves.

Father of the Earth, Master of the Blood

Rosari speculated that Yarrow, which seems to mineralize the soil, may have a mineralizing effect that makes a malnourished person stronger. Another Irish name is *Lus na fola*, meaning "Herb of the Blood." This is almost identical to what I call it, "Master of the Blood." Not only does it staunch heavy bleeding, open the capillaries to increase peripheral circulation and release fever, but it may also improve hemogenesis in the bone marrow.

The English name Yarrow is related to the word "gear," which can refer to arms, armor, clothing, and attire. Other names are Carpenter's Herb or Carpenter's Friend, Herbe du Charpentier, Soldier's Woundwort, Knyghten Milfoil, Sanguinary, Bloodwort, and Nosebleed—the latter from its propensity to cause nosebleed (a "like treats like" affair).

Achillea millefolium is native to Europe and Asia. It is naturalized in the Americas, New Zealand, and the Snowy Mountains of Australia, and the southernmost countries of Africa. In addition, there is a native American strain, *A. millefolium* var. *lanulosa*, which arrived in North America before 1492. It had an extensive popularity in Native American medicine, and was used for wounds just like in the European tradition. A Lakota name translates as "Medicine of the Wounded." An Ojibwa name is perhaps the most cute: "Squirrel Tail."

Cuts to the Bone, and Cuts to the Third Level of the Blood

Back in the days of my herbal youth, at Present Moment Herbs in Minneapolis, there was a young employee named Victor. I've told this story before, but not the latest twist. Vic was hired as a worker, not an herbalist, but he still learned by osmosis and the occasional lesson. One day he came in and announced in a puzzled voice: "I had a dream last night about Yarrow. It said it's for cuts to the bone and cuts to the third level of the blood." We asked, "What does that mean?" He replied, "I dunno." A few weeks passed; Victor cut his finger deeply. Goldenseal wouldn't stop the bleeding, but Yarrow did.

We puzzled for a long time but an herbal friend from Arizona, Halsey Brandt, said immediately when I told him the story: "Oh, I know what that means. The first level of the blood is the capillary bed, the second is the arterioles, and the third is the arteries." Yes, that is exactly what it means. Yarrow is for the deep arterial cuts that bleed freely. But thirty years later Victor had a second insight: "Oh, it's for cuts to the bone—that means the bone marrow." He pointed out that Maria Treben wrote in *Health through God's Pharmacy* (1984, 50): "Yarrow acts directly and best on the bone marrow and thus stimulates blood renewal." It is therefore indicated for "disorders of the bone marrow, even caries." Bone marrow produces white, red, and platelet blood cells; therefore Yarrow would stimulate immunity, red blood, and staunching of bleeding.

The sharper the cut, the better the indication for Yarrow. One of my herbal friends told me a story about her son, who is a budding herbalist. She had a client who had a cut that had spontaneously appeared between the thumb and the pointer finger. She thought it was fungus, but she called in her ten-year-old son, who looked at the condition carefully. He said: "It looks like a cut, so Yarrow is indicated. One drop a day on the cut." (Here was another mini-doser, like myself). "It will get better for a few days, then it will get worse and bleed; then get better again and heal." And that's what happened!

Circulation

All of us who have used Yarrow realize that it affects the circulation tremendously, opening and closing the peripheral circulation as needed, also acting on the arteries and veins. It acts on all the highly vascularized tissue—kidneys, liver, bone marrow, heart, and brain. How can we say this? Herbalism is an empirical art—that is to say, it is learned from experience. This is its chief difference from medicine, which is based on research and statistics—the individual person, the case history, is relatively unimportant; the experience of the practitioner and the patient is intentionally ignored in favor of test results.

One suggestion is that Yarrow is particularly suited to enhancement of the circulation below the waist, easing the strain on the heart by bringing it up from below, when there is poor venous return. So it is a remedy for "low blood," when the blood stays down in the lower extremities—in older people, the indication is a blue dark or black band around the ankles with memory and cognitive loss. I use Rosemary for this, but Yarrow is another potential remedy. It is also indicated for varicose veins when the complexion is red (from capillary congestion) with blue veins. Low blood is also a name for blood deficiency, of which there are many kinds. Kim Dudley considered Yarrow specifically suited to the initial weakness of vitamin B12 deficiency.

I helped a woman, aged sixty-three, who was taking Hawthorn for slow weakening of her heart and circulation. The condition was slowly deteriorating, so I told her to add Yarrow, 1 part for 3 parts Hawthorn. This immediately reversed the deterioration and she eventually discontinued the remedies.

"A patient came to me with cold hands and feet," wrote Kim. "I treated her successfully with Yarrow. It seemed to me she had contracted herself and pulled the blood flow from her extremities into her center."

Having said all this about low blood, we also have to consider Yarrow in cases of high blood, or when the blood gets stuck in the head or the surface. Fire rises, so this is associated with heat. There may be headache—Maria Treben spoke highly of it for migraine. The homeopathic provings brought out an affinity for people of a florid complexion (meaning: lots of blood in the head and surface). When the skin is hot and dry, Yarrow is indicated. Likewise when the sides of the tongue are red and the center blue, indicating stagnation in the center blocking circulation; when the tongue is red on the sides and pale in the center, indicating heat in the surface and cold and blood vacuity in the interior; or even when the center is red and the sides are white. Yarrow seems to always have this imbalance between the center and the periphery. When the perimeter is weak, there is lack of protection of the organism.

Aneurysm

I've already discussed aneurysms in just about all my writings on Yarrow, but it turns out that also entertained a high regard for it in this imbalance. He collected twenty-five pages of research papers suggesting a possible association between copper, faulty production or elastin, vascular weakness, and aneurysm formation. This would explain both the Venus rulership in traditional astrology and the affinity of Yarrow for strengthening arteries and veins. The capillary bed doesn't have elastin fibers to any great extent, but its health is dependent on the bigger vascular structures.

Kim inserted a story. In 1957, the Australian government released a pelletized "wonder food" for turkeys. Guaranteed to grow them bigger, fatter, faster, and deader than a doornail. Over 50% of the nation's turkey crop died that year. When they did autopsies, they found that almost all of them had died of ruptured aortic aneurysm. Further analysis showed that the wonder food lacked copper; when they added this, the mortality rate dropped to zero. Statistics show that four to six of every 100 Americans autopsied have died of a ruptured aneurysm and an additional 40% have aneurysms that have not yet ruptured. Called "the silent killer," cerebral aneurysms cause approximately 500,000 deaths a year worldwide. Women and the elderly are affected disproportionately. Risk factors include unequal distribution of vasculature in the brain (Inagawa 2022; Hall et al. 2023).

My friend Paula Jensen, an herbalist in Santa Fe and Tulsa, had an aneurysm suddenly appear and expand on her arm while she was teaching a class. Everybody, including herself, was pretty concerned. She put Yarrow on it and it disappeared by the end of the class. When she told me, I remarked that it would be a good idea to take Yarrow for a month or two, in case there were internal hidden arteries that lacked tone. She did and she found that the spider veins on her legs disappeared.

It seems likely that Yarrow, Schizandra, and Oak—all excellent astringents—act on the elastin tissues. Indeed, this may be true of all astringents, and they might possibly all pass as warrior remedies since they would be associated with disciplining, toning, and strengthening the tissue.

Kim did a lot of research on elastin. It is found in connective tissue that stretches or is flexible, therefore in the joints, the vertebrate disks of the spine, all the blood vessels, bronchial tubes, and much of the skin. Emphysema can be produced in animals by lack of dietary copper. Kim comments: "There is no current evidence that hemorrhoids are made worse by a copper deficiency, but limited experience leads me to believe that evidence will one day appear." Yarrow is a good hemorrhoid remedy. He also wondered whether "a tendency to cut oneself while shaving, will prove to be correlated" with weak elastin. "If so, this would serve as a good early warning." Ah, I love how empirical herbalists think!

Liver and Vasculature

Since estrogen helps with the uptake of copper, young women have fewer problems with aneurysms or bleeding out than men, except after childbirth, when they have lost a lot of copper helping build the placenta and the baby. Men who die of aneurysms have been found to have as low as 26% of normal levels of copper in the liver.

Mechanically speaking, the liver is more heavily dependent on vasculature than any other organ. It constantly receives toxic blood from the digestive tract via the portal vein. This has to be balanced by a massive influx of clean blood through the hepatic artery and of course there are still veins to drain processed blood out of the liver. But the remarkable thing is that the structure of the liver is entirely dependent on the ramification of the portal vein into smaller and smaller veins, which finally are the only thing holding the liver together. Yarrow poultices are the standard anti-inflammatory application for hepatitis of all types in anthroposophical medicine.

Wounded Warrior, Wounded Healer

Nothing stops a severe hemorrhage like Yarrow. It is also for deep emotional traumas—cuts to the bone. Herbalist Barbara Parke called it the "wounded warrior, wounded healer remedy." It is for the warriors "who jump in, put out the fires, but get cut to the bone," she says, but also for healers and gentle souls that are more sensitive.

Fever

Many of us use warm Yarrow tea (or less often, tincture) as a fever remedy, either by itself or in combination with Elder and Peppermint. This formula came from Juliette da Bairacli-Levy; "from the gypsies," she explained. However, the herb by itself is quite competent. I compare it to homeopathic Aconite as a powerful antifebrile in acute conditions, either from cold and wind or damp, or viral infections. It is good for a sore throat. Kim recalled a teaching from his great mentor, Dorothy Hall. Anytime she got out of bed in the morning feeling feverish or sore and chilly, she drank a cup of warm Yarrow tea. The warmth helps bring the blood to the surface and decongest the interior.

Protection Medicine

Yarrow flower essence was also introduced by the Flower Essence Society as a remedy for psychic protection. Many people could testify to its value here, but I want to give the evidence of a friend who did not know anything about these traditions, but discovered the protective influence of Yarrow on her own.

Kathy was greatly helped by realizing that she was a natural empath. Fate offered her a buyout of her city condominium at a good price and she was able to retire to an island in the San Juans:

I need to live on an island because it has such precise boundaries. There are only 2,000 people here year-round, so the psychic atmosphere is more safe for me. When I leave the island on the ferry, I can feel when the submerged part of the island fades away and I am again vulnerable. I also discovered that Yarrow tea would strengthen and protect me; so I drink that often.

As I mentioned in *The Book of Herbal Wisdom* (1997, 82), Yarrow has a strange ability to make one more aware of sharp edges, tools, and knives, and therefore to avoid wounds. One of my students worked as a bartender in a tavern favored by tradespeople who worked a lot with tools. She found that it protected people when placed in the workshop, but had to be renewed about twice a year with fresh plant material.

Yarrow makes a person more alert, or again, it turns down excessive vigilance when a person is feverish and the brain is overstimulated by heat. It is cooling and restful in such cases. In other situations, it improves blood flow to the surface and therefore animal sensation. It improves, coordinates, and normalizes blood flow into and out of the capillary bed, acting partly through the veins and the arterioles. Therefore, it stops bleeding from deep cuts—to the arteries. By bringing blood and heat to the surface and relaxing the pores of the skin, it is an excellent remedy in fever, chills and fever and heat conditions.

Protection of the Teeth and Gums

Victor had been trained by Bob Gallagher, the owner of the herb store where we worked, more than I had, because I was more of an overconfident young buck who thought I knew a lot. Bob told Victor: "The first line of protection is the teeth." "I was young then," said Victor, "so what did I know about teeth problems? But when I got older, I realized that you did have to protect your teeth." He points out: "When you chew Yarrow, it causes the gums to get numb and tingle, so it is increasing the nerve and blood flow to the gums. Great protection." If the gums are healthy, the teeth will be more likely to be healthy because there will be better blood circulation. And we remember that the "Father of the Earth" may "catch the dust" and have a mineralizing effect. Maria Treben also cited Yarrow as a tooth and gum remedy. Shortly, we will have a discussion of Oak bark and the teeth and gums, another medicine I have placed under Warrior Medicine.

Chamomile is the great remedy for the pain of teething in children, but it is possible that Yarrow should also be considered here. Kim Dudley observed: "Cutting one's teeth in a new situation may affect more than the gums."

The Spiritual Warrior

"To be immersed in Yarrow is to become a soldier of either carnal or spiritual fortune," wrote Kim. "Military battle and the military battlefield are no different from the internal battle on the battlefield that is found within each of us as we come face to face with our own inner enemies."

What constitutes spiritual warfare? Certainly, it is a matter of standing up for what is right in the world and against dishonesty, greed, and tyranny. But what Kim—and I—would particularly think of is the great internal war we fight to become better people; closer to the spirit. Quakers call this the "Lamb's War." We don't always know what we are looking for or how to grow into the spirit, but there is one activity that occupies the time and energies of the spiritual warrior. "Every esoteric healing tradition recognizes the need to recapitulate one's lifetime of experience," writes Kim. "To scrutinize every past event to ensure that nothing has been left unresolved. One shouldn't dwell in the past if nothing is being resolved. But every memory left unexamined may harbor a suppressed emotion, a purposefully forgotten desire, which has to be examined if we are to grow."

This is very hard work. It takes a realistic perspective on life, ruthless self-examination, and discipline. In short, inner processing is one of the greatest endeavors of the spiritual warrior. "Some will procrastinate, to defend themselves against inner change," wrote Kim, while "others will become workaholics." Even the attempt to recapitulate builds spiritual character. "Only in the primacy of battle are some of the noblest qualities of the human spirit occasionally seen—valor, self-sacrifice, and compassion."

Kim saw Yarrow as the ideal remedy here, both for laziness and the exhaustion of hard work. It is also the remedy for those who withdrew from the battle, did not take up the challenge, even missed their calling:

Yarrow is the remedy of the public servant who feels the wasting of his life confronted with the inescapable demands of bureaucracy, his life slipping away on sheets of paper in their respective "in" and "out" trays. It is the remedy of the bank clerk and the remedy of the professional soldier. (Dudley 2012)

There is a similar pattern under the next herb, Schizandra, which is for those who have followed their calling until they have exhausted themselves, as well as those who wake up in their sixties and realize that they have wasted their lives by not following their calling. These indications are also analogous to the next remedy, Oak, which is indicated when the "mighty Oak is broken down." It helps us choose the battles we can win, and not exhaust or hurt ourselves in those that are impossible to win.

The Double Injury

The opposite of the recapitulation is reliving the pain over and over. According to Kim, the name for this in Taoism is the "double injury." Kim repeated the following story from Arthur Waley, *Three Ways of Thought in Ancient China* (1939, 73):

> When Prince Mon of Wei was living as a hermit in Chung-shan, he said to the Taoist, Chan Tzu: "My body is here amid the lakes and steams; but my heart is in the palace of Wei. What am I to do?" "Care more for what you have in yourself," said Chan Tzu, "and less for what you can get from others." "I know I ought to," said the Prince, "but I cannot get the better of my feelings." "If you cannot get the better of your feelings," replied Chan Tzu, "then give play to them. Nothing is worse for the soul than struggling not to give play to feeling that it cannot control. This is called the Double Injury, and of those that sustain it, none live out their natural span."

Beatrice describes the same problem in Dante's *Inferno* (2001, 61):

> *The double grief of a lost bliss*
> *is to recall its happy hour in pain.*
> *Your Guide and Teacher knows the truth of this.*

Kim taught that the remedy for the double injury was Yarrow. The Yarrow person has been cut to the bone. The blood must flow freely and clean the wound. But it also needs to stop. Yarrow doesn't force the wound closed; it cleans it out, reabsorbs coagulated internal blood into the lymphatics, the inner cleansing system; repairs the nerves as best as possible; and allows the regulatory factors released by the wound to naturally bring the lips together.

Kim also saw the double injury as relevant in acute disease. "One example of the double injury is that of rain and wind together," he commented. Cold and damp would also be another double trauma. "Exposure quickly chills the body and threatens to lower the core temperature. The mind becomes numb, the body hypotensive." We see the action on the periphery and the core.

Exhaustion

Kim emphasized the problem of fatigue with Yarrow. He especially highlighted cases where he or his mentor Dorothy felt drained by the person they were working with—a problem of the empath. Or the problem may arise from stress:

> In the subclinical setting the patient complains of feeling run-down after a prolonged period of stress. They may have been involved in nursing a partner or relative through a terminal illness. They may have been under constant threat of losing their job, or been involved in a long, drawn-out legal case. Invariably, they will say they feel drained. They may even feel a particular person has drained their energy.

In some cases, the practitioner is drained by the client:

> I frequently find, after treating or interacting with schizophrenics, that I am left with a feeling of having been depleted or drained. On two such occasions I recall falling prostrate on the clinic floor and needing several minutes to recover. (Dudley 2012)

In other situations, the exhaustion is due to laziness. Kim wrote:

The great Indian saint Shankacharya once said that the greatest obstacle to spirituality, or self-knowledge, is laziness. Sloth is one of the seven deadly sins. We all often have such good intentions. We will study harder, we will be more disciplined in our attendance; we will start eating the right food; we will stop eating too much; we won't let another idle thought cross our mind; we won't gossip any more; we will practice everyday. [But] procrastination becomes a way of life. We just don't feel up to making the effort. Each morning we stay in bed a little longer. It's so cold in winter. We make do. The meals become simpler. We lose the interest to make sure we are always looking our best. He can wait a little while for his money. (Dudley 2012; edited)

Yarrow stops our laziness and brings all that is suppressed to light. It unearths all that has been buried in the catacombs of the past. By removing our laziness it defines our aspirations, the aims we have for our highest good. Yarrow grants us the ability to break away from our old patterns and habits and start each day anew.

Connective Tissue

If Yarrow has such a powerful effect on the elastin in blood vessels—which many of us have observed in practice—then it would certainly have a significant influence on the connective tissue (cartilage, joints, tendons, skin). It has, in fact, been traditionally used for arthritis and "rheumatism" in folk medicine—especially when worse from damp, adds Rosari Kingston. She recommends the dried Yarrow tops, used as a tea.

A British herbalist, Ali English (2019), thinks of it as detoxifying around the joints. The cartilage does not have its own capillary bed; the blood drops off the nutrients and picks up the toxins at the edge of the cartilage. That's why the cartilaginous strip down the chest of a chicken is pure white rather than pink—no blood. The cartilage gets its nutrition by the slower movement of the interstitial fluids. But an expansion of the capillary bed next to the cartilage is sure to help. Comfrey helps pull the nutrients and toxins through the cartilage and maintain the tissue; the allantoin in Comfrey helps regrowth of damaged cartilage, which is very hard to repair. Solomon's Seal and Teasel will strengthen and rebuild when there has been catastrophic injury; apply over many months. When the joints are injured, the muscles inflame and tighten up—Yarrow again, for this. The wounded warrior. Kim cites it for rheumatism, tendonitis, spondylosis, fractures, and exostosis (a benign overgrowth of cartilage on the bone). All of these plants will work better for these conditions when they are applied locally.

Female Reproductive Tract

We should not forget that those who bear children are warriors too. If Yarrow helps blood vessels, improves circulation below the waist, provides copper for the mother and child, and prevents aneurysms (more common in women), then Yarrow is a preeminent female herb—long assigned to Venus, despite its warrior ways. "First and foremost, it is a herb for women," wrote Austrian herbalist Maria Treben (1984, 50): "I cannot recommend Yarrow enough for women." She cites Father Sebastian Kneipp: "Women could be spared many troubles, if they just took Yarrow tea from time to time!"

She recommends it for young girls with irregular menses, older women during menopause, or already past the climacteric, and I would add that it is a remedy for both lack of menses and excess bleeding—I gave some case histories in *The Book of Herbal Wisdom*. Kim adds:

> Yarrow is a universal regulator of the female reproductive system. For irregular menstruation, or to calm the flushing of menopause, Yarrow has few equals. Inflammation of the ovaries, prolapsed uterus and fibroids all respond to Yarrow sitz baths. Spastic conditions of the pelvis and parametrium are relaxed. (Dudley 2012)

The parametrium is the fat and connective tissue surrounding the uterus. Kim also thought Yarrow was an important remedy for candida. In his opinion: "Thrush seems to be associated with an abnormal sensuality, either excessive or deficient." In such cases I would think first of the Water Lilies, White (*Nymphaea odorata*) and the Yellow (*Nuphar lutea*). The former is an excellent remedy for yeast infection, and both are for excessive sexual thoughts.

And like the caboose on the train, we might as well mention men. A healthy vascular system and toned, astringed tissues are necessary for virility, prostate health, and reproductive fitness.

It takes two warriors to raise one child, especially when the village and the neighborhood is no longer intact.

Energetics and Signatures

Yarrow is usually considered cooling and drying—it combines a strongly cooling bitterness with mild astringency that tones the mucosa. Yet it also opens the peripheral circulation to moisten the skin with sweat and reduce fever. Richard Hool (1922) suggested that Yarrow should be used when the skin is hot, dry, and constricted, with restlessness, wakefulness, and delirium. After administration, the skin will become soft, moist, and flexible; the mind "calm, rational, and inclined to sleep." Or the person awakens from sleep with a healing perspiration—the fever "breaks."

The lacy leaves unfurl in the spring; the hard stalk rises afterward, with leaves appearing along the sides. In mid to late summer, the shield-like inflorescence (collection of individual flowers) appears at the top. So there is a contrast of hard and soft—"wounded warrior, wounded healer." The shield so perfectly pictures protection. The leaf has been cut back through evolution until there is nothing but the vessels, a perfect picture of the capillary bed. Yarrow has traditionally been assigned to Venus, the ruler of the veins, but it is so Martial in quality that it is easy to doubt this designation. It seems necessary to attribute Yarrow to both Venus and Mars, as it normalizes between sensitivity and violence. The Scotch ballad "The Downy Dens of Yarrow" contrasts love and murder.

I could never understand the Venusian rulership until I awoke one night and a little voice said in my ear: "You have blood in your kidneys." And sure enough: I soon knew how blood mixed with urine looks and feels. I sipped a cup with a dropper full of Yarrow tincture in it and felt an incredible soothing across my kidneys. *Oh, no wonder*, I thought: *It is ruled by Venus.* I presume I passed a stone. I had one more release of blood in the urine in the day; never again.

Kim associated Yarrow with the "female psyche" and noted that it contained a lot of copper, the metal associated with Venus:

Yarrow is a major regulator of the copper balance in the body. It effectively administers to the soldier's wounds because it heals the soldier's female psyche, which he so pompously ignores while he plays at war. With its usage he tends to yield rather than become the aggressor. Yarrow particularly resonates with copper, especially copper sulphate, the great healing crystal of the Middle Ages. (Dudley 2012)

Kim quotes Steiner, who likened Yarrow to a sympathetic person— Venus is the planet of sympathy and comfort:

Like sympathetic people in human society, who have a favorable influence by their mere presence and not by anything they say, so Milfoil in a district where it is plentiful, works beneficially by its mere presence. (Dudley 2012)

The English herbalist William Coles, in *Adam in Eden*, noted that the feathery leaves looked like hair, "if your fancy will have it" (1657, 556). He says it will stop shedding if the head is bathed with a decoction.

Shamanic Initiation

An herbalist who had an incredibly deep shamanic experience with Yarrow is Christine Dennis, of Port Burwell, Ontario. She was teaching a plant-attunement and plant-journeying class with Yarrow when she got tired, withdrew from the circle, and lay down. As we have seen, tiredness is a characteristic associated with Yarrow. All of a sudden, a large blue being appeared before her. It asked Christine to identify the color. She replied: "Azulene." This is an azure-blue volatile oil found in Chamomile and Yarrow. This turned out to be a "cross-the-threshold" question and what transpired over the next several years was so taxing for Christine that she regretted having answered it.

The immediate impact was so intense that Christine saw stars, diamondlike sparkles, as if in her aura, and understood the "astral body" in a new and intense way. It was like an apocalypse happening within her—earthquakes, tsunamis, battles: "It was more intense than ayahuasca." It was transpersonal; moved her beyond herself, opened her up to what sounded to me like the "wounded warrior, wounded healer" experience. "Then it told me I passed the initiation and gave me a shield of protection, which was very practical on the metaphysical level. It stiffened and thickened my astral body."

The award of the protective shield was followed, for Christine, by a year of aggressive encounters. Each time she was protected. She also experienced her "Achilles tendon" during this period. She dreamed that she "entered a battle that wasn't mine." When she was thinking about this at the kitchen sink, all of a sudden her back went out. "It was my Achilles tendon."

"I do feel Yarrow with me all the time. I'll call on it if I am not comfortable." But she warned us, our little group of herbalists from North America, England, and Ireland: "If you are ever asked a question testing your skill, don't answer it." Christine didn't feel the suffering, scars, threats, and aggressions made up for the gift she received. But that is so often the way it is on the shamanic road, on the spiritual path: with every gift, more is asked.

Preparation, Dosage, and Contraindications

Yarrow is a strong but relatively safe herb; a very small number of people have had anaphylactic reactions, which also occurs occasionally with Chamomile (once or twice out of 150 million doses). It can be used dried or fresh to make a tea or tincture. Almost always the flowering tops are used, though Achilles used the powder of the root. Contraindicated during pregnancy.

⪧ Schizandra, Shizandra ⪦
(*Schizandra chinensis*)

This agent is not for the "wounded warrior" but for the "worn-out warrior": the person who has taken life by the horns and expended a lot of energy doing so. However, it is also for the person who has ignored their calling and worn themselves out fighting against their true calling.

Schizandra is native to the border regions of Manchuria and Russia, down into the Koreas. It is most plentiful in Russia and was used by big-game hunters in Siberia to improve peripheral vision, mental concentration, and stamina. It came into Chinese medicine and was known as Wu Wei Zi, meaning "five-flavored fruit." It is said to possess all five flavors—sour, sweet, salty, bitter, and pungent. The actual flavors, according to my tongue, are salty (in the first instance, as there is some salt on the outside of the berry), strong sourness, and puckering astringency, followed by a nutty and mucilaginous taste in the seeds. In addition, it is defined as warming.

The most important property is the astringence and it is widely used in Chinese herbalism for that property. Russian scientists found that Schizandra contained lignans that have the adaptogenic profile and it moved into Western popular commerce as an adaptogen. "This Chinese herb is now used in the West as an adaptogenic tonic, although in China its chief use is as a tonic astringent," wrote Michael Tierra (1988, 346).

It is important to differentiate between the traditional and modern applications. Too many Westerners ignore traditional indications, uses, and theories, thinking their own science is unquestionable. But this information is important for another reason. The traditional use is associated with the dried fruit and seed, and is the common form found in the marketplace in China and the United States. Some modern preparations contain only the seed or nut.

The Chinese herbalists generally aren't too keen on astringents because they don't want to close off a discharge that needs clearance from the body. Instead they tend to use "yang tonics," or herbs that are warming—to help the yang or active processes regain control over the water. Schizandra is the most popular astringent in Chinese herbalism, probably because, as an herb of five flavors, the astringence is moderated by the other flavors or constituents.

Schizandra is classified as warming but it is not strongly warming. All astringents are slightly warming. When we stop perspiration, which is cooling, the net effect is to warm the organism. The taste is not warming, however, because it is a sour berry, and most sour fruits have a cooling taste and effect. To make it cooling and vastly improve the taste, combine it with cherry liquor. Due to the "five flavors," Schizandra is said to benefit the "five organs," that is, the primary or yin organs: lungs, heart, liver, spleen, and kidneys.

Pharmacology

Schizandra contains lignans (schizadrin, gomisin, deoxyschizandrin, and pregomisin), phytosterols (beta-sitosterols, stigmasterol), volatile oils, tannins, nutrients (Vitamin C and E).

Constitution

When Schizandra is indicated as a specific medicine, rather than just as a general tonic, astringent, or adaptogen, the person is either highly dedicated to some calling for which they sacrifice much and wear themselves out, or, they conform to social standards to such an extent that they don't fulfill their calling and realize that life has passed them by. I learned about this from Swani Simon, an herbalist in Saarland, Germany. "These are people that are working too hard, too active," says Swani, or "people who reach retirement age and then realize that they wasted their life. Schizandra is good particularly for those in the early sixties." She says it is also for people who, though they have goals they are pursuing, feel frustrated because they haven't accomplished anything. They are "set in their ways; inflexible; congested."

Mind

Schizandra is good for anxiety, agitation, and scattered thinking (Tierra and Tierra 1998, 2:231). Astringents are used in Chinese herbalism to bring together the pieces of the mind or spirit that are going in different directions. When the "heart" (physically or metaphorically) has been hit by a shocking blow and the *shen* is scattered, Schizandra will "relocate and rehabituate consciousness to the heart," says herbalist Seán O'Donoghue. Shen is the "soul part" usually translated as "mind" or "spirit"; in terms of this book, it most similar to Jung's "Self" or Steiner's "soul-and-spirit." Schizandra is also indicated in "heart neurosis, when a person thinks something is wrong with their heart," adds Swani Simon.

"Heart not storing the shen" includes the symptoms of attention deficit and hyperactivity. Herbalist David Winston introduced Hawthorn for this problem and I have used it repeatedly. Herbalist Thomas Easley uses Schizandra. He notes that many of the ADD people are kinesthetic learners, like hunter-gatherers caught in the wrong environment, and Schizandra matches them very well. These two remedies seldom fail on their own, but they also make a good combination (see below under the Heart).

Head and Eyes

A symptom called "veiling" may occur, as if something were veiling the eyes and head, with foggy brain and unclear vision (Huang 2009, 467).

Schizandra definitely increases peripheral vision. I found this *very, very* disturbing when I experienced it on a crowded New York City subway platform after sampling the berries. I could see the people around me, but not in front of me. The thing about peripheral vision is that animals have it and hunters want it to be able to sneak up on the animals. So this is one reason Schizandra is used by hunters in Siberia. In addition it improves stamina. It can be used like the pemmican made by American Indian hunters—berries mixed with meat.

Lungs

Schizandra is well established as a lung remedy; it strengthens respiration, deepens the breath, and reduces coughing. This is partly because, as an astringent, it strengthen the kidneys, which "grasp the qi in the lungs." In Chinese medicine the depth of respiration is attributed to the kidneys. Remember that nervousness and exhaustion cause shallow breathing.

As an adaptogen, it has been used to improve stamina and resistance to acute diseases or to reduce the length of the sickness. A formula for when a person is coming down with a cold or flu might be Schizandra, Elder, and Lemon Balm.

Huang Huang (2009) is an empiricist who prefers "specific indications" derived from historical and personal experience and therefore attempts to define the action of medicinal agents according to their most characteristic symptomology. He doesn't discuss the energetics or the "five-flavors" theory; he simply gives a symptom picture, primarily based on the lungs.

Huang says that Schizandra is indicated in cough or "counterflow," where qi ascends in the lungs, and for difficulty in breathing. The patient has difficulty breathing when lying flat, and is better from breathing while propped up. There may be chest distention, "froglike rales" or "wheezing sound in the throat, breathing with an open mouth and raised shoulders." There is no trouble when sitting quietly, but panting may occur upon starting activity. In severe cases there will be fluid loss with sweating, restless sleep, excessive dreaming, confused dreams, flusteredness, palpitations, seminal emissions, aching of the lumbar vertebra and knees, and diarrhea (Huang 2009, 465–67). The kidneys reach up and "grasp the qi in the lungs," which deepens respiration and prevents the "counterflow" of qi in the lungs that Huang mentions— that is to say, difficulty breathing, sleep apnea, or asthma.

My first Schizandra patient was myself. I had gradually increasing urination at night and eventually also during the day, with more and more dribbling, sudden urging, water retention in the hands from kidney backup, drying out of the skin of the hands and forearms (a leak below can dry out above), and finally—partly due to accidents— inflammation, spasm, and drying out in muscles of the back. Lifelong tendencies to insomnia became worse and worse with the waking at night. The kidneys were not able to relax from sympathetic into parasympathetic and I finally felt like I was being driven crazy by the insomnia. In my case the problem seemed to stem from the nervous system—which could not turn off the sympathetic at night. This fits the research on the adaptogenic uses, which show balancing in the nervous system. So far, not a lot of studies have been done on the endocrine.

A client I was trying to help couldn't pay me, so he gave me a quart jar of Schizandra seed and berry tea with honey as an energetic exchange—the most worthwhile exchange I have ever received. I drank about three-quarters of the jar in the first five days. The effects were immediate, deep-acting, and (after a while) long-lasting. It immediately pumped the water out of my hands (and elsewhere?), and when this water had passed, I suddenly went from five to seven visits to the bathroom at night to three, which is slightly above average for my age. My kidneys and my mind relaxed, and the insomnia became less uncomfortable and the hours of sleep increased.

As mentioned, in the Chinese organ/system method, "the kidneys" reach up and "grasp the qi in the lungs." This is held to deepen respiration and—asthma. I've seen this many times.

Kidneys

The first action listed in the Chinese materia medica, and therefore probably the one for which Schizandra is most commonly used, is "deficiency of the kidneys." Since it is a slightly warming astringent, it is specially for yang deficiency.

The kidneys "store the jing," or primal archetypal/genetic material that gives every organism its "essence." They also store the primal yin and yang, water and fire. A deficiency of jing is seen in slow maturation, low reproductive powers, and congenital defects. Schizandra is used to stop "leakage of the jing." This may occur through excessive sexual activity, or giving away one's energy in some way, or it may result from a congenital deficiency. The primary symptoms are excessive fluid loss from sweating, night sweats, nocturnal emissions, premature ejaculation, vaginal discharge, urinary incontinence, and daybreak diarrhea. A signature for the kidneys is found in the two kidney-shaped seeds found in the fruit.

Going deeper, Schizandra is used for spontaneous, uncontrollable perspiration, frequent urination, and what the old Chinese doctors called "wasting and thirsting syndrome" (consumption or tuberculosis). It retains and encourages production of the various fluids of the body.

Liver

Schizandra has a very gentle action on the liver and is certainly more gentle than St. John's Wort. It is indicated in depression, lethargy, heaviness, drowsiness, and exhaustion associated with what we would call "toxic overload" of the liver in Western herbalism. It "supports the liver if the person has drunk or eaten a lot, and expects a hangover," notes Seán O'Donoghue.

An herbalist with a liver that had been damaged by a rabies vaccination (increased liver enzymes in the blood) writes that Schizandra "makes me happy and energetic . . . so I move more . . . and supply myself with natural serotonin, I guess," cutting down on lethargy and depression. "I saw the same with my mom. She was highly lethargic and she started walking, going out feeling more alive, basically."

There is research supporting a possible action on the CP450 enzyme pathway, like St. John's Wort, but more gentle. Seán O'Donoghue has confirmed this in practice. He also considers it blood-sugar balancing in insulin resistance. Schizandra and Cinnamon can be combined for this.

Spleen

The tone in the walls of the intestine is kept strong by the spleen, according to traditional Chinese medicine. Spleen yang deficiency is associated with inability to hold back the fluids, or a shedding of water from the intestinal walls, resulting in diarrhea. The spleen is associated with absorption problems and it may be that the action of Schizandra as an anemia remedy is due to an improvement in the absorption of iron through the intestinal wall.

Schizandra can be combined with Yellow Dock Root and Wild Cherry for heat in the intestines, with diarrhea.

Spleen deficiency can also work the opposite way, in cases where there is "leaky gut." Here is a pertinent case history. A woman writes:

> I'm bipolar and have a lot of digestive and blood-sugar issues that trigger anxiety, and I take schizandra everyday. And it works. I've never felt better, and when I stop taking it, my mania worsens, and it gets harder to digest certain foods. . . . I've noticed over the years that my mood swings get worse when I've eaten too much sugar and gluten. I seem to be able to tolerate them better if I've had my regular skizzy berries (what I call them). It's not any specific symptoms. I have inflammation issues that trigger both the bipolar and chronic pain flare-up points due to old injuries, so I have to be extremely careful with my diet. I also take reishi and spiny date seeds (Suan Zao Ren in TCM) at night to help me sleep.

Heart

Schizandra controls "heart-blood and yin deficiency" symptoms such as palpitation, forgetfulness, insomnia, irregular pulse, and irritability. "Heart-blood deficiency" refers to cases where the mind is particularly affected by blood deficiency, resulting in lack of focus and forgetfulness. There is also insomnia because there is not enough blood to "pacify the spirit," which is "stored in the heart," with waking at two or three in the morning. "Keep on the nightstand by the bed, for when they wake up," says Seán O'Donoghue.

A common symptom in the unvaccinated after Omicron—also found in some of the injected—was rapid heartbeat at night, or positional orthostatic tension syndrome (POTS). The head starts to fill with blood, the feet are cold, suddenly the person wakes with a thump of the heart and rapid heartbeat. Sitting or standing relieves the symptoms but they come back night after night. Four of us herbalists had this symptom, as well as some of our clients. The usual formula was Schizandra and Hawthorn, and I also used Schizandra and cherry liquor. Other agents were sometimes necessary but this basic formula shortened the duration and strengthened people right from the start. Another remedy for this symptomology is *Pilocarpus jaborandi*. Lomatium was too warming.

Reproductive

When the liver is not fully active, breaking down hormones, Schizandra berry can turn the tide. It may have a direct influence on the hormones, since it is an adaptogen. It can be for sexual weakness or weakness from too strong a sex drive. It is probably a normalizer. Australian herbalist Bianca Patel reports that this berry has restored female libido "many times."

Research

Now let us turn to the research on Schizandra, which led to its use as an adaptogen. Russian medical researchers noted that hunters from the tribes in eastern Siberia, such as the Samoyeds, would chew on the berries to give themselves greater endurance while on the hunt. This led them to examine that plant for adaptogenic properties. The Chinese name also suggests wide-spectrum use such as we would associate with an adaptogen.

Donald Yance gives a thorough account of the modern research on Schizandra (2013, 579–83). He repeats the report that the fruit acids in the berry can act on the seeds and destroy the most important ingredient, the schizandrins. The account is quite valuable in other regards, but I asked David Winston about the fruit-acid problem and he said it was a translational error. At any rate, all adaptogenic research has been done on the seed with the berry eliminated because the researchers were looking for the active ingredient—the lignins. For this reason, the following list of indications is divided into "berry and seed" and "seed."

Specific Indications (berry and seed)

Mind agitated and scattered; anxiety, forgetfulness; insomnia, bad dreams; stress-induced palpitations and asthma; stuffiness, congestion, and constriction of the head; hyperactivity; colds (leaf tea); shallow breathing, coughs, weakness, wet phlegm, wheezing, asthma, chronic obstructive pulmonary disease; heart palpitations associated with nervousness, sleep apnea; normalizes blood pressure; frequent urination, urinary incontinence, impotence; vaginal discharge, excessive menstrual bleeding; low libido in women; menopausal night sweats; or other excessive perspiration.

Seed: Strengthens the response of the nervous system and body in general to stress; nervous depression and exhaustion; strengthens the senses; beneficial to eyesight; cardioprotective; normalizes stomach acid; improves gastric motility and secretion; protects the liver and rebuilds after damage from alcohol and drugs; lessens excess febrile reaction; low platelets (combine with *Ceanothus*); preventive and active against cancer (research collected in Yance 2013, 579).

Formulation

Reishi and Schizandra are a natural combination (Seán O'Donoghue). They are both what we could call "shaman remedies," supporting people who have strong spiritual drives and overextend themselves; also for collecting the thoughts and improving the application of the mind.

The taste of Schizandra is a bit nasty so I like to prepare it in cherry liqueur, which moderates the flavor and makes a cooling formula. It combines well with Hawthorn or Wild Cherry or cherry liquor. I have a further modification under Dragon Medicine.

Preparation

Schizandra berry decoction sweetened with honey improves the taste and is an effective medicine. This retains the warm property. Schizandra berry wine or tincture is best made in a sweet medium like brandy. The cool tea favors the kidneys, the wine may seek out the heart, while the warm tea would be more active on the skin and digestion. One can simply chew the dried berry.

℞ Oak ℘
(Quercus alba, Q. robur)

I wrote extensively about Oak in *The Book of Herbal Wisdom* (1997, 409–20). There is a lot of interesting material from homeopathy—from

Dr. Compton Burnett, who used Oak tincture in 25-drop doses—which I quoted. He gives a lot of case histories showing a successful treatment of alcoholism; I have seen this in practice too. Oak, the tree of integrity, re-establishes lost integrity but also teaches us not to try to "out-integrity" the issues of life. So, it "normalizes integrity"—what a great property!

The European Oak (*Q. robur*) is one of the Bach flower essences, though one can just as well use various Oak-bark tinctures in its place—in drop doses. The officinal Oak in North America is the White Oak (*Q. alba*). The Oak genus (*Quercus*) falls into two major subdivisions: the White Oaks and the Red. The former have blunt leaves, the latter have sharp. Any member of the White Oak–half of the genus can be used instead of the official *Q. alba*.

Dr. Bach said Oak was for people who fight on against adversity, never give up, but never succeed. This is for both a weakness of integrity and an overreliance on this trait—people who try to "out-integrity" the issues of life. It is also for those who lack integrity in some part of their life and fight the weakness on and on, without giving up or succeeding. Therefore, it is a remedy for drug addiction and addictions of other kinds.

After Susan had been thrown from a horse and injured, she had swollen blue-black veins all over her chest. This was a good indication for Oak. I gave her this remedy and she said: "I understand now. This is the remedy for knowing which battles you can win." That's Warrior Medicine. Slow-growing Oak may also be a Turtle Medicine.

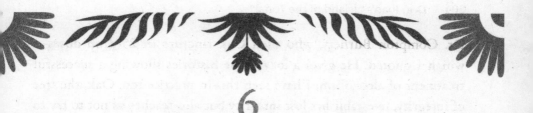

6

School for Shamans

The texture of the branches was so even—the leaves so thick and in that conspiring order—it was not a wood but a building. I conceived it indeed to be the Temple of Nature, where she had joined discipline to her doctrine.

THOMAS VAUGHAN

To understand a proverb and a figure, the words of the wise and their dark sayings.

PROVERBS 1:6

Having made our preparations for the journey, we are now ready for "shaman school." Our education falls into two distinct units: the outer teachings and the inner. The former are explanatory and informational; they are communicated by speech. The latter are internal and can only be learned directly from a teacher (person, plant, animal, stone, or other being) as an inner knowing, by empathy, dream, or descriptions of analogous experiences (example: the parables of Jesus). The reason we need an outside teacher is that we literally don't possess the hardwiring for this knowledge. We are "in the dark."

One way or another, the student finds their way to the kindergarten of shamans. How do we teach kindergarteners? Stories! So, this is the first instrument of instruction on the path. We have already touched on this subject several times, but it important enough to require a formal lesson. Rudolf Steiner explains (1922, 3):

> The first point in occult science is by no means the advancing of assertions or opinions which are to be proven, but the communication, in a purely narrative form, of experiences which are to be met with in the world other than the one that is to be seen with physical eyes and touched with physical hands.

On the shamanic path, one does not begin with dogmatic suppositions or assertions as in conventional medicine and science. One tells stories and describes personal experience in the hope that the student will resonate with them later on, when they have their own experiences.

Of course, there are exceptions to all rules. When we have seen mysteries that are not generally acknowledged in ordinary society, we often simply have to speak as if they were true. This was the case with William Blake. He lived in a time when essentially nobody understood his paradigm. He experienced the world of imagination as the real, the whole, and the true. Because he had no peers or students, except for a few young artists who were baffled by him but valued his eccentricities, Blake made assertions as if what he saw in his imagination was the whole and simple truth:

> I assert, for my self that I do not behold the outward creation, and that to me it is hindrance and not action. It is as the dirt upon my feet. No part of Me. "What!" it will be questiond, "When the sun rises, do you not see a round disk of fire somewhat like a guinea?" Oh, no, no! I see an innumerable company of the heavenly host, crying, "Holy, holy, holy is the Lord God Almighty!" I question not my corporeal or vegetative eye any more than I would question a window concerning a sight. I look through it, and not with it. (Blake 1982, 565–66; punctuation and capitalization modified)

This quotation comes from Blake's *A Vision of the Last Judgment*, in which he sets out a grand overview of numerous spiritual "states" or categories into which souls fall as a result of their relationship to the Spirit World. Indeed, the Last Judgment is a "Stupendous Vision," like a visionary hologram, which people see according to their spiritual position and the character of their vision (Blake 1982, 554).

Late in life, Blake made a few friends who were as eccentric as he, including the astrologer John Varley. This friend reported in his *Treatise on Zodiacal Physiognomy* (1823) about an experience he and Blake had one night. A tiny flea projected itself into a manlike image that, said Blake, "he never anticipated in an insect." He then drew a picture of the face and mouth, staring intently, as if it were modeling for him. When the flea changed position, Blake had to start over again. When he finished the drawing,

> the Flea told him that all Fleas were inhabited by the souls of such men as were by nature bloodthirsty to excess, and were therefore providentially confined to the size and form of fleas; otherwise, were he himself, for instance, the size of a horse, he would depopulate a great portion of the country. (Traill and Mann 1904, 5:xliii)

Later, the flea permitted Blake to draw his entire figure, resulting in a painting called *The Ghost of a Flea*. When Blake finished, Varley exclaimed that the flea was the exact image of a Gemini! I saw this painting at the Tate in London and, indeed, it did look like a Gemini. We're an irritating bunch.

The prominent shaman stories I am familiar with are the seven major stories in Genesis, the Higher Arcana of the tarot deck, and the Scotch ballads that teach us about the faery people. The Genesis stories also show up in Sufism and the Qur'an because they were originally a cycle of stories universal to the Middle East.

What the shamanic educator is trying to do is scatter images along the path so that they will bubble up to consciousness when the student has the analogous experience. The use of analogy is the basis of our language in every way. Herbs are analogies, too.

The Inner Court and the Outer

The outer teachings are those that can be conveyed by speech while the inner are those that can only by conveyed by empathic mind-link or in dreamtime. The former are associated with the reptiles because they don't dream and don't have a warm heart capable of empathy. The latter are associated with the warm-blooded animals, who do dream and possess a loving heart and the aptitude for empathy—as every pet owner knows. These have been called the Outer and Inner Courts of the Temple.

The Reptilian Lessons

Because they don't dream, the reptiles don't have direct contact with the Spirit World. But that does not mean that they cannot teach us valuable lessons. These, however, have to do with preparations that bring us closer to being able to cross over into the Spirit World. That means they are the exemplars of the lessons of the Outer Court. Also, because animal instincts first appeared in the reptiles, we inherit the instinct for truth from them. Because they don't directly reach the Spirit World in dream, they have to do it through the instinct for truth. They also have other faculties that direct one toward Paradise from the outside. In dreamtime we are on the inside.

The Genesis story is based on spiritual seership or imaginal read-outs of the spiritual history of the world. The serpent in the Tree represented the doorway out of Eden. This is actually the Dragon, the grandfather of all reptiles. After the incident in Eden, the karma for the Dragon, according to the narrative, was that it would have to crawl on its belly and eat dust. The oral historian who dictated the story was a master (or mistress, really) of verbal economy. She doesn't say it was a Dragon, but infers it through the curse—or karmic readout. On the one hand, the Dragon lost its limbs and wings to become Snake, in the outer world. On the other, the Dragon itself was exiled into the mineral realm of the Earth ("dust shall you eat all the rest of your days") because it had trapped human consciousness in the material plane and had to stay there with the humans it misdirected. We see this in Michael Harner's vision of the dragon-like creatures that claimed to be the progenitors of all life and the entire planet.

After the end of the dinosaur age, there were four basic kinds of reptiles—alligator/crocodiles, snakes, lizards, and turtles. They represent four paths back to the boundary of Eden. Because we can dream of the reptiles, in the end they can appear in dreamtime and they can operate as a person's familiar or animal spirit.

The cherubim that God set up to block the path back to Eden are the crocodiles. They are stationed outside the Garden. They entered the Hebrew reference system from the Egyptian pantheon and there is more information about them in Egypt than in the Hebrew Bible.

The Crocodile Lords of Death are in charge of the recapitulation of life experiences, which is demanded of the dead when they return from the theater of life in order to "give an account of themselves." The shamans have learned to recapitulate as a method to reduce luggage on their road back to the Spirit World. The alligators and crocodiles help us let go of everything that has happened from the beginning of time down to the present. This is the first method acquired from the reptilian life-wave for approaching the Spirit World.

The lizards are tricksters. The predator grabs the tail but loses the rest of the meal. "Ha ha, ya missed me!" says Lizard. Tricksters help us by teaching us not to take ourselves so seriously, by interjecting humor that reduces morbid seriousness. They help us get to places we would never otherwise have gone, because they can trick the dictator/clown/ego. The lizards help us to see all the things we would otherwise have missed on our path through life. Lizard provides the second reptilian lesson.

Snake is an example of de-evolution or non-evolution, since it regressed, losing its limbs. The consciousness of Snake is spiritual ambivalence. It doesn't care about moving forward on the evolutionary arc. It represents don Juan's "Worthy Opponent," a person who is lawless and tries to take advantage of us. In surviving what they do to us, we learn. This is the third reptilian lesson.

Snake is the guardian of the akashic records and the third eye that can read them, because no other animal can stand to embrace everything that has ever happened since the beginning of time to the present—the good, the bad, and the ugly. The akashic record is more detailed than we need, but it is representative of what we need to see in order to recapitulate.

Turtle stands on the boundary of the cold-blooded and the warm-blooded animals because it has some control over its internal temperature—by pressing its body against its shell it can squeeze out water to increase its internal temperature. Also, the female turtle can hang on to the fertilized eggs for two seasons, until weather conditions are right. This anticipates the warm-blooded animals, who mature the fetus within themselves. Turtle is getting close to the warm-blooded life-wave. It represents the path that brings us right to the boundary of Spirit World: the path of Nature Wisdom. It has reduced every experience from the beginning of time to the present into wisdom. So it finishes the reptilian lesson book.

The Dragons

Cursed to eat the dust of the Earth, Dragon, the ancestor of the reptilian life-wave, passed into the mineral realm. This is why we associate Dragons with treasures, minerals, gems, and metals in the earth. The reason for this was that the Dragons, having caused the exile of humanity from the Spirit World to the materiality of life on Earth, had to take responsibility for their action and remain as the Earth Spirit Dragons, Lords of the Mineral Realm. Not only that, but the Dragons thought of themselves as the true creators, because they had usurped the position of Creator ("Did God really say that?"). This shows up in Michael Harner's vision of the "dragonlike" creatures that claimed to be creators of the planet and all life upon it. They had to remain with their captives (ourselves) in the mineral realm.

The Dragons are our rulers, just as "the mold of man" (Adam) claims to be the True God and commands us to worship him. Both want to immerse us in the material element ("eat, drink, and be merry"). This represents the wedding of the two aspects that caused the rise of the human being as we are—product of the merger of the reptilian brain with human consciousness. The survival instinct merged with human self-awareness to create the self-centered ego, identification with the material world, separation from spiritual vision and dream (the "Tree of Life"), substituting man-made morality and logic (the "Tree of the Knowledge of Good and Evil").

The curse on the serpent or dragon goes on: "cursed art thou from among all cattle, and from among all beasts of the field." The other animals, at least the warm-blooded ones, are not cursed. This is why they still offer a path of return to the spirit land. They remain innocent of spiritual wrong, living their lives on Earth and then returning to join their Elders in the Spirit World; a path we too can take if we become conscious of our own animal self.

Two species fell in Eden: Human and Dragon. When we meet again in the depths of dreamtime, we are both freed from the necessity of staying forever submerged in the mineral realm. The soul becomes an immortal, Eden is restored to the physical-spiritual paradise it was supposed to be, and the hunger of the Dragons for true spiritual knowledge ("Did God really say that?") is fulfilled.

Nobody would ever believe that alternative reality is set up like this, or that we are so far away from the Spirit World that we can't even imagine it, or that Dragons are real, or rule over us. Nobody would knowingly seek these things and nobody could find them—unless the spirit cast upon them the fishing net of magical success. I could only see these things under the influence of coronavirus, which dramatically increased my DMT levels.

There is no virtue in believing any of this. The virtue is in storing the stories in the quilt-work of our memory, so that it is there when we pass through the resonant experience. Then the memory pops up—even deep in dreamtime—and reaffirms that we are on the path. Then we realize that the "shaman story" was true; not necessarily in contemporary human consciousness, but in eternal spiritual/visionary reality.

Alligator Ways

The alligator or crocodile grabs its prey and wrestles it underwater until it can no longer breathe, gives up resistance, and dies. This is analogous to what happens to the human soul after death. The Crocodile Lords of Death grab us and hold on to us until we stop struggling and we recapitulate everything that happened to us.

People that experience near-death report that their entire life flashes before them. According to folklore and esoteric teachings, the dead relive their lives, experiencing everything that was done to them and everything that they did to others. This is not a time for pity but for cold-blooded self-examination and self-understanding. The Lords of Death hold the dead without pity: "crocodile tears."

There are, therefore, three main lessons in the Alligator Way: *facing death without self-pity* ("using death as an advisor," as don Juan would say); *recapitulation* or reliving the experiences of life so as not to be unconsciously controlled by them; and familiarity with the terrible (but useful) *place of no pity*.

The gentle Quaker botanist William Bartram gives us some idea of how terrifying "death by Alligator" would be (1955, 115–17):

Behold him rushing forth from the flags and reeds. His enormous body swells. His plaited tail brandished high, floats upon the lake. The water like a cataract descends from his opening jaw. Clouds of smoke issue from his dilated nostrils. The earth trembles with his thunder. When immediately from the opposite coast of the lagoon, emerges from the deep his rival champion. They suddenly dart upon each other. The boiling surface of the lake marks their rapid course, and a terrific conflict commences. They now sink to the bottom of the lake folded together in horrid wreaths. The water becomes thick and discolored. Again they rise, their jaws clap together, re-echoing through the deep surrounding forests.

Suddenly, Bartram became aware that he was in a dangerous spot:

My apprehensions were highly alarmed after being a spectator of so dreadful a battle. It was obvious that every delay would but tend to increase my danger and difficulties, as the sun was near setting, and the alligators gathering around my harbor from all quarters.

He gets into his boat to try to get to a safer place:

On board, penetrating the first line of those which surrounded my harbor, they gave way; but being pursued by several very large ones, I kept strictly on the watch, and paddled with all my might towards the entrance of the lagoon, hoping to be sheltered there from the multitude of my assailants; but ere I had halfway reached the place, I was attacked on all sides, several endeavoring to overset the canoe. My situation now became perilous to the last degree: two very large ones attacked me closely, at the same instant, rushing up with their heads and part of their bodies above the water, roaring terribly and belching floods of water over me. They struck their jaws together so close to my ears, as almost to stun me, and I expected every moment to be dragged out of the boat and instantly devoured.

This went on in various iterations for the rest of the evening and through an uneasy night with more terrifying reptilian adventures the next morning. At one point, Bartram apologizes to the reader that his account will seem too incredible to be believed. Every once in a while, he stops to catalog the plants and flowers he observed during breaks from the excitement.

Death as an Advisor

Alligator Medicine teaches us not to fear death but also not to forget that we are mortal. We should not waste our precious time while we are sojourning here on Earth, which is itself a precious resource that is being squandered left and right as I write. We should use that time, when we have free will—hard wrought by Adam and Eve—to grow spiritually. Instead, so many people are time- and space-wasters, living a riotous life of self-enjoyment using the Earth's resources.

A chief characteristic of the shaman is the association with death. The shaman is defined as someone who has died and come back to life. A visit to the Land of the Dead is as innate to the shamanic calling as citizenship in the Living Nature is innate to animism. The two are opposite sides of the same coin, Life and Death. The ancient Mayans left us their hieroglyphic descriptions of the "womb-tomb" of the Great Mother (Gillette 1997, 107).

Shamans often work with the dead and the relationship of the living with the dead. What, therefore, do the shamans have to say about the dead, the Land of the Dead, the Lords of the Dead, and the processes of dying and death?

This is a huge subject and we cannot give an answer that reflects all shamans or societies since there are bound to be differences of opinion and experience in a discipline that is so widespread. I think, however, that most shamans would agree with the following basic precept: *If people really understood what awaits them in the afterlife, they would be ready to put down their toys and adopt the way of the warrior, the recapitulation, and suffer no pity as much as necessary.*

This is the essential work necessary for becoming a true shaman—though the work is still outside the Inner Court.

A lot of modern writers avoid descriptions of the afterworld because of a widespread dislike for the pictures of heaven and hell with heavy moral overtones that originated in the Church. Another bunch of writers just want to avoid such a morbid subject. There are also cultural differences. The Indian People from North America don't generally like to discuss this subject. On the other hand, the Day of the Dead is quite important in Mexican folk culture. The ancient Meso-American Indians were immersed in death. The ruler of the land was the shaman king, represented by the Black Jaguar, the totem of the Lord of the Underworld.

The North American Indians generally had a more cheerful outlook on life after death. The botanist William Bartram, "of the tribe of white men, of Pennsylvania," the Quakers, "who esteem themselves brothers and friends to the red men," wrote in 1791 (1955, 391):

> They believe in a future state, where the spirit exists, which they call of the world of spirits, where they enjoy different degrees of tranquility or comfort, agreeably to their life spent here: a person who in his life has been an industrious hunter, provided well for this family, an intrepid and active warrior, just, upright, and done all the good he could, will, they say, in the world of spirits, live in a warm, pleasant country, where are expansive green, flowery savannas and high forests, watered with rivers of pure waters, replenished with deer, and every species of game; a serene, unclouded and peaceful sky; in short, where there is fulness of pleasure uninterrupted.

Colonel Ely Parker, the Seneca secretary for Ulysses S. Grant, looked upon the Christian heaven as a place where the Indian would be freed from the presence of the white man.

There is also the "tell it like it is" theory of "death education." One modern shamanic author who describes her visit to the Land of the Dead is Olga Kharitidi in *Master of Lucid Dreams* (2001). Her mentor in dreaming brought her to that realm. She observed what happened to the dead on the levels of sensation, emotion, and thought. The connection to physical sensation does not automatically end after the death of the physical body. She describes places where sensation is extracted from body parts in tremendous pain because of the attachment to the body the living had during life on Earth. How much more so is the psychological suffering, as the dead slowly give up their attachments to what they loved (or hated) during life. Everyone must relive and let go of their life experiences, or they will get stuck and suffer their personal, egoic attachments endlessly. The dismemberment of the life force and soul is called the "second death" in occultism.

There are several ways in which people can get stuck going through the recapitulation of the afterlife. Many people did not believe in the afterlife while they were alive. For these people, the only solution is the obliteration of the soul. Dr. Kharitidi describes how these souls dissolved forever in the "Lake of Oblivion." No selfhood remains: there will be no reincarnation or existence in the community of souls. Kharitidi realized that it was a act of mercy for these souls; otherwise they would flounder forever in delusion. Her mentor was careful to make sure she did not touch the Lake of Oblivion.

My friend Peter had extensive personal experience with the "Lake of Oblivion." He had HIV AIDS and for six years he wasn't sure if he would wake up when he went to bed every night. He was involved in a prayer group for those with HIV and their partners. Because he had gifts of spiritual seership (and was close to death himself), many times he observed that when a person died who did not believe in the afterlife, they would be dissolved into nothingness in the Lake. Meanwhile, the surviving partner poured their love after them, only to have it dissolve in the abyss, leaving them truly bereft.

The reverse is also true: the love of a partner, relative, or friend can save the dead from dissolution by maintaining the bond of affection. If the deceased person places more energy in that bond than in disbelief in the afterlife, the orientation can change. The living, since they still have free will, can help the dead. In William Blake's picture of souls rising to eternal life in *A Vision of the Last Judgment*, he reserved a place for true lovers who could never be parted. Peter lived for another thirty years (he's not dead yet). After his partner died, he was rewarded with a vision of him waving from the other world.

The novelist Isaac Bachevis Singer said in a lecture I attended when young: "I have seen people on their deathbed, with minutes to live, still yearning for true love." Hopefully, there is an answer for all.

Sadly, the living can be dragged down into death by the dead that they still love. When the teenage stepson of a friend committed suicide, he had a terrible time letting go. I dreamed of the son going down a chute, way, way down into the Land of the Dead. A force then tugged on my friend's feet, trying to yank him down into that world. I warned him. He had a good doctor at the VA; she told him: "This kind of loss often kills a person." One day my friend called me from the park near his house. After a while he said he had a gun in his hand. I didn't know it until he decided not to shoot himself: I guess I talked him into living. I'm an herbalist, not a counselor, but he must have listened. He was a drunk for another five years, but eventually he pulled himself out of that morass too.

A lot of us would like to stay with our loved ones after death, but ultimately, for many, there will be a separation. Only those with a genuine spiritual connection will remain in contact. A. S. Raleigh explained (1932, 17):

> The spirit transcends the personality, and all human relationships are part of the personality. They pertain to the personal plane. The individuality is related to none save those who are of the same Purusha, so to speak; save kindred souls or kindred spirits, and death does not materially affect them.

Some people have hurt others so badly they can't stand to recapitulate the pain they would have to experience, or they want to identify with their ego rather than their spirit. Although they are conscious in the next world, they cannot join the collective world of souls, the Soul World. As Emmanuel Swedenborg related in his account of heaven and hell, it is actually painful for these souls to experience the love that binds together the healthy, intact Soul World, so they have to separate. These people identify with their egos and become the "hungry ghosts" that live in the Outer Darkness.

For the worst of the worst, the *atma* itself will be dissolved in the Abyss of Nothingness. These people did not just commit their conscious self, biological self, and soul, to selfish pursuits that hurt others. They grabbed ahold of the will of their spirit and applied its unbending power to their horrific deeds. So even the primal atom of the spirit, the *atma* itself, has to be dissolved in the Abyss of Nothingness. Perhaps this happens to all who wander as hungry ghosts in the Outer Darkness. I don't know; I only saw it one time.

A lot of mystics seek to dissolve themselves into the cosmic Nothingness. This is a spiritual delusion. As long as we are willing ourselves to go anywhere, including Nothingness, we are acting out of Somethingness. Beyond being a delusion, this is an act of rebellion against the creation itself and Creator who made it, as if the creation itself were a bad thing and their individuality was also bad. This is just more eating from the fruit of the Tree of the Knowledge of Good and Evil—moralizing against creation and Creator, like the Gnostics of old, who thought Creator was evil.

The coils of the Great Serpent or Dragon curl around the Abyss of Nothingness. The Bible speaks derisively of this particular Dragon, but someone has to take out the garbage. It is not the fault of the Dragon of the Abyss if people need to be dissolved down there. Those reptiles get around a lot in the regions of the dead.

In the afterlife, a person has the opportunity to face their inner demons, overcome their challenges, preserve their individuality, and side with the spirit. Of course, we have to have made a habit of this during life because in death we have no other will than that which we bring from life.

The only parts of the soul that survive the recapitulation of death are those where the soul merged with the spirit. This would be the soul that listened to the whispering of the spirit in a greater or lesser degree. "Gurdjieff is emphatic in his assertion that man who does not fulfill his cosmic duties by his own 'conscious labors and intentional sufferings' loses his immortal soul and after death is destroyed forever" (Bennett 1976, 211).

In the dissolution of the afterlife, even the ego ends up having a role. In life it was associated with decision-making and it therefore contains a record of all the decisions—or movements of the assemblage point—during life. In the afterlife it remains as the *shade*, which contains a record of all that occurred during life. In this sense the ego is eternal too, but only as a voiceless, will-less, immobilized relic in the labyrinthian halls of the cosmic library of the Underworld. Here everything that ever happened in time and space is recorded in all its tedious detail. If there were no such record, it would be impossible to maintain integrity in the worlds of time and space. The Creator would be irresponsible if he had not created a mechanism for cause and effect in time and space. The laws of karma and cosmic recordkeeping are built into creation.

If the soul never touched the spirit, the shade would be so boring that nobody would ever want to read the record it left behind. And if it were positively hurtful to others, other people would be repelled by it. But if it were inspiring, remarkable, and unique—reflecting real individuality—it would be like a library book that people would want to seek out and read. So, even in its dark, forgotten eternity, the shade may have visitors—or not.

Witches in dreamtime often use death to destroy their victims. Witches from a reservation in northern Minnesota attached death to my energy body one time. My friend Sondra had to spent an hour and a half getting the curse off. At the beginning of the second hour, I saw and felt death—it looked to me like an enormous raptor-headed man in my imagination. So I thank those worthy opponents for letting me see death so clearly. "Funny," said Sondra, "those witches spoke English, so I had to do the whole ceremony in Tsalagi (Cherokee)."

Those witches don't fool around. I had a friend up on that rez who was attacked by the same set of witches because she was interested in herbal medicine. They threatened her. When she didn't pay attention, they came to her house, hung her from the ceiling of her living room, and left her body there for her children to discover when they came home from grade school. The tribal police were famously corrupt—one Minneapolis newspaper called it the "last banana republic in North America"; they ruled it a suicide.

A century before, this same reservation had numerous serious, careful, well-trained practitioners of herbalism and medicine. This was recorded by ethnobotanist Francis Densmore in 1919. Federal education and healthcare displaced these practitioners. The motto of the Bureau of Indian Affairs was "destroy the Indian to make the man." They destroyed all healing knowledge and authority, all community goodness, that didn't come from the government and the white man's way.

As the healers died out, the witches took over—or were the only ones left with the plant knowledge.

One of my most important teachers of Indian Medicine was a witch—He Who Must Not Be Named. I had to overlook his true orientation, but eventually we went our separate ways. We were herbal brothers though, and he learned a lot from me while I learned from him. "I never learned so much about Indian Medicine since I left home as I have from Matthew," he said to one of our friends.

On the shamanic path, we learn from whoever has the similar energetic temperament, not from who is "good" or "bad." Anyway, we are not to judge and do not know the outcomes for our fellow beings. He also had a love for helping people and in the afterlife I believe the love of others has come back to help him.

Someone once asked this teacher why he used the word "witch" in a pejorative fashion. "You have to understand," he replied. "In your language you only have one word for witch. In my language we have twenty-two."

Because adults are more resistant to psychic manipulation, the witches try to kill the children in the family—or the curses will roll off the parents onto the kids. Witches will even kill children and adults, including their own family members, as they try to expand and clear their psychic field of play. They are often kicked out of the community for its own protection.

A friend who grew up on an Apache reservation told how, during a tribal election that occurred when he was seven, he was warned to be careful and not to venture far from the house. One day he heard a puppy whimpering in the desert. He went to investigate. No matter how far he walked, the sound was always further away. Suddenly he realized with a chill that something was not right. Fortunately, he was able to find his way back to the house. He was greeted with the combination of weeping and remonstrances that a beloved child who has not followed directions will receive.

One of my friends was not so lucky. He liked to go about helping people on several reservations. One of his children, in the bloom of health, died in his sleep. The medicine man explained: "The curses were sent to you, but you are strong; so they rolled off onto your son. This is why I myself no longer live on the reservation."

For the dominant culture, witches are nothing more than fantasies, but in the Indian world they are taken seriously. After the Zunis signed a treaty with the federal government, a group of elders visited Salem, Massachusetts, to congratulate the leaders there for their effective action in combating witchcraft in the community (Jenkins 2004, 31).

We are not allowed to interfere with the will of another being, but if they inflict upon us or a loved one, we have the right to hold their hand to the fire until they let go. This is what Alligator Medicine does: it grabs the prey, wrestles it underwater, and holds on to it until it stops fighting. That is the medicine of the place of no pity.

In his interactions with his literary hero, the poet John Milton, Blake reported that the unfulfilled soul of the great Puritan poet announced his return to Earth so that the unredeemed, misunderstood parts of himself (particularly his relationships with women and sex) could be relived to free himself from these mistakes. Blake considered the deceased Milton to be his artistic mentor, just as Dante's mentor was Virgil, one of the great poets, though a pagan.

"I will go down to self-annihilation and eternal death, lest the Last Judgment come & find me unannihilate," Milton explained to Blake. "And I be siez'd & giv'n into the hands of my own Selfhood." The "annihilation and eternal death" of Milton's "Selfhood" resulted in the "Human Form" of Milton appearing in Blake's garden at his cottage in Felpham, "clothed in black, severe & silent." Strangely, Blake and don Juan use the exact same term for the part of a person that resists the flexibility necessary to process the experiences of life: the human form. Finally, reports Blake, Milton and his female parts are brought together in harmony. The Twenty-Four Cathedral Cities of Albion (Britain) are reawakened to their spiritual tasks, Jesus (the Divine Human Imagination) enters the bosom of Albion (fallen humanity), Blake falls unconscious in his garden and awakens to find "my sweet Shadow of Delight," Mrs. Blake, leaning over him (Blake 1982, 108, 138, 143).

The Recapitulation

Blake was helping Milton "recapitulate" his life experiences. Instead of waiting for the winnowing floor of the Underworld after death, the shamanic candidate recapitulates his or her life while still living, getting rid of illusions and complexes that take psychic energy to keep in place. This frees up energy to seek new goals—the actualization of the spirit being the great goal. It also provides a recapitulation for the Lords of Death, so that they are satisfied when the shamanic candidate appears before them. Most importantly, it is down in the Underworld that the shaman is able to find his or her animal self. That is the goal of the shaman and when this event has occurred, he or she is no longer a candidate or seeker but a baby shaman. Finally, it allows the shaman to be able to help another soul, or souls, and it appears that this is what Blake was doing for Milton.

A full recapitulation touches upon all experiences that left a powerful impression upon the soul. The tape of the experience keeps repeating until it is fully relived and released. It is stuck in this vicious circle until the candidate lays their consciousness upon the matter, feels it in its entirety, and finally can let it go. Recapitulation in waking hours is excellent; in dream, even more ideal.

One night I woke up out of a deep sleep suffering a bout of tachycardia, the first time I had ever experienced that in my life and—for many years—the only time. I was simultaneously aware of some deep feelings. As I lay quietly, they were clarified. When I was two years old, my parents left the only home I had ever known, Ocmulgee village on the Big Cypress Seminole Reservation in the Florida Everglades. I understand Muskogee and English enough to function in daily life, but not enough to grasp an abstract idea like leaving the only home I ever knew. I couldn't imagine such a thing. So it couldn't be explained to me where we were going, or for how long. The life that was all I had ever known just disappeared and I evidently suffered some anguish and confusion and—as the dream made clear—deep mourning for the loss of my home. This was an *event I could not possibly have recollected consciously so it needed to be recalled in dreamtime.*

The average person holds off the recapitulation until after physical death. They want to live and relive the pleasures of the soul and body without having to give them up. However late in life, the recapitulation may start spontaneously. Old folks ponder their lives and are better at giving up attachments than young ones. They are already getting a head start on life after death. People who die in midlife have a much harder time with the afterlife because they were set on many goals or had attachments they weren't planning on giving up. The attachments of children shouldn't run very deep so they are recapitulated more painlessly in the afterlife.

It would seem like recapitulating the diverse experiences of a lifetime would be like a haystack of feelings that would be impossible to analyze. Fortunately, life experiences fall into spiritual "States," as Blake calls them—basic categories. While we could subdivide in great detail, the number seven would be enough. That is why there are seven rungs on the shaman's ladder, seven directions in Native American spirituality, in Ezekiel's chariot, the Throne of God in the *Book of Revelations,* Jacob Boehme's vision of Creator and creation, or the Merkabah of Jewish mysticism. This is what Blake called a "Stupendous Vision" (1982, 554).

Douglas Gillette gives a description from the ancient Mayan standpoint (1997, 40):

These great "star gates" lay at either end of the World Tree/Vision Serpent—one at its foot in the southern sky and the other in its branches in the far north. The southern portal was the White-Bone/Black Transformer/Blacking Dreaming Place, the entrance to the Underworld. The north portal the Maya called the 01 Portal. This was the portal through which the souls of newborn babies enter the earth plane from the Otherworld.

We have to "give the Lords of Death what they want," recounting our life, releasing our attachments, yet retaining for ourselves the pith of our experiences. Here's a warrior story that describes giving them what they want:

My grandfather was Secretary of the War Resisters League during World War Two—that would make him the opponent of the Secretary of War in the U.S. government. He told this story about a war resister from the Vietnam era. A young soldier decided that he opposed the war and didn't want to participate in it. One day his sergeant noticed that he was limping and sent him to the doctor, but he couldn't find anything wrong. The young soldier was cheerful, but continued to limp. Then his commanding officer noticed and sent him to the doctor. Still nothing showed up. Still cheerful, still limping. Then the commander of the base noticed and sent him to the doctor. "Well, I can't find anything wrong with you," said the doctor, "but I'm going to have to give you a medical discharge because we can't have a limping soldier." As he left the camp, he walked without a limp.

Another medicine animal that personifies recapitulation is the noble Salmon. She returns to the water where she was born—from the ocean where she has lived. She traces her exact route, past every rock and waterfall, past angelica stalks, reeds, tree roots, upstream to the quiet headwaters of her creation. Here her species is reborn. In Celtic lore, Salmon represents wisdom, in particular the wisdom of self-knowledge derived from the recapitulation.

The Place of No Pity

There are some pretty hard lessons on the shamanic path. These have great value if they do not destroy the aspirant. On the path of the spiritual warrior, one cannot indulge oneself in self-pity. Ultimately, one has to give all of that up. Therefore we learn to use the "place of no pity" (another don Juanism).

This is something we can apply to ourselves, but not to others without their consent—that would be cruelty. On the other hand, if someone violates our inner space, we have the right to exert no pity upon them in order to get them to leave our energy field alone. One can hold them in the place of no pity until they let go. The same result can be accomplished a lot less expensively by shifting to the focal point of the human spirit. This only works when both the "victim" and the "perpetrator" are willing to forgive. The place of no pity is like the stick, while the human spirit is like the carrot.

Théun Mares makes a very important point. If one is not talented at "seeing" (sensing with the energy body), one can instead use the place of no pity to isolate truth: it forces us to see the truth. The reptiles are associated with the place of no pity and the instinct for truth. Sensing with the energy body and dreaming release problems with less suffering.

The cold-blooded reptiles do not dream, so their address lies outside dreamtime. Yet, they too are creatures of God and therefore, they have the ability to determine truth from falsehood. The warm-blooded animals (including humans) experience the truth of the Spirit World directly through direct bonding with it, but the reptiles have to experience truth indirectly. They do this through the place of no pity. But no human would want to live there with them permanently because we are warm-blooded animals with a warm heart. The place of no pity is, in one sense, the afterlife state that requires the death of all attachments; for those who can't give up their attachments, it is the Outer Darkness.

⊙ ALLIGATOR MEDICINE ⊙

Is there any good that comes out of Alligator Medicine for the individual in the human world? Deer Medicine gives grace, Badger and Bear Medicine toughness. Seminole chief James Billie says in his song "Big Alligator" (1996), Alligator Medicine gives prosperity.

Jim Billie was one of my father's students in 1955—he's a few years older than me. Later he became chief of the Seminole tribe and ushered in a huge prosperity for the tribe—one of my friends estimated that they own about 40% of downtown Miami. The opposite of the place of no pity is the land of milk and honey. I don't know how that gift works, but the spirits told me never to worry about money and I never have, despite being an herbalist.

I only know two Alligator Medicines: Teasel and Burdock. We can tell by looking at the leaf—it is like alligator skin. This is true for Burdock only in the early spring and it is not as strong as Teasel. Alligator Medicine re-establishes the "blueprint of health" in those who have forgotten what health feels like, psychologically or physically.

The leaves of Teasel have warty or horny knobs that look like the scales and blotches on the back of an alligator. Imagine my surprise when I looked up Teasel in Dioscorides, the ancient Greek herbal, and found that he knew it as "Crocodilion." Teasel also looks kind of skeletal.

☙ Teasel ❧
(*Dipsacus sylvestris, D. fullonum*)

This giant "thistle" was long supposed to be akin to the aster family, which includes the true thistles. However, recent work on the genome has shown that it is a member of the Honeysuckle family. Surprise! Shock! Crazy!

Signatures

The "thistle" on the top of the stalk looks like a comb and has been used to "tease" the wool—straighten the fibers. The thistle top has led to the names "Wolf's Comb" and "Venus's Comb." This reminds us of the Lords of Death, teasing the lessons out of the tangle of life experiences.

This thistle looks like a tick biting into the skin, so that we are tipped off that it is a remedy for tick-borne illnesses; it is virtually a specific for many people with borreliosis, or Lyme disease proper.

I always imagined the comb shifting through muscle fibers, straightening them out; Teasel is a tremendous remedy for scar tissue as well as bringing spirochetes out of the muscles and tissues into the blood where the immune cells can kill them. If we put the plant on good soil or care for it, it will grow to nine or ten feet in height and in this form it reminds me of a skeleton hanging on a stand, in an old-time medical school, looking down at me very seriously, as if to say: "What are you doing with your life, young person?" It has a very saturnine presence. Such a boney appearance associates this plant also with the shade, death, and the Underworld. Teasel combines well with Solomon's Seal, which smells like burnt bones.

Teasel has prominent joints, like a Wolf Medicine. The leaves are joined across the stem, like Boneset, so this is a bone-healing signature—the Chinese name translates as "To Restore What is Broken." The way the leaves join around the stem is a kidney signature, since they hold water. It is said in Chinese herbalism that the bones are an extrusion of the kidneys, and Teasel (*Dipsacus japonica*) repairs the bones and joints by strengthening the "kidney jing" (essence) and the "liver blood" that nourishes the muscles. Teasel acts more deeply than the bones, per se; it acts on the essence. That conforms to the idea of Alligator Medicine. It is amazing how these traditions support each other.

The water that collects and is exuded into the pockets by the leaves is another signature for the "kidney essence"—the kidneys hold the primal water. This water is slimy, like the biofilms that form when there is too much moisture; it is likely that Teasel breaks through biofilms that reinforce the entangled fibers.

Recapitulation

Teasel is the medicine of recapitulation. On the physical level it "guards the blueprint of life," helping the body "remember what it was like to be healthy." Both Burdock and Teasel have this property and both have been used for syphilis and Lyme disease (which destroys the blueprint). Another remedy that protects the blueprint is homeopathic Mercury (*Mercurius vivus*). The old alchemical works equate a Reptilian Monster with Mercury. Our genetic material needs to be ruling in our bodies in a healthy way during life, but we have to go beyond the howling power of the genes to discover our spiritual source material.

Honeysuckle (*Lonicera* spp.) was Dr. Bach's remedy for being stuck in the past, but its cousin Teasel pulls us through the past. I know of no other medicine that causes the body to so fully relive its body memories.

Healing from Pain

Not only does Teasel help us recapitulate but it comforts us as we live or relive the unpleasant experiences of life on Earth. When I was taking a class with the late Margaret Colquahoun at Pishwanton, a center for Goethean studies in Scotland—near the home of Thomas the Rhymer—we did a plant attunement with Teasel.

According to tradition, the water in the "cups" that the leaves form around the stems is supposed to aid the eyes. I put the water on my eyes and lay down. Teasel said to me: "Your eyes have seen many terrible things"—meaning the sights I have seen during my sojourn on Earth—"I will soothe them so that these sights will not be so painful for you."

I learned from this that the recapitulation can relieve us of memories that cause suffering or pain. So the place of no pity can take away suffering as well as bring it on.

Rudolf Steiner and Dorothy Hall taught that sharp points on plants indicate the presence of silicon—the sharpest of all the elements. This makes silicon an "externalizing" agent that cuts away the "underbrush" (old polymers and biofilms) to move debris to the surface. This property is found in Teasel: it will draw or push complex splinters, shrapnel, objects, and so forth out of the flesh when used either internally or externally.

Dosage

Teasel is a powerful plant; 1–3 drops is a sufficient dose in Lyme disease, but one can use "cowboy doses." It causes a person to relive the symptoms and that can be a bit forbidding.* I believe this plant would make a good addition to many formulations where the blueprint of health needs remembrance.

---

*See the accounts in my *The Book of Herbal Wisdom* (1997, 233–41) and the chapter on Teasel in Wolf-Dieter Storl's *Healing Lyme Disease Naturally* (2010, 163–82).

Snake Ways

Snake lives inside of us as the kundalini, the magnetic power in the nervous system that favors egotism, selfishness, and sensory addiction through the combination of the survival and reproduction instincts of the reptilian brain and the human frontal brain. Sometimes the reptilian brain has to interrupt the internal dialogue of the human brain and let us know about dangers. Ironically, one of the dangers that triggers this response is seeing a snake!

The Worthy Opponent

This is a term introduced by don Juan; one among the many that this Native genius introduced into our vocabulary through the intermediary of his apprentice, Carlos Castaneda. People who are stuck on whether don Juan was "real" or not miss the point: the teachings are real.

The traditional symbol of the Snake's hold over us in Western mythology is the ouroboros, or snake biting its tail. This represents the self-consuming, contractive, limiting world we live within. It is similar to the Wheel of Dharma symbol of Indian mythology. Until we birth our animal self, we live under the power of the circular serpent. When we see our animal self for the first time in dreamtime, the curse and imprisonment by the ouroboros is broken.

As the party responsible for the start of the self-conscious dimension of human experience, Snake helped initiate the "beginning of time" and is responsible for all the experience that has occurred from the beginning down to the present: the good, the bad, and the ugly. The instigator must assume responsibility. But, of course, Snake is the perfect receptacle for this material because he *is* ambivalent about good and evil, pain and suffering, truth and falsehood. By comparison, Turtle distills wisdom distilled from all the experiences of life, from the beginning of time down to now. Pardon me if I'd rather be friends with Turtle!

Snake is *completely flexible*, able to move its body in almost any direction. This is the signature for ambivalence. Snake can adapt to any shape, any philosophy, any truth. This makes Snake "protean," or capable of continual change and adaptation.

Humanity and the serpent are not friends. The conscious self created by the conjunction of the reptilian brain with the higher cortex is jealous of the power of serpent power, which resides in the sensory organs, survival instincts, genitals, and spine. It wants total control; it does not want to be immersed in the senses and unconsciousness of the reptilian brain.

> I will put hate between you and the woman. Between your seed and her seed. He will strike you on the head, and you will strike him on the heel. (Genesis 3:15)

This is a perfect metaphor: humans and snakes threaten each other and the threat is instinctual. But this also represents the fight within us: the conflict between the conscious self and the unconscious reptilian forces of survival, reproduction, and sensation. Blake named the two forces Urizen ("you reason") and Orc, the energy of life and instinct. Eventually, Orc is so beaten down by Urizen that he assumes the voice of reason and becomes the enticing Snake itself.

Christians, who think they can take anything in the Hebrew Bible and treat it as if they understood it and it belonged to them, identify the seed of the woman with Christ and the seed of the serpent with Satan. But the dichotomy between the seed of the woman and the seed of the serpent is a description of the everlasting fight between the conscious self and the reptilian self—both of which are found in our brain. The Wheel of Dharma, which turns endlessly, binds us to a polarized world of made-up good and evil.

The staff of Ascelpius, the caduceus—a green leafy staff with a snake (sometimes two) intertwined up the staff—represents the kundalini or serpent power in the central nervous system—the vehicle of consciousness and the "Tree of Experience of Good and Evil." This therefore is a symbol of disease and healing—it is the staff of Asclepius and the symbol of the medical world down to the present day. It is also a symbol of our entrapment in the world of karma, but of our potential to be cured of this enslavement.

We hear a lot about "raising the kundalini." This means letting the kundalini rise from the lowest chakra (genitals) to the crown chakra (pineal). This brings to consciousness all significant psychoenergetic contents encased in the body memory of the person, so that they automatically recapitulate everything. For some people, raising the kundalini recapitulates all information from all lifetimes, since Snake is the storage container for all karma. For some, the confrontation with all their addictions and complexes destroys the body or the balance of the mind.

Raising the kundalini sounds very good from the standpoint of psychological self-development, but it must be remembered that Snake is our slave keeper and raising the kundalini does not free us from the Snake or our exile from the Spirit World. It is a deceptive "spiritual event." When Snake raises the kundalini it goes up over the top of the head to the third eye and opens the perception of the psyhic worlds, since Snake is tied to the akashic records. With Turtle, on the other hand, the kundalini goes past the third eye, down to the throat and actualizes the animal self, because the throat is the boundary between the human and the animal. We can expect this from the "main stem" of the warm-blooded animal life-wave. The teachings of Grandfather Turtle are the basis of the Grand Medicine Society of the Anishinabe Ojibwa.

Apologists for Snake usually point to the shedding of the skin as a symbol of death and rebirth. Yes, it is—but this is the unending death and rebirth of the human race stuck in the post-Edenic world. We die in unconsciousness, our ego is annihilated in the afterlife process, and our materials are mixed with those of other unconscious souls and reborn as another unconscious human soul. This is the "Wheel of Dharma": ongoing meaningless lives that do not reach up out of the world to become eternal. The "shedding of skin" is just a metaphor for this meaningless peregrination from life to death to life.

At the end of the day, it looks like Snake is not good for anything, but this is not true either. The medicine of Snake opens the "third eye" of clairvoyant vision, including access to the library of karma and past lives. This, however, is not innately good or bad. It simply is. If we can see into the karma and past lives of people, we can see the origins of their problems, *but we cannot necessarily see their solutions* because Snake does not arise above the Wheel of Dharma. Even this gift of Snake is ambivalent. The sights we see in clairvoyance can also be fascinating and entrapping.

The "gift" of an open "third eye" is the gift of Snake, but it is ambivalent. It was symbolized by the serpent over the brow in the headdresses of the Egyptian pharaohs. As in ancient Mexico, with their shaman kings, the Egyptian pharaohs were not just temporal rulers, but originally they were also spiritual "initiates." Imagine having a ruler that could see everything going on throughout the kingdom.

The ultimate gift of Snake is the lesson of the Worthy Opponent: we lazy humans need to be stimulated in order to accomplish anything on the spiritual path, and that is the job of Snake—to oppose, hurt, trick, mislead, mesmerize, and seduce.

The American Rattlesnake is terrifying in appearance but not terrible in aggressiveness, seldom striking "until he is first assaulted or fears himself in danger," as William Bartram wrote in the eighteenth century. He adds (1955, 222):

> But if you pursue and overtake him with a show of enmity, he instantly throws himself into the spiral coil; his tail by the rapidity of its motion appears like a vapor, making a quick tremulous sound; his whole body swells through rage, continually rising and falling as a bellows; his beautiful parti-colored skin becomes speckled and rough by dilatation; his head and neck are flattened, his checks swollen and his lips constricted, discovering his mortal fangs; his eye red as burning coals, and his brandishing forked tongue of the color of the hottest flame, [he] continually menaces death and destruction, yet never strikes unless sure of his mark.

The Creek are very cautious in their dealings with rattlesnakes, notes Bartram. They would not kill them if it could at all be avoided, believing that the spirit and relatives of the snake would cause them trouble. An illustration of this belief still extending to the present, and its manifestation in her family, occurs in Phyllis Light's *Southern Folk Medicine* (2018, 4).

❂ SNAKE MEDICINE ❂

There are a lot of "Snake Medicines" all around the world: plants that resemble a snake are usually used as snakebite antidotes. The best of these, in my opinion, for journeying and medicine, among the North American snake remedies, is Black Cohosh or Black Snake Root (*Actaea racemosa, Cimicifuga racemosa*). It is an old American Indian female remedy and snakebite antidote. The long flower stalk looks like a spine or a snake, while the black, tangled roots look like a writhing pit of snakes. Other Snake Roots of North America include Senega (*Polygala senega*), Virginia (*Aristolochia serpentaria*), Canada (*Asarum canadensis*), Kansas (*Echinacea* spp.), Button or Corn Snake Root (*Liatris* spp.), Rattlesnake Master (*Eryngium yuccafolium*), Snakeweed (*Plantago major*), and Rattlesnake Plantain (*Goodyeara* spp.).

☙ Black Cohosh ❧
(*Actaea racemosa*)

This plant is not seductive, like some of the Snake Medicines and the Nightshades. It possesses a real internal integrity, so it can attune one to serpent power, the kundalini, without sacrificing integrity. It is a nerve and spinal remedy so it interacts with kundalini.

The "Black Cohosh person" is highly aware of inner dimensions of the soul. One of my clients described herself as a "psychic/intuitive trans-medium," in other words, someone who picks up on other people's feelings and has an intuitive sense for how the hidden dimension of the soul works through love and wisdom. The Black Cohosh person, usually a woman, is highly aware of the depth of the soul and seeks deep relationships. For this reason, she has deep romantic connections that are difficult to disengage when the time comes to end them. All those psychic fibers leave a person "tangled up in blue." Black Cohosh helps to free that energy up and process a person out of stagnant soul connections. It is indicated when there is tightness in the trapezius muscles crossing the shoulder blades, amenorrhea, and PMS with a dark, brooding state of mind. I have discussed Black Cohosh in great depth in my earlier books.

The Way of the Lizard

Lizard is the least appreciated of the reptiles. We don't notice him much. That is part of his strategy. However, Lizard needs to bask in the sunshine like all the reptiles, so he is susceptible to the predator—mostly raptors flying around in the air. Even then, if the predator grasps the tail, it comes off. Lizard boasts: "Ha ha, ya missed me!" He is therefore associated with one of the great archetypes of human culture: Trickster.

Tricksters are thin on the ground in the Hebrew and Christian Bibles, but this is made up by folklore, which supplies many from Reynard the Fox to Bugs Bunny. There are quite a few different Trickers, actually: Coyote, Fox, Rabbit, Spider, Lizard, Cloud, Mist, Fog, and even Snake. The first image in the Higher Arcana of the tarot, after the Fool, is the Magician, Juggler, Joker, or Trickster. He trumps all the regular cards but is trumped himself by all the other Higher Arcana. We all want to invest in the Bugs Bunny Hedge Fund and International Bank sometime or other: *In Wabbit We Twust.*

The first lesson of the Trickster is that we should not take ourselves too seriously. We should be able to laugh at ourselves and our foibles. Whenever I got too serious, Arlo would always start making jokes. The second lesson of the Trickster is also that we are susceptible to being tricked. And rather than being angry—taking ourselves too seriously—we should laugh at our foibles. The third lesson is that we need to develop our own bag of strategies and tricks, so that we can escape dangers that arise here and there on the path of life. In this regard, Trickster is innately connected to the spiritual warrior, who is always looking for strategy. For this reason, Lizard Medicine is connected to Eagle Medicine—connected to its own predator, the raptor. Warriorship is connected with the reptilian brain because war is based on survival skills. In spiritual war, we transfer our attention to a higher goal: we are searching for spiritual enlightenment. This is why spiritual warriorship is associated with the Eagle.

Different tricksters have different functions. They can relate to the big ego (Coyote); the insecure ego (Rabbit); the survivor ego (Rabbit); the cunning mind (Fox); the cunning, secretive mind (Raven, Crow); the cunning and ambivalent mind (Snake); mental connectedness (Spider); the passive delusions of the mind (Cloud, Fog, Mist, Smoke); the trickster (Lizard); and the active delusion spreader or user of delusion (Skunk).

Trickster helps us to laugh at the fallibility of human nature and ourselves, but as a medicine power he might only get the job half done, then walk away. A medicine man in Northern California who counted Lizard as one of his animal helpers told Jaime de Angulo (1950, 341): "Jim Lizard, he sit on rock all day, he pretty clever but not serious. . . . Mebbe he stay and help and mebbe he tell me lie. I can't depend on him."

Some tricksters personify characters who survive by their wits when their society has been completely broken down. A trickster can have no integrity at all. He just survives. Trickster is ultimately out for himself, like Bugs Bunny, Reynard the Fox, or the Wizard of Oz. The alienation, inventiveness, ruthlessness, dishonesty, craziness, and desperateness of the trickster mean he or she is close to the spirit, even if the effect on others is destructive. Trickster can have a lack of integrity and sometimes they have no ultimate purpose other than survival, greed, or selfishness. Even then, Trickster has the protection of the spirit, just as the evil witches do. For a while.

The most dangerous of all tricksters is Snake. This is because he is not only cunning but ambivalent. Snake doesn't care how much damage, suffering, or destruction is inflicted. Snake traps us in delusion and the Wheel of Dharma. And he or she or it is able to do all this with such dexterity and sublimity that people can't even see the deception and suffering they are walking into. But destruction can be constructive. That's the chance somebody took when they let Snake/Dragon loose in the Garden of Eden.

The Contrary

The contrary is like a trickster except that there is a purpose in their strategy: he or she has a goal other than mere survival. The contrary breaks the agreements and taboos of society for some higher goal or strategic outcome. This entails living a life opposite social convention. Like all medicine powers, this is something that can't be controlled. It is like a drive that the person can't deny.

Here is an example of a contrary from the history of the British Isles. It is particularly interesting because the great seer and spiritual voyageur Thomas the Rhymer was involved in the events.

The Scottish succession in the thirteenth century had become a tangle of conflicting claims. This allowed the English to take over. Thomas the Rhymer himself prophesied, after the rebel William Wallace survived torture and an unsuccessful "execution," that Scotland would be plunged into fifty years of war. When Wallace did finally die, Robert the Bruce took over the fight. The first thing he did was kill the only other Scots heir to the throne on the steps of a church. As every Scotsman knew, that was sacred ground, a taboo not to be broken. Bruce had chased him onto the steps, where he thought he was safe. The Pope declared Bruce a reprobate, his lands in Scotland, England, and France were forfeited, his family was taken hostage by the English army, and his soldiers were banned from receiving food or shelter from the hand of a Christian. In a rebellion that lasted decades, Bruce slowly strengthened his hand and eventually he defeated the English at Bannockburn and was acknowledged as the rightful King of Scotland.

To make peace with the Pope, King Robert fought as a Crusader against the Moor in Spain. By this time he was a sick old man. When his troops wavered in battle he said to his standard-bearer, the Black

Douglas: "Cut off my head and throw it forward: the men will follow."
Robert the Bruce won his last battle.

The story of Robert the Bruce tells us that the contrary can have a higher vision but that it can hurt a lot of people. Many of the greatest military and political leaders are contraries that "history cannot control." Examples would include Alexander the Great, Napoleon, and Frederick the Great.

The story of Thomas the Rhymer connected with this event is worth reporting. "True Thomas" was a patriot, but he was also a realist and an empath. Therefore, he was deeply distressed when he heard that William Wallace was still alive. His survival of torture and execution was completely unexpected, and Thomas saw it as an omen. He demanded verification three times: first from the servant of the woman dressing the supposed "corpse," then by the observation of his own servant, and finally he went to see for himself. When he saw that Wallace survived, he was mortified. The rest of Scotland celebrated but Thomas foresaw the social cost of fifty years of Civil War.

The trickster and the contrary are archetypal. They possess power that is supernatural because they have received it from a source outside conventional society. It does not matter whether their motives are good or bad, selfish or selfless; they will be borne up by the spirit because they dare to go beyond ordinary human social norms.

Heyoka and Hi-ya-ka

In Lakota the word for a contrary is *heyoka* (hey-YO-ka). These contraries do everything the opposite of everyone else in society. Sometimes they even walk backward. They can't function as ordinary people. Sometimes they function as clowns at social events, imitating white people or acting in other bizarre fashions. They can't help themselves: they are possessed by contrary medicine. Another definition I heard was that they were the juvenile delinquents who couldn't fit into society, so the Indian People made a separate society for them. My definition is that they "laugh at death" and "frown at life."

A few years ago a man taking classes on herbal medicine from my friend Paul Red Elk noted that there was a technique used by the Marines—he was a retired career Marine—when there was no logical way out of a situation. It was to act in an illogical way and it was called "HI-ya-ka." Now he understood where the word came from. Sondra, who served with the Special Forces, commented: "Yes, we were taught to use this strategy in extreme circumstances but we called it 'distraction.'"

❂ TRICKSTER MEDICINE ❂

Some plants can be tricksters. A good example is Poison Ivy: it looks like other plants so that it can blend in among the surrounding vines and leaves. It grows on ground that has been trampled down—Nature's way of saying: "Don't go there or I'll set up an inflammation." So it is the remedy for overuse.

☙ Poison Ivy ❧
(Rhus toxicodendron)

This is the homeopathic remedy for overuse of joints and connective tissue. The part is stiff and sore until limbered up. The pain is not generally sharp.

In one of the funnier cases, my boss came into the herb store and wondered if I knew of a remedy for a rash on his scrotum. It wasn't an STD. I knew he had just started a relationship with a new girlfriend who was sexually very, very intense and I figured: *overuse of the part.* *Rhus tox.* cleared it up in a few days. The relationship was good, too—it lasted a few years.

I had a client who was a businessman but was terribly bored with his job. He too had a rash on his scrotum. He had been happily married for quite a few years, so I figured this was something like trampling down of the imagination from a boring job rather than "overuse of the part." *Rhus tox.* cured it shortly; he went back to college, got a

Ph.D. in business, and became a professor in business school. He was happy.

A middle-aged woman had been coming to the herb store for several years for minor complaints. This time she came in and complained loudly about how bored she was with her job and how much her hip joint hurt. I asked what her job was. "I work in the interoffice mail, delivering mail between two buildings the offices are located in." Wow! I couldn't believe it: the perfect Gemini job, delivering messages between two buildings! I was ready to quit being an herbalist right then and there but instead I gave her *Rhus tox.* and it cleared up the joint pain and the boredom. When you're bored you need a trickster.

I use the low potencies of 6x, 12x, and 30x. As an antidote to Poison Ivy or Poison Oak, I recommend tinctures of Comptonia, Grindelia, Boston Ivy, and Plantain.

☼ LIZARD MEDICINE ☼

This is not a subject I know a lot about from experience, so I am only going to touch upon it lightly. There is a small family of plants called the Saururaceae or Lizard's Tail family. There is one representative in Southeastern North America (*Saururus cernuus*) and one in the Southwest (*Anemopsis californica*). Others are native to Southeast Asia; one of them is *Houttynia cordata*, the famous "Chameleon Plant" of Chinese herbalism. The Lizard's Tail of the Southeastern United States has a bit of use in folk medicine as a calmative. This caused it to be named "Yerba Mansa" by the Spanish of Old Florida: the word *mansa* means "tamed" in Spanish. It tames the mind and emotions; a skill needed by the warrior.

When the Spanish arrived in California, some botanist or herbalist among the early invaders recognized *Anemopsis* as a cousin and transferred the name Yerba Mansa to this plant. Ironically, it has the opposite effect: to rouse a person from lethargy of tissue or attitude, rather than to relax.

Houttuynia seems to live up to its animal association: it is for mischievous diseases that are hard to get a handle on. It is an antiviral; used by some in covid.

It looks to me that if one used all three of these plants, one would have an excellent command of Lizard Medicine: to calm, rouse, and outsmart. Since I have not used these herbs, except for Yerba Mansa, I am not going to elaborate on them.

The Way of the Turtle

My friend kept on badgering me that evening, saying I had to go visit a certain medicine man to get a naming ceremony. When I finally said yes, rather indifferently, I immediately felt a sensation like a tube breaking in my throat: *Thunk!* From that moment on, a medicine man poured into my consciousness. He was smoking his pipe and the smoke went all through me. He studied me and knew me. Several nights later, I had the dreams about Wolf Person and the automatons. Finally, I wrote him a letter (this was before the internet) and asked if I could visit. I didn't receive an answer but I brought a food plate and gifts and tobacco and set out.

After I had made my decision to go, I saw in my mind's eye a little turtle sitting at the bottom of my scrotum, facing outward, but lifeless as a stone. As I headed out of the Twin Cities, I saw it alive now, climbing up my spine—it was at the bottom of the thoracic vertebra.

It was after dark when I reached my parent's cabin on the Snake River, in central Minnesota, halfway to my destination. The river has that name because it was the old boundary between the Anishinabe Ojibwa in the forested north and their enemies ("snakes"), the Dakota, in the savannah to the south.

The cabin was newly purchased; I had never been there before and I didn't know the layout of the land. By my headlights I found the door. Inside I found a bedroom that I figured must look out on the river.

All that night I lay in a trancelike state. For hours, I saw Grandfather Turtle sitting on a rock in the middle of the river. He had a gentle smile and friendly, dark brown eyes. I knew that those eyes were conjunct; the Living Nature and that Grandfather Turtle knew all the wisdom that had occurred since the beginning of time down to the present. I also knew that his dark eyes were conjunct; the dark eyes of the Indian people, and that the Living Nature was conjoined to their soul.

The aura of the white man rips at the soul of the Indian people. "What? You can see that?" exclaimed Arlo. Another time he told me: "Everyone I went to grade school with is dead now. I'm the last one." He was thirty-six. "Invader," said my friend Percilla.

In our eye contact, my soul merged with Grandfather Turtle and we were one. Little Turtle had passed up my spine, to the top of my head, and over, to my brow and eyes. I had eye contact with Grandfather Turtle. Hours passed. Just before dawn, my eyes finally moved away from Grandfather Turtle, across the river. On the forest floor beneath the woods on the other side, I saw a faint path, barely visible. The leaves of many summers covered the trail, so it looked like nobody had taken it for a long time. A voice said, "That's the Old, Old Path that few take anymore."

As the sun broke through the woods in the morning, the trance drew to a close and I could see out the window. The river was set back further from the cabin than it was in the vision. Instead of a stone in the river, where Grandfather Turtle had been, there was a stump. It was another fifteen feet to the river's edge. I went out to investigate, and on the stump I found a turtle shell. I still have that shell.

As I drove away, I had one more vision:

I saw Grandfather Turtle sitting on the earth. Suddenly, he flipped up, like a door on a hinge, and I saw that he was a doorway to the Underworld and that I had access. After a moment a slavering wolf

came up to the doorway from below to make sure that the unworthy
did not enter. He didn't go one iota beyond the doorway. Suddenly,
the Underworld became a real place for me. I knew the process that
began with the little stone turtle was complete.

Later a friend pointed out that the "tube" in the throat was called
the "Way of the Turtle" in the *Yoga Sutras of Patanjali*. Very appropriately, she was a descendent of Ma-Gish-Gee-Bo, the Anishinabe chief
that had been forced to sell the pineries in central Minnesota.

I was informed by another Native teacher that the channel in the
throat is one of the four points the Ojibwa anoint with sacred oil when
the baby is born, to protect it against outside interference. Since we
can't share the name of the oil or how to make it, we can try Sunflower
seed oil instead to annoint our own points, even as adults, in this
treacherous world.

Turtle marks the boundary between the human (in the head) and
the animal (in the body). That is why, when the Place of the Turtle
breaks open, the animal consciousness flows into the human and we
meet our long-lost ally, the animal self, and become conscious in the
Spirit World.

Whereas Snake raises the kundalini to the third eye and opens
the psychic vision, Turtle brings the energy down from the crown of
the head, past the third eye, to the point on the neck, the Way of the
Turtle, where the human self (head) meets the animal self (body). It
therefore actualizes and brings to consciousness the animal self. It is,
anyway, the ancestor of all the warm-blooded animals. What Snake
does only empowers the human self because it does not connect to the
Way of the Turtle, but only opens up the mind's eye. My friend Jolie
had an experience of Grandmother Turtle:

In my dream I saw a beautiful big brown-green tortoise. I had to slow
down to make eye contact with it. Then I had to slow down even
more, and then even more. I felt my whole being slow down to a
completely relaxed, altered state and I was able to meet the grounded,

slow, wise, patient turtle and lock eyes with her. She transmitted the felt sense how it is to relax and at the same time have slow but steady purpose and dedication. It was the slow wisdom of the elders that is the opposite energy of a puppy, chasing her tail. Slow and steady, efficient, without a calorie wasted on nonsense. Our eyes locked, we merged, and I felt her and she felt me. Then she bowed down to honor me.

At the same time that I was connected to the tortoise, I saw some animals passing behind me out of the corner of my eye. At first, I thought they were dogs. When I left the tortoise, I looked toward where all the dogs were headed and realized they were wolves. There was a circle of about twelve wolves all neatly arranged like divisions on a clock with all their heads facing in and tails facing out. I felt like the pack was building and sharing wisdom; plotting, working together.

One of the characteristics of Turtle is the number thirteen. There are thirteen big scales on the back of a turtle shell. Twelve is the number of solar months, while thirteen is the number of lunar months. Wolf howls at the Moon, to call—as I have said—the human race back to their brothers and sisters in the Land of the Animals. Jolie is now an accepted citizen of that world.

Star Woman marked all the star essences on the back of Elder Turtle. Both the solar and lunar year are pictured there. I have never seen a turtle that didn't have thirteen scales, except for the scaleless sand turtle. While the thirteen large scales represent the lunar calendar, the more numerous small scales around the perimeter represent the solar calendar. The whole thing is a circle with four basic directions represented by the four feet. The head and tail represent the direction of time—birth and death—and the doorways in and out of life within the mundane shell.

Turtle can adjust his internal temperature somewhat. By pressing against his shell he can extrude water to warm up, while by jumping back in the pond he can pick it back up and cool off. Therefore, Turtle is the "most evolved" of the reptilian life-wave. Evolutionary biologists say that he is the "main stem" from which the warm-blooded animals arose. For this reason, Turtle is seen as the foundation upon which the Earth rests, or again, from which the Tree of Life arises. I like to believe that my friend Turtle sits on the boundary line to the Inner Court and the Outer and touches upon Paradise.

Turtle is the representative of the path of Wisdom: both that which is gained by living and examining life, and that which is embedded in the Living Nature—the Wisdom of Nature. As for me, the Wisdom of the Turtle would be enough to give me satisfaction on the spiritual path but it also led me to understandings of these other mysteries of the Outer Court. Thank you, Grandfather Turtle.

The Old, Old Path

When Star Woman descended to the Earth, she set her foot on the back of Original Turtle, upon whom the earth was gathering. The stars of the heavens were imprinted upon the emergent rocks, plants, and animals, so that each one had an essence that guided their formation and manifestation in the world. First Turtle was present at the beginning of creation, the beginning of time and space, but instead of simply preserving a record of everything that has transpired in our creation, Turtle reduces all that experience to Wisdom. So in some ways, lowly Turtle is not the least of the medicine animals, but perhaps the greatest.

Turtle leads us back to the knowledge of Star Woman. This is the Old, Old Path. In the Old World, where Star Woman is known as Sophia, knowledge of the archetypal markings inscribed upon creation is called the *Natura Sophia*, or Wisdom of Nature. This term was originated by Jacob Boehme. The "light" of wisdom that shines forth from within the creation, through their signatures and marks, was called the *lumen naturae*, or Light of Nature by Paracelsus.

The English word "verity" is narrowly defined as "eternal truth," but it infers the contentment found in the contemplation of eternal truths or first principles, also the life of the imagination and creativity, which further hearkens to eternal beauty. Each star essence that appears to us through the looking glass of the intuitive mind is a verity, so Star Woman is eternally true and beautiful and the source of contentment. Who would not want to partake of this vision, this wisdom?

The "Old, Old Path" is the original path to the Spirit World implicit in Nature. Making the shift from the exiled world we live in to the Spirit World, through the actualization of the animal self, is easier when we have knowledge of the archetypes and the Green Tongue; they help us to think in the parallels, parables, analogies, and archetypes necessary for us to be able to recognize and articulate the discovery of the Far Distant Shore of the Spirit World. The Old, Old Path leads to the door, but is not actually capable of bringing us across the threshold. That is the prerogative of the spirit.

On the Old, Old Path of Original Turtle, we see that Earth Wisdom is built into the creation, for every stone and mountain, plant and animal, is a personification of a verity that emanated from the supernal archetypes in the Spirit World. The wisdom shines forth through the signatures marked on all creatures. It is a spiritual wisdom innate to that world. It is a slow path, like Grandfather Turtle himself. If we follow that path, we will draw right up to the door of the spirit, the boundary between the human and the animal. This point is the culmination of the Way of the Turtle.

☯ TURTLE MEDICINE ☯

I have mentioned in my books several times that the upper shell of Turtle represents the natural world, in which we learn to appreciate the outer world of Mother Nature; while the underside represents the hidden side of the natural world, in which we see the signatures of creation. The living body of the turtle within the shell represents the Living Nature within the shell of the material world. On the mundane level, Turtle Medicine helps to balance water and solid, and has a natural affinity to the kidneys and bones.

ᘒ Gravel Root ᘒ
(*Eupatorium purpureum, Eutrochium purpureum*)

This plant grows on the edge of the water and the upland, so it balances water and solids. That, obviously, makes it a kidney medicine. But it balances throughout the body. Through clinical experience I have come to the conclusion that Gravel Root opens the capillary bed to release water into the extracellular matrix. This is why it can bring movement to a frozen shoulder or joint. This is also how it keeps the peritoneum clean when there is pus from colitis or Crohn's disease or typhus (in the old days) in the abdominal area. It was a major remedy for sepsis in the nineteenth century. By opening the capillary bed for the blood plasma to flow into the renal tubules, it becomes a powerful diuretic. It almost certainly has a direct influence on glomerular filtration and it has been used for water retention. It also washes out excess calcium depositions and kidney stones. We (my friends and I) have confirmed the old folk-medical uses for "gravel": stiffness from calcification in the muscles, and regrowth of damaged bone. When I discussed this with Tsalagi medicine woman Sondra Boyd, she added an additional insight: it not only opens the capillary bed to discharge serum in the matrix, it also opens the tight junctions or pores in the lymphatic capillaries to drain the matrix. It operates at both the inlets and the outlets of the great Mother Ocean of the extracellular matrix. Now we can see another reason why Gravel Root "hates pus." It cleans out the matrix, removing waste material. This ought to make it a good liver remedy as well, because 25–50% of the lymph plasma originates in the "space of Disse" (the extracellular matrix of the liver).

The ability to balance water and solid not only reminds us of the turtle as a land and water animal, but also of its ability to adjust the water it "carries" on its back by pressing itself against its shell to remove water.

Gravel Root squeezes in and out.

This plant is also known as Joe Pye Weed because, according to the botanist Amos Eaton, the Indian medicine man of that name gave it to Zachariah Moore, the president of Williams College, in western Massachusetts. Williams was connected to the Stockbridge Reservation in western Massachusetts through shared clergymen. Joe Pye was an important leader there in the middle of the eighteenth century and a medicine man who studied under the Rev. Samuel Occom, an older Stockbridge minister, chief, and medicine man. There are still members of the Occom and Pye families on the Stockbridge Reservation—which is now in Wisconsin. In the late 1780s, the Stockbridge Indians were driven by greedy settlers from Massachusetts to upstate New York, and on to Wisconsin, where they reside today. It is possible "Joe Pye's Weed" (as some of the accounts read) was given to Moore by a successor to his knowledge.

A serious lifelong problem for Susan has been Crohn's disease. Bob, the owner of Present Moment Herbs and Books, where I worked at the time, stopped it completely for ten years with Calamus rhizome, but it didn't work after ten years. The gastroenterologist said, "You have two or three weeks to get a handle on this with prednisone to suppress autoimmune disease. If not, you're going to have a full colostomy, with a colostomy bag." After three days on prednisone, Susan said, "I can't take this stuff, it eats my soul."

Solution: Go on a camping trip with your dog. The dog got into a ground wasp nest and Susan got bit sixteen times getting him out. "The funny thing was, I didn't have an allergic reaction, like I usually do. Sixteen bites should've killed me." I laughed once again at Susan's ability to survive near-death. "That's because you still had the prednisone in your system."

Back at home, Susan reached a conclusion: "If God can't save me, I'm ready to die." She was at the end of her rope. She couldn't take the prednisone and she couldn't take another operation—last time, her wounds were open and needed dressing for six months because of the inflammation from the autoimmune disease.

We talked on the phone. After I hung up (a good time to watch for magical thoughts), an herb popped into my mind. I remembered another case of Crohn's disease halted by Gravel Root. So, I brought her some of the roots from the herb store and told her to just munch on little bits every day. When she was a little better, we visited a small swamp near my house where the Gravel Root grew. Actually, that root had mineralized crystals on it that prevented consumption—but it is important to get to know a plant when your life depends on it. Slowly, Susan got better.

The Crohn's never grew again until twenty years later, when she went through a period of stress. We have X-ray proof that it didn't expand in all those years. That's not just because of the Gravel Root but because Susan changed. She's had a whole life since then. Married, new family members, farm. Susan put her life on the line when she put the health of her soul and spirit above life itself.

A few years later, Susan was at the hospital after being bucked off a horse. The doctor asked, "What happened here with this Crohn's disease, where the medical record just ends?" "Oh, I took herbs," she answered. They didn't want to hear any more of the story because biomedicine is a routine (not a "science") and if anything lies outside the routine, it is *terra incognito*.

It took eighteen months for Susan to pull out of that deep pit of inflammation and weakness when she defied the gastroenterologist and the prednisone. She needed Gravel Root and spiritual healing in the sweat lodge with medicine men. One of them said: "Keep taking what the doctor is giving you." He didn't know that the "doctor" was an herbalist!

Susan had a low fever that consumes strength. That's the kind of fever for which this plant was originally used by Joe Pye. It is for Crohn's because it is like an autoimmune version of typhoid. It's mostly used as a kidney medicine however—hence the name Gravel Root.

⚘ Goldenrod ⚘
(*Solidago canadensis, S. virga-aurea, S.* spp.)

This is another member of the aster family. It has a bitter, pungent, savory taste, like Gravel Root, and it also acts on the kidneys. It is an upland plant and its Turtle Medicine signature is different from Gravel

Root: the leaves appear early in the spring, it grows slowly through the whole summer and finally flowers in late summer. So, it advances slowly, like a turtle, and in fact herbalist Lise Wolff has found that it is good for slow growth and retarded bone growth in children.

One of my Native teachers pointed out that in the fall the roots suddenly thicken out into a bunch, as if it were saving its strength through winter, for the next year. So it is also a stamina remedy, and it is especially a remedy for people who feel like they are too tired to make it to the goal, to fulfill the vision, to get to the finish line.

I taught Lise Wolff about this when she was first learning herbal medicine with me—she's been a professional for decades now—and she and I have flushed out the picture of Goldenrod pretty well. I described this plant (and Gravel Root) in *The Book of Herbal Wisdom* (1997, 269–81), so there are details there I have left out here.

The Goldenrod person feels the goal in the distance is too far away, or is so tired they can't see the goal anymore. The feet are tired, the lower back and maybe the kidneys too (urine dark and scanty, copious and stinky, etc.). The motto is: "Where's the nearest chair?"

Lise found that it is for slow growth in children; it "pops them up." It can thicken the bones. In Chinese medicine the kidneys store the "jing" or essence, which is in charge of unfolding the blueprint of life, and they are in charge of the development and health of the bones. "Jing deficiency" is marked by developmental sluggishness, slow closure of the fontanelles, teeth problems, "drops out the baby teeth" says Lise, a thin frame, lack of tenacity and stamina. She's found that it can sometimes stop miscarriages. One woman she helped said: "I always thought I could never have a baby, could never make it to the end." Goldenrod acts on the male reproductive system too: a Canberra herbalist taught me that it can reduce prostateinflammation.

Our dear friend, the late William LeSassier, used it to thicken the mucosal layer of the digestive tract; it also strengthens the respiratory tract. I use it when the viral infection is drawing to a close and, just as the person thinks they are getting better, bacteria set in—the discharge gets yellow and thick. The kidneys are too overburdened to remove the protein debris from the dead cells. William used the leaf as a stomach bitter to increase secretion in the stomach—Gravel Root can be used the same way.

⚘ Lady's Mantle ⚘
(*Alchemilla vulgaris*)

This member of the Rose family is native to the low mountains of Europe, easily cultivated, and long used in European folk medicine—less so by professional doctors. I don't think it would have much of a profile today if it were not for the treatment afforded by Maria Treben in *Health through God's Pharmacy* (1980, 29–30).

It came as a great surprise to me that Turtle claimed Lady's Mantle as one of his medicines. The roots look like cat's feet so she has been known as Lion's Foot. She acts on the heart muscle, according to Maria Treben—I have confirmed this a couple of times. The heart fits the profile for a Lion Medicine as well as a Sun Medicine. However, Turtle told me Lady's Mantle was one of his medicines and indeed, she shows that characteristic liquid/solid balance of the Turtle Medicines. The leaves extrude fluid and collect dew so that there are little droplets with the defined edges that is characteristic of water organized by living tissue (H_3O+/H_2O_2-, as compared to H_2O). These droplets remain in the folds of the leaves until vaporized by the heat of the sun later in the day. The alchemists gathered this water—thus the name *Alchemilla*—and Dr. Bach also sought the special powers of dew in his preparations made in dew and sunlight. We do see a connection with Sun Medicine in this water, which can only be made by exposure to sunlight—see Gerald Pollack's research on the properties of "living water" (Pollack 2013).

It was during Omicron and I'd been sick off and on in 2022. It would attack and close the top of my head, isolating me from the "spirit star." This felt quite awful—no creativity, no heart, no spirit, no good dreams. Turtle showed his protective shell was all around me while he was merging more deeply with Earth for my protection. On the third day, I was shown Lady's Mantle in my mind's eye and understood that she would carry on the protection for Turtle.

Up to this experience, I had been calling our friend Lady's Mantle "Female Protection Medicine" because she is a woman's remedy and protects women who are subject to abuse or violence—see my write-up in *The Book of Herbal Wisdom* (1997, 113–24). That's a property that incarnates the name "Lady's Mantle." Now I understood that the protection extended to negative psychospiritual influences that had nothing to do with one sex or the other. I would say, however, that Lady's Mantle connects with the Goddess—one of them, but I'm not sure which: Mother Nature or the Queen of the Faeries or who?

Lady's Mantle was originally used for cuts and wounds, which have an analogy to assaults on the psychic periphery of the body. It is particularly good for rips and tears. In recent centuries it came to be associated with female conditions including vaginal injuries, torn abdominal muscles postpartum, and restoring the tone of the breasts after lactation. It has a specific affinity for tissue in sheets: some muscles, mucosa, skin. Treben used it for hernias and to strengthen the atria of the heart.

When I told Susan about this, she suggested that I combine Lady's Mantle and true Solomon's Seal "because they like to grow together." And indeed, the former protected the outside, while the latter soothed the mucosa and respiratory tract.

Nature Speaks

After Susan recovered from the ulceration of her colon, she held a *uwipi*, a sweat lodge, to thank all the people that had helped her. I was there. Deep in the ceremony, when my time came to talk, I thanked Gravel Root. Almost immediately, the plant spoke to me as clear as day:

> *You can tell I'm a Turtle Medicine because, just as Grandfather Turtle rose up out of the sea in the beginning of time to create the first earth, so too do I rise up out of the swamp to create the first soil.*

That's the way it is with silent knowledge. The communication comes to us in very exact words. The words are usually arranged in such a way that they strike the inner mind as "perfect" in their brevity, sincerity, and meaning. The Speech of Nature does not make an assertion, but paints a picture, a parable. It does not demand belief: we can believe or not.

7

The Animal Self

Even a man who is pure in heart
And says his prayers by night
May become a wolf when the wolf-bane blooms
And the autumn moon is bright.

Curt Siodmak, *The Wolf Man*

Scholars now knew that the "Hidden Lord" hieroglyph did
not stand for normal sleep states. Instead, it carried the
sense of a menacing, subterranean consciousness. . . . The
symbol of the jaguar that is hidden within the person of the
shaman king could now be read with sobering clarity. It
was the verb "to sleep," "to dream," and "to transform into
an animal spirit by enchantment." It was also the noun
"shaman," "sorcerer," and "animal companion."

Douglas Gillette, *The Shaman's Secret*

Don Juan once said to Carlos that one struggles for a lifetime and
the reward is a moment of clarity that will guide one for the rest of
one's life. I used to think: *Geez, what a waste of effort—there must be*
more to it than that. I thought enlightenment was a permanent state
of consciousness. The shamanic model turned out not to be equivalent to my stereotype of enlightenment. It has more in common with

fundamentalist Christianity, which claims that a single realization brings lifelong change.

For the shaman, the revelation of the animal self answers the great questions of existence, establishes personal wholeness, makes one an authentic human being, and ignites the senses on the spiritual plane. It does not happen twice. There will still be dramatic reckonings and lessons to be experienced on the shamanic path—Wolves, Dragons, and faeries may talk to us—but there is only the one watershed moment.

The Actualization of the Animal Self

This event is so crucial in the shamanic experience—it is the defining experience of shamanism—that I feel obligated to describe it in detail referring to my own experience and that of my close friend, Susan. Here is the transformative dream I had at age thirty-one, initiated in me by a visit to an Anishinabe Ojibwa medicine man in northern Minnesota: This is the central pivot of the entire book. The actualization that alters us permanently and deeply. Here is my experience from deep in dreamtime.

> *I was in the underworld. I was looking at the Lord of the Underworld; his face was just a darkness. He pointed toward my right and said: "I want you to meet one of my Captains." I followed his outstretched arm and saw the Big, Bad Wolf, half-animal and half-man, standing upright, leaning on an inner city lamppost. He was illuminated by a circle of light shining down from the streetlight. He had the head of a wolf, his arms were folded over his chest, and he was standing on two wolf feet. He had on an old dark blue sweater. He was smirking and I heard him chuckle "Heh, heh, heh," as if to say: "What do have we here?" He exuded a predatory aura.*
>
> *While I was still looking at Wolf Person, the Lord of the Underworld spoke: "And now we are going to make a psychic link between you and the Wolf Person."*

That jolted me into survival mode. "Wait, wait, WAIT a second!" I called out as I started to wake up. "I've studied occultism and shamanism for years, but I don't want a familiar spirit in the Underworld. That's, that's . . . going too far!" A part of me was shocked and terrified while another part was making a simple, unruffled observation: Wolf Person is the one who dares to go too far. *I had done that. I was experiencing the results of explorations of consciousness. I had always admired and loved the wolf—now I was one.*

The scene disappeared and my awareness shifted as I was waking up to a more superficial level of consciousness. I felt a bandlike sensation around my head. The band turned into a snake biting its tail: the mouth was clamped on the end of the tail over my "third eye." Then the mouth opened, and the snake flopped out the back of my head. I woke up with a lurch and a shudder, desperately looking for a snake in my bed. A feeling came over me: I am freed of an ancient curse upon the human race.

One thing that is absolutely characteristic of the animal self is that it is a wild animal and we are domesticated beings, so that when we experience our animal self, it is quite threatening. To contact the animal self, we must return to the wilderness within. Some have called it the "wild self."

The terror one feels in this experience is twofold: the encounter with the wild, undomesticated animal self and the first meeting with the completely alien spirit being that has no earthly genetics or reference points. The latter is more terrifying because the Lord of the Underworld and his realm belong to the inorganic beings (remember, he is the spouse of the Queen of the Faeries). They are the lords of dreamtime and in that world have the power to trap us. It feels like they can make us cease to exist because they are merged with the realm of the uncreated. In other words, it can obliterate the primal atom of individuality, the *atma* of individual existence. After we meet them, these beings take after us like the proverbial demons out of hell because they are attracted to the juicy realm of the soul as much as we are—we who need to have feelings all the time to be human. Castaneda talks often about the terror inspired by the inorganic beings in the latter books in his series.

Notice that in my dream the Lord of the Underworld, who we refer to as the "Keeper of the Animals," didn't use the word "animal" but referred to his Captain as the "Wolf Person." He found the distinction between humans and animals artificial, distasteful, and inaccurate. In our language, the distinction is fairly recent. The Greeks did not have a word for this difference until a generation before Socrates. We were often known in ancient times simply as the "talking animal."

Jaime de Angulo was conversing with one of his Indian friends in Northern California. He was trying to get Bill to differentiate between animals and people. They were talking about the Creation Story. The anthropologist understood his friend to mean there were animals in the world, but no people had appeared yet. Bill vehemently disagreed.

> "Whad'you mean there were no people? Ain't animals people?"
>
> "Yes, they are . . . but . . ."
>
> "They are not Indians, but they are people, they are alive . . . Whad'you mean, animal?"
>
> "Well . . . how do you say 'animal' in Pit River?"
>
> ". . . I dunno . . ."
>
> "But suppose you wanted to say it?"
>
> "Well . . . I guess I would say something like *teeqaade-wade toolol aakaadzi* (world-over, all living) . . . . I guess that means animals, Doc."
>
> "I don't see how, Bill. That means people, also. People are living, aren't they?"
>
> "Sure they are! that's what I've been trying to tell you. Everything is living . . ." (de Angulo 1950, 372)

I hadn't read de Angulo when I had this dream so it is interesting that the Lord of the Underworld preferred the word "person." What did he mean when he called Wolf Person one of his "Captains?"

Wolf, Cat, and Human are at the pinnacle of the predatory pyramid. Therefore, in a sense, they are rulers of the animal kingdom. In the ferocious pre-Columbian Mayan shamanism, the glyph for the Hidden Lord and the shaman who units with him is Black Jaguar.

Wolf often appears as a "Captain" of the Lord of the Underworld, just as Dog appears as the servant of the human. Wolf is in charge of the boundaries and not infrequently a person will meet Wolf in dream-time before they are ready to enter. Dog is the representation of the human world, which is domesticated, while Wolf is the representative of the untamed wilderness and, therefore, the ferocious Underworld.

The curse I felt released from was the one laid upon humanity when our ancestors consumed the fruit in the Garden of Eden. Snake was with us from the start and is still with us, holding us in our delusions of good and evil until we reawaken the warm-blooded animal-self part of us that is not under the domination of Snake. It took me twenty years to accept this—it was "going too far" to claim such a distinction for myself.

The ongoing dominion of Snake over captive humanity is represented by the ancient symbol of the serpent biting its tail. The Greeks had a word for this symbol, so they too had seen it: ouroboros. The actualization of the animal self breaks the curse of involution and contraction, graphically represented by the ouroboros.

The ring around the head actually occurs when one is "losing the human form," to use don Juan's expression. When the top of the head opens to Creator above, the resistances in our mind break up and slowly move down the body.

Susan had a dream similar to mine, but she was one of those unusual people who experience the actualization of a reptile, instead of a warm-blooded animal. The element of terror comes out even stronger in her dreamtime experience. She allowed me to share this with readers:

> I was at a peace conference for all the species in all the worlds in the galaxy. I was in the human booth—and let me tell you, we are

a pretty boring bunch. The King of the Alligators was marching from the distance up to the booth. He arrived with his retinue of Alligators following behind him. They went on for miles and miles. Thousands of them: walking on two feet. They were fanatically loyal to him. At his command, they would tear anyone apart in a second—and the King looked ferocious. He stopped in front of the booth. His eyes were obsidian black. I knew he was trustworthy, but his appearance was so terrifying all I could feel was the calm of terror.

Susan turned to me and asked, "Have you ever felt that?" Her eyes flashed in their obsidian depths. "No, I haven't," I answered meekly.

I thought I had to save the humans, so I said to one of them: "Get the gun." Instantly, I was strung up on two poles in front of all the species of all worlds. I had committed a Big Mistake: it was a peace conference! They all stared at me.

Eventually, I was let down from the poles. I thought, I should give the King a peace offering. *I figured rubies were the prettiest gemstone, so I carried a ruby necklace over to where the Alligators had set up their Court. The stones were as big as golf balls. He didn't really care. He said: "If you pull a gun, you'd better use it."*

There was a Snake Woman there with her tail darting back and forth, sticking out from under her skirt. She was screaming, "Kill her, kill her!" Nothing was working for me. I was missing the point of the whole thing. Finally, she screamed "Kill the bitch!" and I woke up.

Each medicine animal has a "motto," so to speak. As Susan came out of dreamtime, she knew the motto of Alligator was "I'll kill you if I have to." It came to me a little differently; I told Susan: "You have that *I-might-have-to-kill-you* look in your eyes." She said: "Oh, I never actually *killed* anybody; I just shot 'em in the legs."

Snake Woman was actively condemning Susan, who felt she was committing all sorts of mistakes, whereas in my dream Snake simply threw in the towel. Susan's experience was different because she had a long history of feeling like she was doing things wrong. Snake was trying to keep her imprisoned in self-judgment.

The opening of Susan's eyes in dreamtime, signified by her eye contact with the King, meant that the curse of the Snake could no longer hold her. The blackness in the eyes of the Alligator King is like the dark face of the Lord of the Underworld in my dream.

Susan had a deep connection with horses: over the years she kept horses and dreamed with them. She was sensitive, like a horse. Before the thought became conscious in your own mind, she would know what it was. Susan could travel—move her assemblage point—to the farthest ends of the galaxy. Sensitivity and traveling are Horse traits.

A few weeks after her experience, Susan went out on a date and the poor guy had a dream that night in which she emerged out of a lake, half-woman and half-alligator. "We never went out again," observed Susan solemnly. "Just when you think this stuff is all a bunch of crap, it ruins your sex life."

When the cold-blooded animal self dominates our dreamtime, our lucid dreaming lacks emotional context. It took Susan several more decades for her warm-blooded animal self to become more powerful than the cold-blooded. People with a Horse animal self travel far in dreamtime.

My neighbor at Sunnyfield Herb Farm had Alligator Medicine too. Sam lived with his mother in the guesthouse on the farm. She had a life estate. She had been an astrologer, palmist, and occultist in younger years. Sam was raised in South Chicago. He was the only white kid in the private school he went to. He was 6' 7" tall and had a scary look in his eyes. After he graduated, Sam went out to Berkeley and dealt drugs until he was thirty. "I don't know why I'm still alive," he said one day. "Everybody else got killed when the Colombians took over." Twenty years later, he was in his fifties, taking care of his elderly mother. "She used to change my diapers, now I change hers."

Sam only ever attended one sweat lodge in his life. However, during the ceremony he had a vision that showed him the Crocodiles—the cherubim—guarding the Garden of Eden. One day, out in the yard at Sunnyfield Herb Farm, I said: "You know, Sam, you have Alligator Medicine. The motto of the Alligator is: *I might have to kill you.* You have that look in your eyes." He slowly turned that over. "Oh," he replied, "I'm sorry, I thought I got rid of that a few years ago."

When Susan first came to visit me at Sunnyfield, she noticed Sam's hands. They were smooth because he worked in a restaurant with animal fats and oils. "His hands were soft but I knew those were hands that could kill." Sam couldn't stop talking about hallucinogenic mushrooms with Susan. The two Alligator People recognized each other.

Sam's vision reveals why Alligator might have to kill somebody. It is the protector of the sacred precincts and has the responsibility for keeping the unready and irresponsible out. The Alligators form a protective boundary around Eden. Because they don't dream, the reptiles don't have direct access to the Spirit World. In fact, they are the doorway out, as the story of the serpent in the Tree shows us—actually, it was the father of reptiles, Dragon.

It was twenty years before Susan started to have emotions in her lucid dreaming. This followed an outstanding ceremony in which the warm-blooded animals blessed us and told us they would protect us. Then they felt sorry for the human race—I guess we are in for it in the future . . . or else they just feel sorry for us all the time. Then Creator came and there was a direct interpolation of Divine energy into Earth. Something serious is afoot . . .

A week later, Susan saw a buck just standing in her horse pasture; not moving, fifteen feet away from her. That night I saw a buck along the road; not moving, five feet from my truck. It was shocking. My friend Tracey was with me: we both thought it was a statue until we turned around and drove back up to it. Well, there are several "zombie deer" diseases, but I prefer to believe it was a Divine interpolation into Earth reality.

Castaneda's account of his encounter with his animal self is recounted in *Journey to Ixtlan* (1972, 250). His experience occurs in "alternate reality." First Carlos saw a man in the distance. Then he heard a sound like a jet plane. Then he saw a coyote walking toward him. At first, he was afraid of the coyote: he thought it might be rabid. But when it came up close, Carlos saw that it was calm and safe, and he had a conversation with it and felt at ease with Coyote; but he didn't want to approach the figure in the distance.

The next day don Juan interpreted the experience for his apprentice. Coyote is the "animal companion" that would be with Carlos for the rest of his life. Don Juan notes that, unfortunately, Coyote is a trickster that is not reliable. The man in the distance was the "ally" Carlos is going to have to wrestle with in the future in order to complete his lessons. Carlos was extremely fearful about having to fulfill that requirement. This is normal and understandable because the spirit-beings are in fact terrifying until we get to know them. Only when the aspirant has completed the appointment with the ally will he become a "man of knowledge," don Juan explains to Carlos.

The ally is equivalent to the Lord of the Underworld who appeared in my dream. Notice that I saw him before I saw Wolf, just as Castaneda saw the indistinct manlike being before he saw Coyote. This is because the Lord of the Underworld is also the Keeper of the Animals. In that guise he was the one to whom the old hunters prayed for success in the hunt. He co-rules the Spirit World with his companion, the Queen of the Faeries. The experience of the animal spirit comes first, then the experience with the faeries.

In the later Castaneda books, the allies are described as "inorganic beings," or the inhabitants of dreamtime. The word "ally" reflects the teachings of the witches and sorcerers who used the plants as allies to gain occult powers. This is not only a lesser perspective, but the use of plants to gain powers over other people is a corrupt practice. Don Juan had to use the term "ally" because "inorganic being" (whatever the original Spanish) was impossible for Castaneda to understand at first.

Beyond the terror of the sudden appearance of an alien being and a dangerous animal, we feel great love for the animal co-walker that we are associated with. When we merge with our animal self, we realize that we have always loved that animal. It is like we have always known it for what it was—a part of us—and finally it has been revealed to us, to our soul—the part of us that loves—and we love it and in that love we remain permanently merged with it. In addition, the spirit self now has a reliable channel to our awareness, since the animal self never lost that connection to the Spirit World.

What is the part of us that is terrified by both the animal self and the spirit being? It is the reptilian self. What it cares about is survival, the next meal, reproduction. The fearful reaction to the animal self and spirit-being shows how different the reptilian self is from them. However, each gives us an important spiritual instrument. The reptilian self gives us our survival instincts, which we carry with us into the Soul World and the Spirit World, where it helps us to discern what is safe and what it not safe. It gives us our survival instincts that eventually morph into our instinct for truth. The reptiles are bound by the laws of creation, so they can at least be a source of truth-knowing. Plants are also bound by the laws of creation, but they are the source of "patterns of energy" and "patterns of chemistry" rather than instincts. We can therefore use them to heal and transform. To use the reptilian and vegetable life-waves for personal gain would fall beneath our highest calling.

The Automatons

The newly awakened eyes of the dream self look back upon the human world to show us that we human beings, in our unawakened state, are in an unconscious condition with regard to the Spirit World. Shortly after my dream of Wolf Person, I had the following dream:

I was in the Underworld. I knew there were different levels and I was on one of them, but I didn't know which one. It was like a parking garage with a low ceiling, underground, with nondescript gray-yellow walls. Human beings were walking in all directions, like robots, like wound-up toy soldiers, blindly marching in straight lines until they hit a wall and bounced off. I recognized one I knew in the world to be an intelligent, kind, and sophisticated person. I grabbed his sleeve and

yanked on it, trying to wake him up . . . but he was groggy and
unaware of anything in the trans-automatonic world.

Susan had the same experience in dreamtime:

You had to go down to get there. There were human beings marching
around like wind-up toys. They marched in a straight line until they
hit a wall, then bounced off in a new direction. It was like they were
asleep. I was terrified I was going to be stuck there and woke up.

Until we wake up in dreamtime, we have no true will of our own:
we only think we do. Every impulse is thwarted by our masters—Snake,
Dragon, and the human genome—who have ruled our race since the
beginning of time. This is a pretty glum assessment of the state of
human affairs. But let's not paint too gloomy a picture: as long as we
are listening to the whisperings of the spirit, there is a force within us
that can protect from the worst monsters the galaxy can throw at us.

We're not in Kansas anymore, Toto!

Toto was an animal spirit too.

The Wild Self and the Human Spirit

We bear the shape of a human being, but within our human body, an
animal shines forth. This makes a person look like an animal, as well
as a human, so that we say the person looks like a bear, deer, wolf, coyote, bird, hawk, ferret, rabbit, snake, and so forth. Pugnacious Winston
Churchill looked like an English Bulldog or a Wild Boar. Josef Stalin
had the predatory gleam of the Wolf in his dark eyes. Ariel Sharon,
Yasser Arafat, and Saddam Hussein all had the big stomach and pushy
personalities of Badger. Poor little King Hussein—a graceful Deer—
was stuck between them all.

Unlike the mammalian genomes, the human genome is not connected to the Spirit World. This is due to the "incident in Eden," when
our genome rebelled against our Creator and decided to become its own
God. The animal genomes are still conjoined with their animal totems

in the Spirit World, but the human genome is not conjoined with the human spirit.

The human spirit did come down to our level to reconnect with us—that's the whole Jesus thing, in a nutshell. It is therefore now possible to gain access to the Spirit World through the human spirit—though the human genome remains its own god: "Eat, drink, and procreate." The human spirit operates in the imagination. That's why Jesus taught in parables or word-pictures. On the shamanic path, on the other hand, we work through the animal spirits, and that means we have to go through dreamtime to get to the Spirit World. There is no conflict between the imagination and dreaming—they are different facets of the same thing, day and night.

The awakening of the animal self is our "enlightenment." We move from the darkness of the physical senses, which can never accurately represent the spirit realm—except in the instance of a "rare" spiritual intervention—to the awakened eyes and ears of our newly minted spirit body. This is how Rudolf Steiner defines "enlightenment" (1947, 52):

> The organs thus formed are spiritual eyes. . . . The spiritual world with its lines and figures remains dark as long as [the student] has only attained what has been described as preparation; through enlightenment this world becomes light.

This event is life-changing. Steiner continues (1947, 57): "After enlightenment, under all circumstances, the union of the soul with the spiritual world is effected." This is a dramatic step, but not by any means some kind of conclusion. So many of the foibles of our human self remain, providing material for a lifetime of self-work. And so many challenges remain: dealing with the faery people, the rulers of dreamtime, the Dragons, rulers of the material world.

The reason the Christian principle of being "born again" is similar to the shamanic is that it occurs through the human spirit, which is analogous to the animal spirit (each being a "totem"). However, it occurs in the imagination and is concerned more with awakening to the ability to be a human and getting back in alignment with Creator and the laws of the creation as a human. It is a wise idea, if we have experienced the actualization of our animal self, to pursue our human nature because we are innately human, and human rule over the animal within fulfills our destiny more completely. One of the drawbacks of the shamanic path is that the animal self can dominate over the human. This is not the same as being "dedicated to evil" or something like that: it is a personal choice at best, a habit at worst.

A characteristic of the shamanic path is alienation from the human genome. This tends to arise naturally in some people since the genome is dissociated from the Spirit World and the human spirit. This alienation makes it harder to feel and be human. A major problem with the shamanic path is that one has to actually try to be human, while it comes naturally to other people.

The advantage to this situation is that it causes the shaman to be more conscious in making life choices. This situation explains the two "techniques" that don Juan outlines for working on the spiritual path: *dreaming* and *stalking*, or increasing awareness in dreamtime and in the "human situation," that is, ordinary life.

One problem with the path of the human spirit, a problem we see in so many naive Christians, is that they judge the animal self as bad. This is seen in the long, drawn-out history of the monastic movement, which does not have anything to do with Judaism or Jesus' teachings. (There is no parable that says "The kingdom of heaven is like a monk who turned his back on the world," or anything like that.) A widespread and deplorable doctrine among fundamentalists is that the "heart is bad." There is no parable about that either.

We possess both the reptilian back brain and the animal midbrain. The reptilian back brain/self can operate as an entity independent of the midbrain, sometimes united with it, sometimes opposed to it. It is concerned with survival and reproduction only, and therefore with the most basic drives. The midbrain is associated more with social skills such as bonding, parenting, relationship, and community. The bad reputation of animals mostly comes from the reptilian side.

Amphibians aren't that concerned with survival. They just sort of exist. We kick over a dead log and find a salamander and it just sits there. We pick up a frog and it doesn't really look that disturbed. It doesn't seem to anguish, like a snake that is threatened. In comparison to amphibians and lower orders of animals, the reptiles have noticeable survival mechanisms. They fight against death.

The actualization of the animal self automatically triggers the actualization of the reptilian self because the survival mechanisms have to always accompany any part of us that becomes conscious—so the kundalini rises after the fact, if not before. Even at this point, after all the work necessary to bring the animal self to consciousness, it is still possible for one to be dominated by the survival and reproductive instincts of the reptilian self. Castaneda himself was a debaucher. Since the actualization of the animal self happens virtually simultaneously, we don't always notice the identity of the corresponding reptilian animal companion.

Strengthening the Animal Self

Animal instincts come to the surface and are communicated from the autonomic nervous system through the solar plexus—a little nerve ganglion below the sternum, associated with the stomach. This is where we feel our instincts. When they are intense, we feel a "thump on the belly" or even a burst of stomach acid, and we can even be hit with a burst of adrenaline.

There are remedies that strengthen the solar plexus and we often have to use them in ordinary herbal practice because of the importance of the stomach and the autonomic. On a practical level, they strengthen the stomach muscles and secretions to improve digestion. More generally, they "help things go down." On the shamanic level, these medicines improve the "gut level" or "animal instincts," so they are also important for establishing a strong foundation for development of the animal self.

The chief animals that I think of in terms of strengthening the stomach, solar plexus, or gut-level instincts are Badger and Dog.

❁ BADGER MEDICINE ❁

Many Badger Medicines hit a person with a punch in the stomach. Anyone who has ever smelt or tasted Goldenseal knows what I'm talking about. Gentian hits us with a jolt due to its bitterness. Badger Medicines often have yellow roots and strengthen the autonomic nervous system and the muscles of the GI tract that it innervates, and they improve peristalsis or gut movement. Yellow Dock Root is also a member of this group. It has yellow roots that look like a little badger. Its cousin Rhubarb is another member of this family—the root looks like a big badger.

Paul Red Elk pointed out that Badger is fastidious about his food and therefore associated with the principle of making herbal preparations—and is also considered knowledgable about herbal properties because he lives in Earth.

✎ Goldenseal ✎
(*Hydrastis canadensis*)

Goldenseal powder, if sniffed, will cause a thump on the belly. It is a bit shocking. Goldenseal is a cooling bitter that increases secretion from the mucosa, especially of the stomach. It feels like it runs a current through the mucosa, evidently prompting the internal linings to greater movement and activity. It strengthens the autonomic but has little direct effect on the central nervous system.

Goldenseal is used for stomach ulcers and external ulcers, diabetic ulcers, bedsores, and torpid skin and mucosa generally. The powder can be put on herpes and shingles—but there are cheaper, more available members of the buttercup family that can be used here. The tongue is often wide, apathetic, with poor tone and sometimes ulcers in the tooth-marks on the side.

The yellow color is associated with the Earth in Chinese herbalism. Goldenseal does not disappoint us in carrying through on this signature. A sixty-year-old woman had a strained neck and right shoulder—too much work and a previous injury. Doctors said: "irreparable disk damage," "strained neck," "surgery." Their ideas didn't even make sense to her. Her usually reliable chiropractor made it worse. From the way she held herself, the evaluation was clear to me: the tissues had been forced (Blue Vervain) and she was "writhing in agony" (Prickly Ash). When she received Goldenseal for injured disks she felt a current go through her body, her spine straightened, and she felt "connected to the Earth." The pain soon abated and function returned. Later we added magnesium and Ashwagandha powder for muscle spasm and atrophy.

Pinches of the powder and drop doses are all that are needed— even a fraction of a drop is powerful. Goldenseal is environmentally challenged and has been for more than a hundred and fifty years, so it should be used in moderation. Twenty years ago, a professional wild-crafter told me: "You can't find it within a mile of a road anywhere." If one is using berberine, the so-called "active ingredient" that is an antibiotic, one should not use Goldenseal but Barberry or Oregon Grape Root. One cousin, Yellow Root (*Xanthorhiza simplicissima*), has close to the same properties and the aboveground sticks are harvested, making it environmentally safer for use. I am not experienced with it.

☙ Gentian ❧
(*Gentiana lutea*)

This bitter root is one of the central plants of traditional European medicine, the indications for which were established centuries ago and have not been significantly improved upon, except for the addition of mental indications by Dr. Bach.

Discovery of the medicinal properties of the plant was attributed to Gentius, king of Illyria (modern Bosnia and Montenegro). The official species, *Gentiana lutea*, is found in the mountains of Europe, but Dioscorides (ca. 70 CE) notes that it grows both on the tops of mountains and in swamps. This indicates that he was including a lowland species as well as the high—a flexibility that was long allowed in herbal medicine but was eventually abandoned in favor of the mountain species.

Gentian illustrates the Wolf/Dog polarity since it acts on the gallbladder/stomach axis, especially when the stomach is weak or the gallbladder is overbearing. The connection to angularity we note in Wolf Medicine is seen in the placement of the leaves, which are opposite on the stem. This is found in many of its relatives, like Fever Root (*Triosteum perforatum*)—here the leaves merge together across the stalk. Gentian has yellowish roots, a signature for Badger Medicine, an analog of Dog Medicine.

Gentian is similar to Werewolf Root, but here the opposition is between the animal self (gut-level instincts, stomach) and the ego (gallbladder), instead of the ego and spiritual will (kidneys).

Various Kinds of Gentian

The European herbalists and physicians originally used many different kinds of Gentian, before the yellow-flowered species became officinal. This flexibility carried over to America. The early nineteenth-century physicians tended to use native members of the family, such as *Frasera carolinensis* (Columbo), *Sabbatia* (American Centaury), or *Triosteum perfoliatum* (Horse Gentian, Fever Root, American Gentian). With improvements in herb commerce, the European Gentian came to predominate in American practice and the cousins are now only of historical interest. All of these plants were used by the Eastern Indian people, who also valued bitters, and presumably by black practitioners as well.

"The Great Bitter"

Yellow Gentian is an intense bitter with an affinity to the "golden arc" of the digestive viscera strung together by the portal vein: stomach, duodenum, gallbladder, and liver. The bitterness stimulates the salivary glands, taste buds, appetite, hydrochloric acid, pancreatic enzyme secretion, and bile production. This powerful action strengthens the innervations of the "enteric brain" presiding over this region. Sir John Hill noted that Gentian "is the great Bitter and Stomachic of the modern

Practice" (1755, 159). It is still used in European medicine as a bitter to increase digestion. It is very reliable in this role, but stereotyping of use is not useful in establishing its deeper and wider applications. We need to understood the mental and emotional correspondences of the stomach-gallbladder axis, which pits the instincts (stomach, wild self) against the egoic will (gallbladder, gall, tame self). This touches upon the polarity of the Dog and the Wolf (the tame and the wild). For some reason, although Wolf is associated with the wild and Dog with the tamed, the medicines of the Wolf relate to the gallbladder; those of the Dog to stomach.

The intense bitterness provokes secretions from the stomach, so that Gentian improves appetite and digestion and strengthens the gut-level instincts. By increasing secretions from the stomach and gallbladder, it also facilitates the lubrication and movement of the stool. When the food is sitting in the stomach or fermenting in the gut, Gentian is also often indicated.

In her unpublished notes, Dorothy Hall thought of Gentian more as a gallbladder remedy, but in her published work she puts the emphasis on the stomach and digestion, as it is normally portrayed in Western herbalism (1988, 164–67). In Chinese herbalism Gentian is also associated with the gallbladder. It is really a remedy for both, increasing secretion from both stomach and gallbladder, and improving the timing between the two as well as the intensity of secretion because the gallbladder depends upon a signal from the pyloric end of the stomach to release bile and digestive enzymes.

Intermittent Chills and Fever

In the days when malaria was common, Gentian was used for intermittent chills alternating with fever. Today these symptoms may appear with influenza and Lyme disease and its various co-infections. Perhaps Gentian should be considered. Alternating chills and fever wreak havoc on the autonomic. Bitters are often suited to this problem because they cause a "chill" or shiver to run through the involuntary nerves. Persistent chills lead to the exhaustion of organs innervated by the autonomic—digestive tract, liver, and gallbladder. The timing between the different structures is damaged.

Digestion

Gentian is primarily thought of as a digestive remedy in Western herbalism. In her book Dorothy Hall emphasizes that the Gentian person reacts to emotional stress by losing their appetite. They have little appetite, and what they have is easily lost, so, as she says, these people are "tyrannized" throughout life by their digestion. Those seated at the same table or cooking the meal may feel tyrannized as well (Hall 1988, 164–67).

The Portal Vein

This vein drains the golden arc of digestion and metabolism. Dorothy Hall found Gentian to have its most prominent and deepest effects on this region, which she calls the "yellow system" (1988, 164). She was clued to its use by the personality (more about that later) and the iridology. It was indicated by a swollen, twisted, dark vessel in the sclera, adjacent to the liver area, which she interpreted as an indicator of serious portal congestion. This is visible even to a non-iridologist, but in addition, the late herbalist Michael Moore pointed out specific indications for portal congestion: varicosities of the veins behind the left knee.

The Portal Vein and the Heart

Congestion and enlargement in the portal vein will back up into the liver, gall ducts, and even into the veins entering the heart. Dorothy considered this an important remedy to prevent and reverse some kinds of heart disease; Culpeper says it "comforts the heart" (1850, 83). Gentian is an established hemorrhoid, varicose vein, and portal vein medicine. Other remedies that act on portal congestion are Stone Root (*Collinsonia canadensis*) and Horse Chestnut (*Aesculus hippocastanum*), which are stimulating astringents—so they have a completely different modus operandi. Because it is for feeble blood circulation, Gentian is for bruises (externally) and putrefaction or sepsis.

The Bitter Person

In her unpublished notes for students, Dorothy Hall drew correspondences between the portal system and the emotions. Just as the blood is congested and blocked in the portal, these people are not able to allow their emotions to freely flow, but block them. They might be caught in the wrong relationship and don't feel able to leave. This is like Werewolf Root, another gallbladder remedy. This turns them into a bitter person, whereas the Werewolf Root person becomes weak and can't break out of the domination of another. One thinks here also of Black Walnut hull: "too much under the domination of another." Also of Centaury, a cousin of Gentian: the doormat who is weak-willed and allows others to dominate them.

The "Gentian person" feels deprived of the basic needs for a happy life. They relive all the bad breaks that have been meted out to them rather than processing their emotions and going through them. They talk about a bad event long ago, keeping it current and unresolved. Worse yet, they try to undermine other people's happiness with negative comments that spread doubt. When they are opposed, rather than admitting their own problem or trying to work through it, they stir up emotions or intentionally create anger. They frequently turn to alcohol or cigarette smoking to block their emotions.

Dr. Bach's Indications

Dorothy Hall and myself were much influenced in our view of the Gentian person by the account of Dr. Edward Bach's flower essence. He used *Gentiana amarella*, which is interchangeable for physical and psychological purposes. He considered this a remedy for self-doubt: when the person is progressing well, but there is a setback and they lose confidence; when they suffer chronic depression from inability to cast off doubts. In another presentation, the person asks repeatedly if the remedy is going to work, and needs continual reassurance—even when they already feel better from it. Most irritating are the people who back off when the instinct of the healer kicks in and we are certain about the remedy. "Oh, I was just wondering theoretically what remedy you would give." They are afraid of your instincts as well as their own. Give the remedy then and there to reassure these autonomically challenged individuals.

Moxie
This is the perfect word for a person with a strong, balanced gallbladder. It means courage, stamina, and will. A soda pop by this name is made from Gentian root extract and is still found in New England. A piece of the root is worn in Appalachia to increase courage and stamina.

Energetics
Because of the widespread use of Gentian, the energetic indications have been well-established from the most archaic times. In traditional European medicine it was classified as a warming remedy for cold, phlegmatic conditions (Culpeper 1850, 83). However, this remedy is also useful for a hot, dry choleric or bilious constitution, not weak but tough and strong—often with an overbearing gallbladder. We see, therefore, that it is for two opposite conditions. This is often found in herbs, which tend to normalize between opposing states.

Angostura Bitters
I had a client I had been helping for over fifteen years. She was now seventy-six. For three years she had a blocked tear duct causing lack of secretion in the left eye. We tried everything. Eyebright was slightly helpful but slowly it got worse and worse. Now her conjunctiva looked like "chopped meat" and it hurt her terribly. The doctor said: "Lots of people your age have symptoms like that; we can cut open the tear duct to remove the blockage." She didn't like that option. Finally, she also complained: "I'm losing weight. My boyfriend is worried. I don't have any appetite and I don't even like the taste of food." Her mouth was dry; I figured she was drying up, as older people sometimes do. She was naturally tall, slender, and strong—a "choleric" constitution. I recommended Gentian for the lack of saliva and appetite. (She had

Angostura Bitters in the house, which are made from Gentian.) In the next week scum started coming out of her eye, then secretion, then the conjunctiva improved. The heat had been baking down the fluids and causing the blockage in the eye. Her appetite came back and she started to gain weight. This woman had the habit of starting out by intimidating me: telling me how she wasn't getting better. Then she would reverse gears and tell me what was really happening. After I got the Gentian for her, I realized this was the overbearing side of the Gentian personality.

Anaphylactic Shock

I learned from one of my students that Gentian is an excellent remedy for anaphylactic shock. The person turns white and feels threatened, like they are going to die. On the way to medical help, try this and probably it will blow over.

This is a good remedy to keep on hand. I've had only one ana-phylaxis in thirty-five years of herbal practice: a woman turned pale and exclaimed she was going to die after sniffing corn silk! Gentian flower essence immediately brought her back to earth and we continued the class.

I publicized this usage and a nurse from a Waldorf School contacted me and told me she had used it this way for years. She had the parents sign whether they wanted the remedy to be used while the emergency-response team was being called, or even before they were called. She had many successful cases.

I see the anaphylactic shock as a reaction that "separates soul and body," or the egoic will and the animal self, so this usage is a logical extension of the other uses of Gentian.

☙ Dragon Gallbladder Root ❧
(*Gentiana scabra, G. triflora, G. manshurica, G. regescens*)

This is the Chinese Gentian; it is used in a fashion similar to the European. I doubt that they have properties that are intrinsically different. Both work on the gallbladder/stomach axis and that means egoic will/animal instincts. Both have yellow roots.

The uses of Gentian in Chinese medicine are almost identical to those of the European officinal species, and I thought I would discuss the Chinese to deepen our picture of Gentian. There is one major difference, however: the Eastern plant has a better name. Maybe it is a Dragon Medicine.

Damp Heat

In China, Gentian is classified as a cold and bitter remedy used to clear heat and dampness from the liver and gallbladder, in "excess liver-fire syndromes." It is applicable for swelling and pain in the region of the liver, for jaundice and hepatitis. If the fire flares upward, it causes redness of the face and eyes, tinnitus, headache, and hypertension. Or, if it is conjoined with dampness, it can flow downward along the liver meridian, which curves around the external genitalia. It can therefore be used for swelling and sores in the lower part of the body. It is a remedy for genital herpes. The circulation of qi and blood stagnates to cause "steaming of the testicles"; intolerable itching of the scrotum; in women, "steaming of the vagina" due to damp heat, with yellow, foul leukorrhea and severe itching pruritis (ouch!).

⍩ Yellow Dock Root ⍩
(*Rumex crispus*)

Herbs can even help us understand the spirit more fully. A member of the *Rumex* clan native to the Upper Missouri Basin is used by the Indian People to increase understanding of spiritual experiences. It is mentioned by Melvin Gilmore in *Uses of Plants by the Indians of the Missouri River Region* (1991). This is called "Medicine of Understanding." We use the common *Rumex crispus* in Western herbalism.

I had a peculiar experience with this plant that showed its relationship to its cousin. One of my long-term clients called me from the hospital. Her colitis had flared up. She was on 55 mg of prednisone a day but was having fifteen to twenty bowel movements a day. This occurred five weeks after the birth of her third child. I thought that she possibly got thrush from her baby. She had to stop lactation—a real trauma for her little daughter.

I arrived at the hospital in the evening. Sarah's big, extended Jewish family had gone home. We talked easily. I wasn't very worried about which herb to give. She had a sort of reddish/brownish complexion with spots of yellow, like inflammation with serum coming up to the surface. Evidently, this was what was going on in the intestine. I already knew of yellow and red as a complexion indicating Yellow Dock Root.

A nurse came in and asked who I was. I didn't think it was particularly her business so I said: "The witch doctor." She scurried out of the room and about fifteen minutes later a doctor came in to investigate who I was, surreptitiously. "Oh, my son has Crohn's disease, what would you do?" and so on. "Every individual is different so you just have to use what's appropriate for the case," I replied. It was amusing.

We got witch-doctor results. Sarah was on 55 mg of prednisone a day and she still was having diarrhea all day long. The doctor mumbled, "If this doesn't stop, we'll have to operate." I had a quarter-ounce of Yellow Dock Root tincture with me. I gave Sarah a dose and left it with her. She was constipated for the next two days. The doctors didn't ask what I gave, of course. They weren't sincerely interested. But they did start taking down the dosage of prednisone rapidly. Then something happened. The doctor noticed: "Hey, you're blessing people." Sarah answered back: "Well, what do you want me to do, curse 'em?" She was diagnosed as having "religious ecstasy" from the prednisone withdrawal and put in the psych ward for three days. She did, in fact, have visions of God and her life and how it all fit together, and she helped a person in the lockup with her who was suicidal. Afterward they put her on a regimen where they reduced the prednisone by 5 mg a week. She was weaned off the drug after several months.

Everything went well for a year and then I got a call. Sarah was having diarrhea again. "Take the Yellow Dock Root again," I said. She called back: "Every time I take a dose, I have a blip of religious ecstasy."

In the intervening year I had heard about "Medicine of Understanding" so now I realized that Yellow Dock Root had some kind of similar effect. I explained that somehow the religious ecstasy was part of the disease and stirred up by the Yellow Dock. "Take one drop a week and slowly the diarrhea and the religious ecstasy should go away." And that's what happened.

Later, Sarah said, "Now I am more down-to-earth about spiritual issues. When someone tells me they've had a spiritual experience, I say: 'Yes, but what are you going to do about it?'" She is well twenty years later.

☉ DOG MEDICINE ☉

Another animal associated with gut-level instincts is Dog. When the stranger arrives, Dog instincts kick in and Dog barks. I don't count myself as the last word in shamanic herbalism (though maybe I am the first!), but it appears the Badger Medicines rely more on bitterness and the yellow bitters, while the Dog remedies act more on the innervation of the solar plexus. Wood Betony and Bryonia, which I have placed here, actually seem to be Human Medicines in some measure—the human and the dog are bound together.

⚲ Black Hoarhound ⚲
(*Ballota nigra*)

This is the less-known cousin of White Hoarhound (*Marrubium vulgare*); they are both in the mint family, both native to the Old World, both "furry." That explains the "hoary"—like a hoarfrost. The spelling "horehound" is more common, but not correct. Originally, I thought the furriness was why they were "hound" remedies, but more recently I became aware that *Ballota* was used as a rabies remedy in Europe. This may have been due to the doctrine of signatures: the fur indicating its use for dog bites.

This medicine plant came late into my apothecary, but when I adopted it, I found that it covered a niche that was really needed.

David Hoffmann is one of the few contemporary herbalists who mention it. He writes in *The New Holistic Herbal* that *Ballota* is "an excellent remedy for the settling of nausea and *vomiting* when the cause lies within the nervous system rather than the stomach" (1992, 181). In other words, the stomach is not itself irritated or full or disordered; the problem lies in nerves acting on the solar plexus. He recommends it for motion sickness, the vomiting of pregnancy, or nausea and vomiting due to nervousness.

I misinterpreted this somewhat. I did use *Ballota* a few times for nervous tension reflexing to the stomach but eventually discovered that it was a specific for nervousness and anxiety centered in the solar plexus itself. In other words, it is a solar-plexus medicine.

A mother I had been doctoring now and then over a decade or more brought her daughter to see me—I mean, they flew in from another state. The daughter was suffering from low-grade but socially debilitating problems, with anxiety and nervousness felt in the stomach. She didn't like to go in department stores because she felt trapped by the layout—which is intended to trap a person. The symptoms were subtle but the location in the stomach was the best hint. Black Hoarhound cured this and she married a nice guy a year and a half later.

David Hoffmann reflects the English herbal tradition. I think the fount of tradition on this plant may be attributed to Richard Hool, who said he learned about the remedy from his mother. From him we learn that *Ballota* also acts on the gallbladder, which is so intimately tied to the stomach—as mentioned under Gentian. In *Health from British Wild Herbs* (1918), he explains that Black Hoarhound is one of the best remedies for "biliousness, bilious colic, and sour belchings," what we now call esophageal reflux. It acts "as if a current of electricity had passed into the stomach, allaying all the symptoms momentarily."

Hool extends the use to spasms throughout the body, reminding us that spasms are accompanied by "a disturbance of the equilibrium of the blood circulation and the nerve force." It is therefore a remedy for coughs, bronchitis, asthma, and chronic respiratory problems. It "resolves the viscidity of the mucus secretions, and acts as an alterative tonic upon the mucous follicles," cleaning and healing them. In holistic medicine we think about what is happening in the tissues; biomedicine thinks in terms of molecules.

Ballota is also for excess or lack of menstrual flow. "It may seem contradictory to the ordinary reader" that the herb may be used in "opposite conditions," comments Hool. However, the problem is due to a "loss of equilibrium," which *Ballota* restores.

This generalization is true for many, many herbs because they normalize between two extremes. Sometimes tradition or experience only tells us about one side of the imbalance; then there is more to be learned about this herb, lurking in the background. As I read back over this account, I wonder if Black Hoarhound would be remedial for the dystonia and vagal problems that follow in the wake of covid and other problems that distune the autonomic nervous system.

⚘ Wood Betony ⚘
(Stachys officinalis, Betonica officinalis)

I cannot honestly call this a Dog or Badger Medicine because its effects on the solar plexus (and brain) are tonifying rather than stimulating; it is more gentle than the herbs in these categories.

Wood Betony is a wonderful remedy for strengthening the innervations of the brain of the head and the brain of the stomach—both the central and autonomic nervous systems. It is for slender, ungrounded people—it helps connect the brain to the stomach and the brain and stomach to the Earth. It is excellent for the elderly. The aboveground parts are safe: a mint nervine of the highest order.

As a shamanic herbalist, one might be called upon to cure all sorts of things. Wood Betony is the remedy for "alien abduction" problems. There are a lot of different "aliens." I gave some interesting case histories in *The Book of Herbal Wisdom* (1997, 165–78). Seán O'Donoghue says it helps people who feel they themselves are aliens or alienated from their community.

One time when I gave Wood Betony for a man who had been abducted by aliens, I had a vision:

As I was driving down the street at dusk, my consciousness projected out of my head through a hole in the clouds. I heard voices singing "Holy, Holy, Holy is the Lord God Almighty." I found myself in front of the throne of God. I could see up to his knees—about three stories high. He boomed out: "I have made a covenant with the Earth, that I will not allow the Earth to be destroyed." Wow, that's great, I thought. *Then he added: "And I'm not relying upon the human race to help me."* Of course, we're the problem. *"They're a weak reed to rely on."* Wow, this sure is Old-Testamenty, I thought. *I asked what would happen to the human race, but he faded away.*

At two in the morning, I was awoken by one of those gray aliens with the big black slanted eyes. She put a probe in the inner canthus of my left eye to communicate with me. "The Earth is dead. Therefore, we are going to launch an evacuation, and we'd like you to be a leader because people are so terrified by us." End of transmission, pulled the probe, gone. I felt nothing but terror the whole time.

I tossed and turned until morning. I couldn't figure who was right: *God or the aliens?* That's the way it is with some visions—you are so removed from normalcy that it takes a while for common sense to kick back in. I called and asked a friend at eight in the morning. "Well, God, of course!" she said. *Yeah, that makes sense,* I thought.

☙ Bryonia ☙
(Bryonia alba)

The true Mandrake (*Mandragora officinarum*) of the Middle East and Central Asia was much esteemed as a fertility medicine within its range and even finds its way into the Hebrew Bible. The stories about Jacob in Genesis are filled with magical references, among them the use of mandrake by his wives Rachel and Leah in their contest to have the most children. The name seems to come from the words "man" and "drake" (dragon)—whatever that means. During the homeopathic provings, one chronically infertile woman got pregnant.

The Mandragora is not native to Western Europe, but the English herbalists noticed that the big, plump root of their own native White Bryony (*Bryonia dioica*) sometimes looked like a man, so they called it "Mandrake," not having the exotic Mandragora. This plant is not known as a fertility medicine; it is a hydrogogue or a cathartic so intense it drains the fluids out of the colon. It had to be moderated by admixture with gentler appropriate agents. This was in centuries before the appearance of cathartics like Rhubarb and Senna. Making mandrake usable was a trade secret closely held by the herbalists and herb guilds of the time.

Not only the formulation but even the digging of the root became a special affair. The old herbalists concocted a ritual to maintain their secrets. It was said that the root screamed when it was pulled out of the ground so they would dig it out almost entirely, tie their dog to it, walk a long distance away then call for the dog, who would rip it out of the ground. This led to the stories surrounding Mandrakes told in the Harry Potter books.

Not only did people harvest the root in these crazy rituals but they would grow them in molds or carve them to look more like human beings. William Turner writes in his *New Herball* from 1568:

> The roots which are counterfeited and made like little puppets or mammets, which come to be sold in England in boxes, with hair and such form as a man hath, are nothing but foolish feigned trifles, and not natural; for they are so trimmed of crafty thieves to mock the poor people withal, and to rob them both of their wit and their money. (Turner 1996, 2:437)

Magical beliefs piled on top of others, so that it came to be believed that Mandrake that grew under the gallows where condemned men shed their blood or sperm was the most powerful. Turner also opposes this belief (1996, 2:437):

But it groweth not under gallosses [gallows], as a certain doting doctor of Cologne in his physic lecture did teach his auditors; neither doth it rise of the sede of man that falleth from him that is hanged; neither is it called Mandragoras because it came of man's seed, as the forsaid Doctor dreamed.

Meanwhile, the herbalists still turned it to their purposes. At country fairs, the fortunate herbalist who possessed such an item would raise it on a staff to identify himself as a guild herbalist. And later, when herb shops began to appear in villages and towns, a Bryony root would be placed in the window for all to see. For more details on this subject, see C. S. J. Thompson, *The Mystic Mandrake* (1934).

All this would be entirely academic were it not for the fact that Chris MacPadden, one of my students (and now one of my co-teachers), dreamed of the rites by which Bryonia was harvested and used by the English herbalists. I told him: "Well, I guess that means you are a qualified herbalist." What was rather odd about this was that Chris is part-Ojibwa and Métis, speaks Ojibwa, and has studied with his elders. In dreamtime there is no such thing as "cultural appropriation." That only belongs to those who can't dream.

In homeopathy, Bryonia is used as the opposite of the old English herbal use: it is for dried out membranes that have lost all their fluids, hence the keynote: worse from movement—because there are no lubricating fluids. I've also found that it is good when people are forced to move from their homes, and the moving process has taken a heavy toll on them. To my knowledge it doesn't help the animal instincts (like the other Dog and Badger remedies), but works with overly strong emotional attachments. I helped one woman who had a red, inflamed, dried-off tongue who said she felt like she had to make a pact with the Devil to get out of the religious cult she was raised in. She needed to know it was okay to feel like one is ripped out of the ground.

Bryony is a member of the Pumpkin family, so it has this great big root like a Cucumber or Squash—but underground.

It is rather fun to have Mandragora or its American namesake, *Podophyllum peltatum*, in the garden. They will actually move, screwing themselves deeper into the ground or out of it. I was once teaching a class at Kate Gilday's Woodland Essences, in the Adirondacks. I mentioned this in front a class of over ten people (only counting the ones that were paying attention) and the American Mandrake moved in the ground. "It shifted!" exclaimed Kate. This is a powerful medicinal plant.

The Way of the Turtle and Self-Actualization

As I already mentioned, the "Way of the Turtle" is a name for the boundary in the throat between the human and the animal, as well as the lessons that can be learned there. It is also a place where the teacher can examine the student. The moment I said "Yes" to visiting a medicine man, I felt a sensation like a tube breaking in my throat. Immediately, my inner space became filled with the smoke of his peace pipe. This was his way of examining me: he "smoked me." Castaneda described the exact same experience: a sensation of the breaking of a tube in the neck, followed by being "smoked" by his teacher. Rudolf Steiner describes this point in *Knowledge of the Higher Worlds and Its Attainment* (1947, 133):

> Thanks to the spiritual organ situated in the vicinity of the larynx, it becomes possible to survey clairvoyantly the thoughts and mentality of other beings, and to obtain a deeper insight into the true laws of natural phenomena.

This "spiritual organ" is usually called the "throat chakra," in Western occultism. It is usually described as a flower with sixteen petals. Steiner continues (1947, 136):

> In the sixteen-petaled lotus, eight of its sixteen petals were developed in the remote past during an earlier stage of human evolution.

Man himself contributed nothing to this development; he received them as a gift from nature, at a time when his consciousness was in a dull, dreamy condition. At that stage of human evolution, they were in active use, but the manner of their activity was only compatible with that dull state of consciousness. As consciousness became clearer and brighter, the petals became obscured and ceased their activity.

In other words, these "petals" of consciousness were developed in the animal period of evolution, as part of animal awareness. Although Steiner calls that form of consciousness "dull and dreamy," in fact it is a doorway to lucidity in dreamtime. It is just dull and dreamy here, in the conscious world of the humans.

Eight of the petals have reference to the human and eight to the animal. So the original eight were where we were at when we were closer to the animal world.

The approach taught by Steiner involves the development of awareness in the eight human petals, which, when finished, actualize the eight animal petals. "Only eight can be consciously developed; the remainder then appear of their own accord" (Steiner 1947, 137).

Each of the eight human petals relates to what we might call a "human virtue." According to Steiner, the first involves the development of (1) *conscious thinking*, so that the person does not entertain and follow random thoughts, but those that are constructive and useful. We can see that this is in fact one of the primal differences between animals and humans: we can concentrate and self-reflect. The second pertains to (2) the *making of resolutions*: a person should agree to proceed only after careful consideration and self-reflection. This is an extension of the previous lesson and also relates to the ability to keep a focus or return to it. The third relates to (3) *intentional speech*, which should not be casual, but carry the weight of self-reflection. The ability to speak is a crucial characteristic of the human life-wave and a doorway through which the spirit manifests. The fourth lesson moves beyond speech to action. It pertains to (4) *conscious action harmoni-*

ous with the outer world. We tend to "stick out" in the natural world in unnatural ways. It becomes necessary, therefore, for us to leave the least noticeable footprint in the forest. The fifth petal involves (5) the *management of the whole of life,* so that the student attempts to live in harmony within the outside and the inside worlds. The sixth petal is named (6) *balanced self-knowledge,* meaning that "he attempts nothing beyond his powers, yet seeks to omit nothing within their scope." This sets the stage for the seventh petal, which involves (7) *learning as much from life as possible.* On the spiritual path, we value all experiences and attempt to extract meaning, value, and background from each of them. We don't ignore even the fleeting images in our mind, much less the scars burned into our souls. The eighth and final petal involves (8) *continuous self-reflection.*

All of this must be done in a way that is not "irksome" but flows naturally from within the person as established habit. When these eight "petals" have been actualized, the other eight will "reappear of themselves" (Steiner 1947, 143).

We can see that this is a prescription for a very well-set out-spiritual training program. Steiner notes that it corresponds closely with directions given by Buddha to his students. It also resembles the seven virtues associated with the middle bundle of sweetgrass. This is the kind of behavior we need to be good citizens of human society as well as students on the path of spiritual knowledge. Thinking about the Werewolf, Alligator King, Snake Woman, the Lord of the Underworld, and the ouroboros is not so challenging; but experiencing them, without our defenses, naked in dreamtime, is terrifying. For this we need the sobriety of the warrior. Remember Christine's experience after "answering the question."

The properties of the eight petals relating to animal consciousness are not described by Steiner, but this is where we obtain our "deeper insight into the true laws of natural phenomena," which he also mentioned. Both the channel and the knowledge received there are called the Way of the Turtle. An education in natural law, the Wisdom of Nature, and the opening to the Spirit World are all engraved on our neck, like some kind of spiritual collar. Little Turtle raises his head up to show us this spot. Wolf raises his head upward to let out his mournful cry—the cry of the whole Animal Kingdom for their lost human brother.

Premature Actualization of the Animal Spirit

Steiner comments (1947, 143): "faulty training may easily result in the re-appearance of the earlier petals alone, while the new petals remain stunted." That means that animality rules the person instead of humanity. This is not a completely unknown problem on the Old, Old Path.

The emphasis on rational teachings and self-government described by Steiner is a good educational program, but I experienced a more ancient method. "That old man," said another medicine man, "could initiate a person into the medicine lodge in one day."

The fact that the dream self developed in prehuman times, along with the warm-blooded heart and powerful animal instincts and sensations, hints at the great debt we owe Animalia. I was reminded of this when I was attacked by a young self-described "witch" who, surprisingly, possessed a fully developed (but abused) familiar spirit. This person was addicted to viciously hectoring people online if they didn't agree with her absurd views and personal needs. She had obnoxious ideas about herbalism, which I opposed, so she attacked me and set her cyberbully accomplices on me.

Black Bird Flies

After I didn't knuckle under, she resorted to attacking me in dream-time. I woke up in the middle of the night with a black bird flying at my face. It seemed real for a second but it woke me up and I immediately understood that it was a familiar spirit so there was no reason for me to be afraid. Spirit animals are as likable as physical animals.

I had been thinking about this person during the day and she had even threatened me online, so I knew the identity of the attacker.

Besides, she was a Crow in the way she hectored everybody. Nothing much followed this aborted attack, but two weeks later Black Bird asked if it could stay with me because the witch "was so mean and you're nice." I'd never encountered this kind of question before, so I followed my instincts. They told me I had to ask for spiritual guidance. Separating a person from their animal self can be fatal. Jesus had popped into my mind earlier in the day, so I asked him. He said it was okay to keep a familiar spirit as long as it wanted to stay with me. So it stayed with me.

This experience was valuable. I learned that Jesus was the incarnation of spiritual law in a human being. This law has been incarnated; it is not written on stone or paper, as in the tablets of Moses, Confucius, Asoka, Justinian, Napoleon, or the American Constitution. It is not "blind," like our Justice. I suppose this is exactly what a Christian would say, but there is a difference between thinking of something and having the experience. That was well worth having, so I can thank my worthy opponent for that lesson.

I also came to understand something about witches. Most of them operate as laws unto themselves, deciding who will live and who will die, as if it is up to them to determine the fate of their fellow creatures. This is an incredibly arrogant position to assume.

This lack of awareness shows the vulnerability of witches. They are so imprudent that they will attack people without understanding that they themselves could end up on the losing end of the kerfuffle. To set one's familiar spirit against another person, with intent to do harm, could cause death, mental illness, or damage the spiritual life of the other person; equally, it could damage the sender terribly.

My new animal friend preferred to be called "Black Bird," identifying with a general group rather than an individual species. I don't really know what goes through the mind of an animal totem; they may draw their species and genus lines differently than humans. There is no doubt there is a big difference between ravens, who hang around in small flocks, and crows, who are much more sociable, talkative, and even hectoring.

I also understood Black Bird's desire to stay with me rather than to be "returned to the wild." The Animal Kingdom yearns for association with us, especially for the eight lessons that Steiner described. The animals desire to see, know, and live in association with the integrity, sobriety, and law-abiding conscientiousness that humans can incarnate.

There is always forgiveness for every kind of spiritual offense, but the more serious the crime, the more change is required from the offender. Black Bird's co-walker cannot be given a blank check to happily prance along the path of life, oblivious to the destruction she is causing. It is serious business to damage the spiritual life of another individual, or even their physical body, or inflict on their free will, or (if nothing else) to waste their time.

A few weeks later, a little cohort of witches who were also part of the group sent against me launched their attack. The leader was a dilettante by comparison to Black Bird's co-walker; she was an unworthy opponent. She didn't use a familiar spirit, but instead practiced the usual sort of petty witchcraft based on building up emotional energy and directing it according to images that she focused upon.

The purpose these people had set up was to stop my forward momentum in the world so that I would cease to have influence. This included attacking my voice so I couldn't speak. A friend pointed out the contours of what was going on. I had a few hours' drive with nothing better to do than talk to the chief witch in my mind. I told her she couldn't do this kind of stuff to people and she was going to have to take responsibility for her actions. She was quite upset by the idea of taking responsibility because it turned out she didn't like work and she was happy with the place on the dial where her ego was already set and she didn't want to change. I also noticed she was not sexually disciplined. How anybody with so little willpower and self-control could think to practice witchcraft is beyond me.

The woman needed to take responsibility for her actions but I didn't want to have to monitor her. Just then Black Bird showed up and said, "I could do that for you." "Oh? How would you do that?" I enquired. "Every time she tries to abuse psychic powers, I'll send her a nightmare until she learns responsibility."

This taught me another important lesson. Now I understood that the guardian, the Dweller on the Threshold, actually is a person's animal self. Because animals have excellent instincts, they are aware of psychological wrongs and react like a dog with bared teeth. Until we bring our animal self to consciousness, it operates as the Dweller on the Threshold, keeping us from unhealthy exposure to energies we are not ready to face. It does this by sending us dreams. If our own animal self has been suppressed and overridden by the ego, another animal spirit can take up the task. Now I understood what the witch meant when she said Mullein could be used to send people nightmares. I was grateful for this experience because it taught me, step by step, about the meaning of nightmares.

When a person abuses psychic powers, the animal self—which has healthy instincts (unless it has been abused)—disapproves of the actions of the ego. It bulges up from the unconscious as a nightmare. When, in the fullness of time, we bring the animal self to full awareness and equality with the human self, then at last we see it in its fully developed form. The smug setting on the egoic dial becomes movable, our automatonic existence is ended, and we assume responsibility as a citizen of the Earth—rather than remaining a tramp.

A few years passed. I never saw Black Bird again. Then, one morning I woke up with the Beatles song "Blackbird" playing in my mind. Black Bird was back! A few nights later, I had dreams about being confused and not being able to teach about herbal medicine. As I came out of the dream, I understood that these were curses against me, intended to stop me from teaching my life vocation, and Black Bird was showing me what the curses were. She was bringing them back to me for release. I was grateful for the protection. She checked me out, to see if I needed any help, then flew off to some other project. Like Jesus said, I have to respect the independence of Black Bird.

❂ BLACK BIRD MEDICINE ❂

I count crows, black birds, and ravens together. Because they feed on carcasses, I consider their medicines to be the anti-putrefactives and antiseptics. For me, the signature is a black mark on the leaf or some other structure, or the sudden turning black of an injured part. The plants in this category overlap with the Snake Medicines (Black Cohosh, Baptisia) and other plants with black marks or blackening on the injured leaves—Knotweeds and Viburnums, for instance.

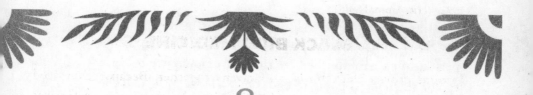

8

The Spirit Self

*Magic is a great, secret, sudden and disbelieved-in wisdom,
out of this world, and opposite.*

PASCHAL BEVERLY RANDOLPH, SEERSHIP

*Dreams, hitherto confused and haphazard, now begin to
assume a more regular character. Their pictures begin to
succeed each other in sensible connection, like the thoughts
and ideas of daily life. He can discern in them law, cause,
and effect. . . . Now there appear before him pictures of a
world he has hitherto not known.*

RUDOLF STEINER, KNOWLEDGE OF THE HIGHER
WORLDS AND ITS ATTAINMENT

The spirit does not take volunteers. However, it is always peeking
through the clouds looking for associates . . . and the impossible is its
favorite ground for action. It knocks on the door of all people, all the
time—when it doesn't knock the door down—advertising a jump into a
river whose destination none can foresee.

It is impossible to dedicate oneself to the spirit because the ego
will never willingly give up its power. That's the nature of the ego and
nobody can change it. And that's why volunteers always have an egoic
agenda the spirit doesn't trust. So the only recourse it has is to trap the

ego in an unwinnable situation. How does that happen? It drives the person to an extremity where they have no choice because life for the ego or the body is going to end. Only to save itself will the ego submit itself to another power.

Mircea Eliade penned the classic characterization of the person who experiences the shamanic calling (1964, 33–66). They become physically or psychically ill to the point where life is despaired. At their lowest extremity they are given a choice: stay where you are and die, or join the spirit and live. The person who is in the best position to accept the offering of the spirit is one whose life is forfeit and this is the kind of person who has lived up to the edge, over the edge, or never had a chance to live a "normal life." That is why Jesus loved the sinners: they were the only ones able to dedicate themselves to a radically new life. People leading a safe life are not ready to give everything up.

When a person chooses the spirit over death, the spirit can at last step in. Afterward the person will be a prisoner of the spirit, and yet they will also be free. How could that be? It is because the spirit allows us to be exactly who we are. That which traps the person also reveals them.

Although the spirit sneaks up on us and takes our free will away, it is the absolute respecter and guarantor of free will. It will not force people to follow it because this would violate its very nature. The spirit requires absolute freedom to operate fully and unconditionally. As the guarantor of freedom, the spirit hates slavery in all its forms. It thoroughly respects the free will of human beings, even though we are automatons with only an illusion of freedom, controlled by unseen forces. It will even allow itself to be taken prisoner and abused by dark magicians.

Although the ego must succumb to the spirit, after it has recognized the hegemony of the spirit, it still has a job: it remains as the protector of the island of the *tonal*. The spirit would drive a person to exhaustion, so the ego, the soul, and the physical body have to learn to stand up for their own needs. We are reborn in the spirit but we also remain in the world. There is a period of adjustment, during which tensions remain, but eventually the three selves should come into a peaceful coexistence.

The spirit is not only the absolute respecter of free will: it is ruth-less by nature, so that once the choice to join the spirit has been made, revocation is impossible. It is the foundation of truth and reality, so we cannot lie to it or retract our vow. We make what Ronald Weasley called the "Unbreakable Vow."

The Big Choice

Those who see this choice coming are not always happy about it. It means they are going to have to give up a lot of convenient things that make life easier for them. Susan recalled:

I remember when I made the choice to follow the path. I was camping. I knew what my life would become. I didn't have a choice. I had to give up all that "out-there stuff." I was going to have to be spiritual. I was literally kicking and screaming because I had no choice. I didn't want that life. It looked like a life of suffering. Then I saw this old, old grandfather sitting by me in the tent. He shook his head, as if to say, "What a spoiled little baby. She's having a temper tantrum."

Knowing Susan, it is hard to believe she wanted to cling to her old life. She ran away from home when she was thirteen, lived in the sew-ers of Minneapolis (literally, *inside the sewer system*), survived a gunshot wound with an exploding bullet when she was fifteen, and was dying from Crohn's disease when I first met her twenty years later. Still, she didn't want to give up that life.

One day Susan washed up at the herb store where I worked—dying. She was trying to pretend she was a normal person with a nor-mal job, but the owner of the store and I laughed at her. We were standing behind the counter, leering at her like two Big Bad Wolves. It was not just because she was good-looking, but because we could feel the wild, undomesticated spirit within her. She was streetwise and inner-city to the core. Bob, the owner of the store, gave her Calamus Root (*Acorus calamus*)—even though it's on the FDA "bad herb list."

That stopped the Crohn's disease for ten years—so stick that in your eye, FDA!

Later, Susan started coming to sweat lodges with me, and later attended the Sundance once a year and walked the "Red Road" of Indian spirituality. She got into that more seriously than I did. It fed her soul. This path took care of the reason Susan had gotten sick in the first place. Nobody supported her spirit when she was young and nobody supplied her with the spiritual education she needed. She didn't run away from home due to abuse, but due to disgust with the culture she was raised in—ordinary American society—and the lack of true spiritual aspiration at home. She was a dedicated spiritual warrior even before she knew what it was. Still, she needed to almost physically die to pass into the hands of the spirit.

A few years later, the spirit sent Susan a test. I guess it still wanted to make sure she would put her life on the line. After ten years, the Crohn's disease flared up again. She decided: "If God can't cure me, I'm ready to die." But we found the right herb—see the full account under Gravel Root.

That hasn't been the end of her suffering, either. She was paralyzed in bed with Lyme disease, so exhausted she couldn't cross one leg over the other. "The spirits came to me and said they would cure me as an act of grace." And they did. Her latter years have been overshadowed by her husband's death and a stroke.

Most people put off making the Big Choice. They want to live the riotous life of the ego and the physical body that we choose as a species when we ate the apple in the Garden of Eden, in the beginning of time. The resources of the Earth are here for us—not to support our pleasures, but to provide a place for us to grow as spiritual beings. Earth is the safety net of Eden, giving us a second chance.

The riotous life of the ego and the body can become such a habit that eventually it becomes the Choice. Or again, some people consciously make the decision to oppose the spirit and exalt the ego. Some people stumble on, trying to find the right path, without guidance. One day they find the spirit because their habits have been moving them in the right direction. Some people don't really make a decision, they just keep on doing the best they can until, one day—because they have been trying to do their best—they cross an invisible line and enter the territory of God. Others don't make a decision, they just keep wasting Earth resources until they slowly start to circle down the toilet bowl. Ultimately, there are only two choices. According to Gottfried de Purucker, the Sanskrit words for these are (1932, 158):

Pratyeka-Yâna ("everyone for himself" path)
Amrita-Yâna (immortal path)

Fertile Ground for the Spirit

There are several different kinds of people that the spirit hoovers over, like the spirit brooding over the waters on the first day of creation. Here are a few of the better-known types:

The Straight Arrow
A small number of people have innate integrity. Male or female, they are naturally disciplined, honest, straightforward, and willing to put others first, even in the face of death. Some people do not need to be cornered by the spirit, they just need to see it in action firsthand. When they see it, the instinct of truth within them recognizes it for what it is, and they drop what they are doing and follow the spirit. This is what they have been waiting for without necessarily knowing it.

The True Heart
The old Arabic physicians taught that the heart had three valves. The names for them are "Mercy," "Justice," and the "Peacemaker." The first one opens up to bring love and mercy to the world. The valve of Justice closes against those who do not deserve our love. The Peacemaker adjusts the balance between the two, so that they open and close in correct balance—not too tight, not too loose.

True hearts are the ones whose hearts are genuine and sincere. Their love is true; they possess the straight arrow of the heart. They love those who deserve to be loved. Because their heart is true, they also learn to know when not to love. They can't love unless the object of affection is worthy. The spirit appreciates this tempered soul.

Since both straight arrows and true hearts make fine partners, husbands and wives, reliable workers and managers, and good members of society, there are not a lot of free ones hanging around for the spirit to latch onto. Without them, society would probably collapse, so it is necessary that most of them remain in the social arena. Many of them learn to operate in both the ordinary world and the spiritual world.

The spirit is always following these people around and "helping them." That is why they have a certain "charm" that gets them out of problems, as if they had a "guardian angel" on their shoulder, or a "love medicine" that made everyone fall in love with them. There is a kind of charm that comes from the spirit. It deals with these people as they deal with others: fair and square. At the right moment it reveals itself to them and there is nothing in them to resist it.

> A month before the appearance of the coronavirus, I had a dream. I woke in the middle of the night feeling as if there was a spasm in my chest, heart, aorta or something. I examined my emotions. Was this because I was processing a deep emotion? No. Was it an emotion I had taken on from someone else? No. Was it a psychic attack? No. After I had eliminated what was not happening, three spirits came and one of them said: "All that is required to enter the new spiritual age is to have an open heart." Of course, I thought. My heart was blasted open. I lay in bed for the next hour. Within the next three months coronavirus made its appearance and would affect the heart of everyone, emotionally and sometimes physically. I had my heart or upper chest tense up and then blast open about a dozen times.

The Lost Cause

Finally, there are the lost causes: the ones who have nothing to live for—junkies, drunks, and failures—and those who have made big, bad mistakes—the "sinners" that Jesus loved so much. These people have nothing to lose and are therefore excellent candidates for the spirit. Remember, the spirit is attracted to the impossible. These people are picked off the wide, wide path, right in front of the eyes of the Adversary.

The religious leaders and seers of our world have given a decent account of the workings of the spirit. It is said to be innately merciful, a property that stands as the battered rock of our conventional religions. The spirit is inalienably attracted to the desperate, the downtrodden, the sinner at the end of the rope, the forlorn hope. Even the fool has a chance. It "is the finder," wrote Jacob Boehme, "who from eternity continually finds where there is nothing" (1920, 17).

Most people are not true hearts and straight arrows. Many are of the forlorn-hope variety, so lost in the wilderness of the world that they don't have any idea they are lost or that there is a spirit. But the spirit will irrepressibly press forth wherever it has a chance. Those who doubt themselves, who regret, who make mistakes, are welcomed by the spirit as much as anyone else.

The Satisfied

These are the people with the least chance of being touched by the spirit. They are content with their lives, with the social world they live in. Probably they are sympathetic to the homeless or less fortunate, but those people also remind them of how successful and important they are. There is one symptom that always marks these people: they have the approval of conventional society. They have been following the siren call of convention and social approbation rather than listening to the still, small voice within.

Possessed by the Spirit

The Indian People, wrestling with the spiritually lame language of their invaders, took up the word "crazy" and applied it to the effect the spirit has on a person. Someone whose life is owned by the spirit is "crazy." The Native words represented by this English term have connotations on the order of "undomesticatable," "wild," "ruled by the spirit," or "possessed by a dream or vision."

A good example of this kind of person was the Lakota war chief Crazy Horse. His name denotes someone who is wild and undomesticated—like a wild horse. That's the way Crazy Horse was. He was the heart of his people—remember the relationship between the heart and the horse. The name of the great Seminole war chief "Wild Cat" should really be translated "Crazy Panther" or "Crazy Tiger." Another such leader was Tecumseh, the Shawnee leader, whose name meant "Springing Panther."

An example of a crazy person in the white man's world is Oskar Schindler, the German war profiteer who saved thousands of Jews during WWII. Before and after the war, Schindler was a failure, but during the war he was probably the only person who dared to save Jews right in front of the Nazi SS.

After the Nazis overran Poland, Schindler came to Cracow as a member of the Nazi Party, intending to scoop up industries and make a fortune. He seemed to have no scruples. However, he was appalled when he realized that the Nazis were embarking on a campaign of genocide. Switching his priorities, he masqueraded as a Nazi industrialist while resisting the destruction of Eastern European Jewry. He had all the skills that were needed for the situation. He was a cunning black marketeer, a master of bribery, a bald-faced liar, an alcoholic who could drink his SS "friends" under the table—and a procurer of women. He was a courageous bearlike giant who commanded the respect of the SS men—the "good German" with a "Jew-loving" fault. He partied with people that would make most of us throw up—to save thousands, hundreds, handfuls, individuals, even Jews that hated him.

But there was something more to Schindler than the right set of skills for the situation. It was as if he was possessed by a power greater than himself. When some women prisoners were brought in to work in his factory, he told them: "If you work here, then you'll live through the war."

The promise had dazed them all. It was a godlike promise. How could a mere man make a promise like that? But Edith Liebgold found herself believing it instantly. Not so much because she wanted to; not because it was a sop, a reckless incentive. It was because in the second Herr Schindler uttered the promise it left no option but belief. (Keneally 1993, 91)

When we attach ourselves to the chariot of the spirit, destiny can be changed. Schindler modified it to his own ends—not selfishly, but to save others. Because of his generosity in putting others first and trusting to . . . whatever it was he trusted in . . . in the face of relentless personal danger, Shindler was protected . . . and they were protected. He attuned to the power of destiny and from the beginning of the war to the end, the spirit was with him. Edith Leibgold felt that definitive reality:

All the time she pondered Herr Schindler's promise. Only madmen made promises as absolute as that. Without blinking. Yet he wasn't mad. For he was a businessman with a dinner to go to. Therefore, he must know. But that meant some second sight, some profound contact with god or devil or the pattern of things. But again, his appearance, his hand that reached for the wine; it was a hand in which you could somehow sense the latent caresses. And so she came back to the idea of his madness again, to drunkenness, to mystical explanations, to the technique by which the Herr Direktor had infected her with certainty. (Keneally 1993, 92)

Madness . . . in other words: crazy. When the times are lawless, a crazy person is in his or her element. When the times are conventional, there may be no scope for them. After the war, Schindler would never again be a success at anything to which he turned his hand, but he was gratefully supported by the men and women whom he had saved—and immortalized in the book and movie *Schindler's List*. One is struck not only by the gratitude of the people he saved, but the sense many of them had that they had participated in a miracle.

Witness for the Spirit

Although many times Schindler was threatened with death or imprisonment, he never doubted that he would survive. Furthermore, he felt that he had been designated to be a witness. This was also felt by one of his right-hand men, Leopold Pfefferberg, a Jew who served as an officer in the Polish army but became a captain in the hidden war Schindler was fighting against the Third Reich. Although a Jew, Pfefferberg did not worry about his mortality, but knew he also had been appointed to be a witness to the events of his era. It was Pfefferberg who convinced Thomas Keneally to write *Schindler's List*, fulfilling the job of witness.

When I received my license as a "true physician" from the hand of the Living Nature, in a vision, I understood that I had the right—the obligation—to practice natural medicine according to the laws of Nature. Those laws flashed across my mind as I received that visionary parchment license: the Wisdom of Nature; the doctrine of signatures; the law of similars, the law of contraries; regard for spirit, soul, and body as sacred. But something I did not expect was also communicated to me. I was told that after the death of the body I could be called on to be a witness against those who were self-appointed physicians. Their occupation was man-made—founded on money, prestige, and corrupt science, at the expense of empathy, intuition, inspiration, truth, and spiritual principles. The real doctors and nurses will be respected, no matter what.

When we clear our minds out, so that we can tell the difference between our own thoughts and those that are "sent," we do not doubt them. I was young then, but the pictures and thoughts I received were strong and remain vividly engraved on my mind now as they were then.

Truth be told, I had no interest in being a witness against false-faced medicine until the holocaust of the mRNA injections, with the corporate takeover of regulatory agencies, disinformation and misinformation, suppression of scientific and popular opposition, denial of real injury, and over and over again the lies, lies, and more lies.

The Spirit Star

The story of Noah's Ark is a description of the psyche, with three levels, four directions, and all the animal forces in Nature on board. The Ark only has a window on top. This signifies the opening on the top of the head, through which each human being has a connection to their Creator. The three levels, four directions, and all the animals in the world represent the complete inventory we need to make in order to clear out that door on top of the head.

I first read about the opening on the top of the head in Frank Waters's *The Book of the Hopi*. My father gave me the book the year it came out as a Ballantine paperback (1969); I was fourteen. A few years later, I found out about the opening on top of the head in Vedic, New Age, and Theosophical literature, although this was not quite as vivid, and more philosophical in tone than the Hopi stories. In my adulthood, I learned about it from experience. The opening at the top of the head can occur on one's own, but it is much easier "wherever two or more are gathered."

The spirit is connected to us through the top of the head, like a golden cord reaching from our world up to infinity. There is a "bulge" or glowing star up the cord that corresponds to our spirit self. The usual name for this star in Western occult or New Age teachings is the "soul star," but this is not the best term since it is actually the personal spirit self, not the soul. The golden thread can also be seen as a pathway rather than a cord—Dorothy's "yellow brick road." Paschal Beverley Randolph described how the golden cord of some people can appear in a scrying glass (1930, 108): "I know of cases wherein that identical spot of golden light has resolved itself into an ethereal lane through which magnificent supernal realities have been seen."

It would be more appropriate to call it the "spirit star." Sondra Boyd—also a reader of Theosophy—concurred with me about this. Here is a dream I had about the spirit star on October 5, 2017:

I had been feeling psychically attacked for several weeks in my waking life. I wasn't sure if it came from a specific enemy or a general social movement. In the dream I was feeling and recognizing this same energy. I was living in an old Victorian house with a bunch of roommates, like when I was young in college. One of them was attacking me. I fiddled with the door until I finally got it closed and latched. At that second the irritation ended and I instantaneously turned and looked out the window. The stars were falling from the sky, although they looked more like falling cinders. As soon as I saw that, I knew: the world is ending.

Instantaneously, my consciousness shot up the golden cord to my spirit star. I was in a group of spirit stars—a bit less than a dozen. We were all trying to work for the betterment of the planet, but there was no coordination between us and some of us were even fighting against one another because we didn't understand the others' work. All of a sudden, as if a switch had been clicked, we were all coordinated and humming as one. (My conscious mind intruded from the ordinary world to comment, "It seems that the Guardians of the Planet have total control of evolution; they could change everything in a moment if they chose to do so.")

As I woke up further, I wanted to look down from above to see what was going on in the world. I saw an ocean of wild, thrashing waves of chaos. I saw a world leader; he was just an especially big wave.

When I told Sondra about this, she said: "Oh yes, I remember that. It was last October. I was out in my yard. The stars were falling out of the sky. All the little animals were glued to the sight like I was."

Another friend added an important interpretation: "The falling stars were the soul stars of the people who have been neglecting to develop their spiritual life all this while. They have been cut out of heaven and fallen to earth." I knew she was right. As the dream said, it was the end of the old cycle and the beginning of a new one. This concurs with the Hopi stories, which report that at the end of each spiritual age—we are at the end of the fourth—the people with tops of their heads open to Creator were led to safe places where—to their surprise—they met others who also followed their "spirit star."

From one perspective, we see chaos everywhere and coarseness and lack of spirituality. From another, we feel the solidification under our feet of a new world. This reminded Susan and I of something the spirits said to us in ceremony shortly after the turn of the Mayan calendar: "New path under the feet. Don't look to the right and don't look to the left."

The Tree of Life

The image of a Tree of Life is found throughout the world. The name Arbor Vitae is attached to the Northern White Cedar (*Thuja occidentalis*) in Western culture. The mythic Tree represents all life-forms woven into a single living being. It also represents the golden cord that connects us from the Earth under our feet, up through the top of our head to the spirit star, and on to the infinity above. And that means it represents the imagination and dreamtime that connect us to the Spirit World. The Tree of the Knowledge of Good and Evil, on the other hand, represents rational and materialistic thinking which divides and separates all things, and which shuts us off from the All-Life.

In many pictures of the Tree of Life, the roots rest on the back of an enormous Turtle, while an Eagle sits in the top branches. Turtle represents the foundation of the world, from the beginning of time down to the present, while Eagle represents aspirations toward the heavens. He also represents the spiritual warrior, who is always reaching for the highest for himself or herself—and all others. And finally, he represents the perceptive organ for the golden cord, the pineal gland, which is sensitive to light and non-ordinary consciousness.

◉ EAGLE MEDICINE ◉

We already touched on spiritual warriorship, learning that it depends upon survival instincts and therefore upon the reptilian self. That means that it is pretty much limited to activities associated with earthly existence. While we are struggling with the challenges of life on Earth it is commendable to be as disciplined and well-organized in our spiritual and daily lives as we can be. After a while, the warrior's way should become habitual; we don't need to think about it.

As long as we remain in exile from the Spirit World, our warriorship is commendable but it is not as essential to our well-being. When we step across the frontier into dreamtime it needs to be so ingrained in us, on a deep level, that it kicks into operation in dreamtime automatically because we can't use the rational mind in the Spirit World.

The pineal gland is poised in the "top branches" of the human neuroendocrine system. It is attuned to light, penetrating all the way in from the eyes, and it is also associated with the inner experience of light, as in dream, imagination, and awareness.

The pineal gland is therefore in charge of changes of awareness. It releases melatonin, which puts us to sleep, and it responds to DMT, which puts us in the dream state.

I learned a lot from the Delta coronavirus. It caused me to have lucid dreams; it could not do anything to me without causing me to dream about the change. It was like an entity, not a virus. As with many other people, it told me what herbs to take. The lucid dreaming was so strong that when the disease began to ebb, I had symptoms like drug withdrawal. Finally, when I had the last relapse, I felt the virus go through my brain from the frontal cortex, through the middle, where it lit up the dream centers, to the back brain—probably from there to the brain stem because then my heart and respiratory rates slowed down for about fifteen minutes. It was tracing its mental course in me. Omicron, on the other hand, caused me to spend lots of time in the consciousness of the Tree of the Knowledge of Good and Evil, until finally I had to discipline my thoughts.

The lofty, tall White Pine is an Eagle Medicine. In general, I think all the conifers can be included here, but the White Pine in eastern North America and the Douglas Fir in the West are particularly notable in having a relationship with Eagle. In addition to Pine, medicines that seem to operate on the pineal include the Smoke and Cloud Medicines, which we will pick up on later.

❧ Pine ❧
(*Pines* spp.)
❧ White Pine ❧
(*Pines strobus*)

Dr. Bach introduced Scotch Pine (*Pinus sylvestris*) as one of his flower essences. Since Pines don't have flowers, he made the essence by mild boiling of the tips, so it is also not unlike a gemmotherapy preparation. Pine flower essence was Bach's remedy for shame and guilt. That is an emotion that is going to cut us off from ascending the Tree of Life. I am not the only practitioner who has seen it work nicely. However, I prefer to use a preparation of White Pine made from the young needles because it grows in my region and is so noble in appearance.

I originally thought Pine was the remedy for guilt and shame because it is the most tall and lofty of the trees and lofty ideals, shattered, become the stuff of such emotions. The loftiness is less true of the Scotch than the White Pine. I wonder, however, if our alienation from the Spirit World does not, in itself, generate some amount of guilt and shame.

Another signature is the viscid, green sap—which is analogous to deep, viscid, green mucus adhering down in the lungs. Ben Charles Harris points out this signature in *The Compleat Herbal* (1975, 144). This is a good indication; though generally I prefer Elecampane for green mucus. Guilt is like a viscid substance, clinging to our soul.

During the original coronavirus pandemic, when Delta was the main form of the disease, Phyllis Light pointed out to me that we "needed to protect our pineal gland," and she recommended Pine because the pineal is named for the pine. The top of the caduceus, with the two snakes climbing up the leafy branch, has a pine cone between them to represent the pineal, it appears.

I took White Pine needle at the end of my coronavirus episode— three and a half months—and it was very good. The use of the "Five Finger Pine" was also known throughout the Native world. Then the internet got ahold of it. Pine and many other plants contain shikimic acid, which is an "intermediary model for the production of drugs effective against the influenza virus" (Singh et al. 2020). Star Anise is a particular example used as a precursor to an influenza drug. I personally would need more specific information than "influenza," like specific symptoms or regional affinities to use a remedy.

Initiation

The European occult tradition speaks of "initiation." This refers to the transmission of silent knowledge from one person to another, especially in a graded and systematic form. The idea is that the occult lodge holds silent knowledge that is handed out in careful grades from the older to the younger "initiates."

In my experience, silent knowledge is transmitted between people of similar temperament and is unstoppable when the similarity is present and whether the giver and the receiver are ready or not. It even passes between those who are dedicated to the good path and those on the dark side, and vice versa. So, I can't help but think that the idea of "graded and systematic" transmission is an idealization. Reality is a lot sloppier than that. Remember the motto of the human race: "Oops."

If a teacher has a distinct boundary line set on the inner plane and a student crosses it, knowingly or unknowingly, a transmission will occur. This is what happened when I said "yes" to seeing a certain medicine man and I felt a *thunk!*—like a tube breaking in my throat—followed by an empathic link to him.

Transmission can also occur from animals and plants to humans. This is actually much more reliable because humans are so changeable and ego-bound. This is probably how shamanism got started in prehistoric times.

One of the less fortunate methods of transmission occurs when a person who is not ready tunes into the silent knowledge of a medicine holder and asks to be taught about it. The holder can refuse, but after the third request he or she has to teach the aspirant. This is not a man-made rule; it is just how the energy works. If the aspirant is not ready, both parties may be injured by the resulting mess. It's happened to me—on both ends of the transmission.

Every transmission of silent knowledge passes through the psycho-sexual band (don Juan's "shift below") to get from the teacher to the student. That means one has to stay pretty conscious in the sexual sphere. This state of affairs favors committed relationships. Eliot Cowan, who introduced "Plant Spirit Journeying," was told by his Indigenous teacher that he had to be in a committed relationship for the duration of the apprenticeship if he wanted to be a student. So he asked his girlfriend if she would marry him for seven years, or maybe it was twelve—I can't remember. She told him she'd marry him for life.

Secret Tradition

Secrecy is natural to the shamanic tradition. Some say this is the case because it would be dangerous if shamanic practices were revealed to the wrong people. Unfortunately, it has proved impossible to keep this knowledge out of the hands of the "wrong people," so this is not the primary reason why the knowledge is secret. Anyway, it should be obvious that "we have seen the wrong people and they are us."

About a year or two before my initiations into the silent knowledge of the Turtle and the Wolf, I had the following dream:

I was a member of an occult society. There was great joy in the air because we were meeting again after many years of separation. I was on the front steps with some of the other members, some of whom were dilettantes while others were serious, dedicated occultists. Suddenly, a young boy about eight years old came up the stairs from the neighborhood. He wondered what was going on. "We're having a meeting," said the owner of the house. All of us stood in suspense to see what would happen. We couldn't deny him entry if he wanted to come in. No sign of comprehension crossed his face, but suddenly he said, "Okay," turned around, and walked down the steps. There was an almost audible sigh of relief and an intensification of the feeling of joy. It was considered a great omen that he did not press his way in. We went inside, met old friends, talked and took our seats. The lights dimmed as the stage lit up and we settled in to watch the history of our society reenacted.

This dream signified that I was getting ready to enter the occult fraternity. And I did, several years later, though it was through the medium of an Indian medicine man, not a Western-style occultist. "That old guy could initiate you into the medicine society in one day," commented one of his peers. I choose not to be a member on the outer level, because it was not my community. Or maybe there is some society I belong to that only allowed me that one beautiful dream.

Another factor making the teachings secret has been persecution. Western shamans have been exposed to everything from witch burnings to intellectual belittlement, exclusion from occupations, and imprisonment. By the nineteenth century, the witch burnings had stopped, but it was still dicey to be an occultist. William Cheney, the popularizer of astrology in nineteenth-century America, was imprisoned for two years without charges in a New York City jail with his mentor, Mark Broughton. When psychology was introduced about 1900, English astrologer Alan Leo reinvented astrology as a form of psychological analysis, in order to evade the fortune-teller laws.

Even as late at the twentieth century, the life of an occultist in America was still dangerous. A rather weird incident occurred in the career of Albert Sidney Raleigh (1881–1932). On April 7, 1911, the *New York Times* reported:

CHICAGO, April 6. Albert Sidney Raleigh of the Order of Melshisedec and its prophet and leader is suffering from a beating by James B. Knoblock, who manifests a distinct objection to the doctrines taught his wife.

Mrs. Knoblock refused to agree to spend her next life with Mr. Knoblock. He got mad and gave her teacher a beating. Raleigh, noted the *Times*, advocated nonviolence, vegetarianism, and abstinence from alcohol. However, the convalescent occultist admitted from his hospital bed that alcoholic spirits were useful for pain relief.

In 1932, Raleigh died from a sunstroke on an Arkansas prison farm, awaiting trial for teaching unconventional religious doctrines.

More commonly, the persecution only affects one's reputation. The day Rudolf Steiner declared himself an occultist was the last day of his long career in German academia. Michael Harner's distinguished career in anthropology was ended by his decision to advocate shamanism as a way of life. Shirley MacLaine was branded as a "crazy New Ager" when she stepped out of her role as an actress.

It was, of course, even harder for Indigenous people. In the mid-twentieth century, a Hawaiian would have been sentenced to a thousand-dollar fine and a year of hard labor under Hawaiian territorial law for "pretending" to be a kahuna. Both Hawaiians and American Indians were prevented from practicing their own religion until the passage of the federal American Indian Religious Freedom Act in 1978. The practice of astrology was not free from criminal prosecution until 1986.

I remember the 1970s. Getting alternative medical advice was subversive. From Minnesota one had to travel to Nebraska or North Dakota to find the closest practicing herbalist. Dr. Christopher was arrested more than thirty times. Maurice Mességué, in France, had been arrested thirty-six times by the time his autobiography appeared in 1970. The old Amish farmer Solomon Wickey was arrested just once, but fought a long and hard trial. That was in 1982. The last attempted prosecution in Minnesota was in 1996.

I started my practice in the herb store in 1981. I think they ignored us largely because we were a bunch of counterculture nutcases. It was when one "pretended" to be "scientific" that the establishment took note. In 1992, Minnesota dairy farmer Herb Saunders was met in his front yard by helicopters; local, county, and state police; the state Attorney General's office, the USDA, and the FDA. He was selling colostrum from cows injected with the blood of the sick person. The Attorney General's office dropped charges for medical fraud when they found this immunological technique was patented by the University of Minnesota and medically proven. Dr. Robert Gallo was prepared to defend the technique in court—this was at the peak of Gallo's influence as an "AIDS doctor."

"Ya' got cows to milk?" asked the judge when Herb was presented at court that afternoon.

"Yep," replied Herb.

"Then you're free on your own recognizance. Go back home."

Bail was not necessary for a dairy farmer who would lose his herd if he left home. His defense lawyers—volunteers whose lives had been improved by alternative medicine—argued that Herb's clients had the freedom to choose their own medical care. Two juries were hung because first one and then all members refused to convict. The frustrated state Attorney General and County District Attorney gave up. The time had come when juries, following their own conscience, refused to enforce an outmoded law.

But the Minnesota Board of Medical Practice still had independent powers. Now they went after Helen Healy, a prominent naturopathic doctor in St. Paul. This incited a near-riot in the CAM* community since Helen was actually licensed in another state and had the best credentials of anyone in Minnesota. We went to the legislature and changed the law, so that the Board no longer had dictatorial control over alternative practice. It dawned on the legislators that consumers did not have access to their therapies of choice, so the bill we passed was crafted around consumer access. Practitioners' protection came second.

In the 1990s, I was the most prominent herbalist in Minnesota. Persecution for being true to my spiritual calling is as real to me as the palm of my hand. For the first fifteen years of my practice, I felt endangered every day I practiced.

As I write, spiritual and shamanic experiences can only be fit into pathological categories in psychiatry. E. Grahame Howe was one of the only psychiatrists in the mid-twentieth century willing to openly advo-

*Complementary and alternative medicine.

cate in public for the place of spirituality in human psychology. Once a rich Harley Street doctor in London, he was shunned and died in obscurity as the noose of conventionality increasingly overtook medicine.

Howe, by the way, claimed to have asked Freud about the place of spirituality in psychology and received the answer that the world was not ready for that yet. Freud paid a huge price just for advocating the existence of the unconscious. Throughout Central Europe, his ideas were rejected as a "Jewish weakness." Carl Jung was his "golden boy," the first gentile to advocate for the unconscious, but the two had a permanent falling-out. Jung was also persecuted for this version of psychology and today his ideas have been eliminated almost entirely from higher education in American psychology programs. On the other hand, his terms and ideas have won a place in popular speech and thought.

A more negative reason for secrecy is that many experts in the occult and shamanic fields in fact know very little about the subject and therefore have nothing important to say. It is easier to pretend to knowledge than to actually know it—but this is true in every field.

Ultimately, however, the real reason this knowledge remains secret is that the deeper contents can only be perceived and learned outside of physical reality, in that "disbelieved-in, out-of-this-world" dimension of magic mentioned by Randolph. Such experiences are not only innately personal and subjective, but cannot always be adequately described by available vocabulary. This is why shamans use the Green Tongue. As Terence McKenna said (2010c):

A secret is not something untold. It's something which can't be told.

It would not be impertinent to say, also, that sometimes experiences can only be explained when the spirit allows the words to flow in one's mouth. Michael Bastine couldn't talk about the "Land of the Elders" for many years after his experience. In the Celtic tradition, the "bardic tongue" has long been enumerated among the gifts granted to those who have been to the otherworld and returned to tell the tale. And Christians, who are not always bereft of spiritual experience, talk about words flowing in the mouth under the influence of the Holy Spirit.

Finally, when we herbalists and shamans have shaken off the law, we have become a fad and a bunch of whining politically correct missionaries persecute us for "colonialism" and "cultural appropriation," as if spiritual experiences are not universal but only cultural.

The Green Tongue

The only way to communicate about an experience that is invisible is to speak about it by inference, analogy, and contrast. This is true of the shamans, who are universally associated with a "secret language" (Eliade 1964, 96–98). Rudolf Steiner refers to this as the "occult script" (1947, 82), but my favorite name is the "Green Tongue," introduced by David Ovason (in Hedsel 1999). I discussed this at great length in *Seven Guideposts on the Spiritual Path* (2021). Jesus "spoke to them only in parables" (Matthew 13:34–35).

The imagination can only speak in the language of analogy, contrast, and wordplay. One must learn to speak and hear that language. The "occult script" is "traced in the spiritual world and remains there for all time." It can only be revealed to the soul when it has attained "spiritual perception," which is founded upon imagination and intuition (Steiner 1947, 82).

David Ovason writes: "*Senzar* is described by Blavatsky as the 'early hieroglyphic cypher' of the Mystery Schools. She says that this form of writing was invented by the Atlanteans," and that "the forefathers of the Toltecs understood it as easily as the inhabitants of lost Atlantis" (Hedsel 1999, 477). The Toltecs were a culture descending from the Atlanteans and the ancestors of the nagualism to which don Juan belonged.

One of the petals of the throat chakra, according to Steiner, is related to learning to control outward speech. "The student should utter no word that is devoid of sense and meaning." This includes the "usual kind of conversation, with its promiscuous discussion of indiscriminately varied topics" (Steiner 1947, 138). That is a high standard.

This does not preclude the use of mindless conversation when one is with mindless people, in order to deflect their suspicions about one "being different" in some way. The spiritual warrior needs to be strategic and careful: there are a lot of dangerous forces and people out there. Steiner himself did not possess much "charm." Of course, he was not in a situation where he needed to escape enslavement and death, like Randolph.

Discipline of speech was required of Thomas the Rhymer when he was in the Underworld with the Queen of Elfland. This eventually enabled her to give him a gift: "the Tongue that Cannot Lie." Of course, that gift is also a curse—a characteristic of shamanic skills.

The casual reader will think that the Language of Nature is like some alphabet or writing system, but that is a misunderstanding. True, an "alphabet" of esoterica exists in the astrological system or the Higher Arcana of the tarot, but it will be noticed that these are both fixed and constantly in flux: the position of the stars and planets change or the deck is shuffled.

Learning to read the Language of Nature is not like ordinary schooling. It involves the development of a lyrical sensibility—not just for words, but for the Forces of Nature through which the spirits behind Nature form and change the universe.

> The signs of the occult script are not arbitrarily invented; they correspond to the forces actively engaged in the world. They teach us the language of things. (Steiner 1947, 83)

When we perceive through eyes and ears trained to read and hear the Green Tongue, we see everything in the natural, social, and human worlds to be expressions of archetypal forces churning and changing in a constant panorama of spiritual evolution.

Dreamtime

When the shamans actualized their dream self and journeyed to the far-distant shores of dreamtime, they discovered the spirit. One does not become a shaman by growing, integrating, or changing one's soul, nor by spiritual warriorship, nor via the Wisdom of Nature (lovely as that path is), but by dreaming of the animal self and that's that. All these things help; they nudge us along the path.

The shaman considers the peregrination of human consciousness in dreamtime to be a very important basis for the acquisition of knowledge, but this is not generally the case in science, religion, or even most spiritual practices. Science considers dreaming to be a physiological phenomenon of importance to health, not a guide for life. Religion and mysticism largely ignore dreaming. The psychologist grants that dreams can have great meaning. However, only the shaman conceives of developing awareness in dreamtime. A friend of mine asked a world-famous meditation teacher about dreams and was told to ignore them.

Some Sufi and other groups emphasize dreaming. An account of such a group in Samarkand is given by Olga Kharitidi in *Master of Lucid Dreams* (2001). These dreamers established a colony on the Mediterranean. The father of the great Sufi Rumi moved from Samarkand to Anatolia. The Turks called this part of Asia "Rum" (Rome) and that is how Rumi got his surname. These two centers of dreaming are still active.

The Dream Self

Shamanism teaches by experience, not by theory. Therefore, in this section on dreamtime, dreaming, and the dream self we will try to help the novitiate learn to recognize the edge of dreamtime, as it sticks out into the conscious world. It is like the corona of the sun in a solar eclipse: we do not see the sun, we only see its emanations. At first we do not experience real dreamtime, we only experience its corona.

Dreaming and waking are two mutually exclusive states of consciousness. We know this because, when we awaken from a particularly pleasurable dream, we feel the tug to remain in the dream against the tug to re-enter consciousness. Then when we do awaken, we can't easily recall the dream. This shows that the two selves of waking and dreaming are so fundamentally different that they are competitive (Barford 2010, 87–112).

This "stubbornness" in not wanting to leave the dream state is the first inkling we have that there is a specific and different consciousness while we dream. From this small beginning, we can develop the dream-self. However, most people ignore such small signals. The scientist and religionist are so involved in the search for meaning in conscious life that they overlook the small tugs felt at the edge of dreamtime. The occultist tries not to ignore any experience, including the shimmers of the occulted sun. He or she is rewarded by the discovery of another world. Only the shaman is interested in all human experience, not rejecting some of it as "unreliable" or even "unreal."

At first, dreams are confusing. Some are completely meaningless, some seem to be related to completely meaningless events in life, and some seem to touch upon important events, but in an unclear manner. Rare, at first, is the starkly clear, unambiguous dream. The reason dreams are so murky at the beginning is that there is no dream self because we don't have a sensorium or body on that level. Instead, dreams have to come through the sensorium of the physical body so in reality they are part of that world. So they might be helpful for dealing with the issues of that world, but that has nothing to do with the world of dream.

During this initial period, we can use some of these dreams to help understand ourselves and integrate the conscious and unconscious, so that they work together in harmony. This improves the quality of dreams in terms of meaning. It also clears a space away so that the dream self can be birthed, but on the other hand, as long as we are expending a great deal of energy on the life of the conscious self, or frustrated elements of the unconscious, there is no space for dreaming.

Dreamtime is not the same thing as the unconscious. The waking self consists of two sides: conscious and unconscious. This is also the same as human and animal, ego and id, mind and body. Animals are not conscious like we are, but they certainly are awake. Therefore, the animal self is a part of the waking world—but unconscious. In dreamtime it is the whole waking self that is unconscious. That includes the animal self at first.

316 The Spirit Self

In order for the dream self to have its own sensory system, independent of the physical body and the ego that operates through the physical organism, the dream self needs to come into contact with the animal world as it exists in dreamtime and the only way it can do this is in dreaming.

We have only one animal per dream self in dreamtime. However, a lot of shamans or sorcerers like to collect medicine powers or medicine animals. This gives them the ability to look through the lens of that particular animal and gives them the powers of that animal. Like all medicines, the more one pursues powers for their own sake, the further one moves from the path of good medicine, the path with heart, the path of self-realization, to the opposing path.

For every animal there is a corresponding animal spirit that holds the genome and archetype for that species. Each animal spirit possesses the genome for the sensory powers that help the physical-plane animal survive in the niche they occupy in the natural world. Animals survive by their senses. The human world, on the other hand, is the realm of consciousness, and humans prefer to think that they survive by their consciousness and free will.

Just as there is a different animal spirit for each animal species, there is a human spirit for the human species. Instead of a different one for each person, there is one human spirit for everyone. That is just like it is with the animals: each genome has a spirit associated with it. However, the human genome and the human spirit had a falling-out when the genome plucked the fruit in Eden. Individual human souls have to choose between the genome and the human spirit, between "Eat, drink, and be merry" and a meaningful spiritual life.

Medicines to Strengthen the Spirit Self

The reptiles have to sit in the sun to warm up, but the warm-blooded animals carry the sun within them. Therefore, it is the solar remedies that are helpful for increasing awareness of the spirit self. I have already mentioned how Angelica opens the imagination. It is actually one of the most powerful medicines for the spirit self. It is variously classified as a Sun, Bear, and Elk Medicine, because it is warm and drying, with a brown and furry root and, with antlerlike branches. Use it as a smudge.

☼ SUN MEDICINE ☼

Jung identified the astrological glyph of the Sun as a symbol of the Self. Steiner identified the human "Ego" (higher self, soul-and-spirit) with the heat in the body and therefore with the blood that raises, carries, and spreads the heat. Medicines of the Sun are gently warming, like the beams of the sun, elevating our temperature and circulation gently to warm us up and drive out phlegm and water that are bogging us down. It is like the sun vaporizing a puddle on the sidewalk or drying out the phlegm in our brain. They are similar to the "yang tonics" of Chinese herbalism.

The idea of the solar herbs goes back at least to Thessalus of Tralles (ca. 50 CE), who claims to have gotten the idea from Hermes Trismegistus. In his *Astrological Practice of Physick* (1671), Joseph Blagrave gave a basic list of "solar herbs" including Rosemary, Angelica, Calendula, and St. John's Wort (2010, 3–4). Steiner considered Rosemary, widely used as a circulatory stimulant, to be a remedy for increasing the incarnation of the spirit into the body.

Blagrave started every case with three of these four solar herbs before going on to something more precise for the person, according to the astrological chart. However, he lived in England, which is notoriously cool and damp, where such a therapeutic method sounds rather brilliant, actually. One could add Sunflower, Turmeric, Orange Peel, fresh Ginger, Galangal, and many other herbs to this list. Cayenne might have to be considered an herb of Mars.

᦯ Rosemary ᦯
(*Rosmarinus officinalis*)

Those who live where this plant flourishes are fortunate. "The Sun claims privilege in it, and it is under the celestial Ram," wrote Nicholas

Culpeper, so it possesses "warming and comforting heat," which is beneficial in all "cold diseases" (1850, 155). Shakespeare mentions "Rosemary
for remembrance"; it is an old remedy for increasing circulation to the
brain and improving memory. The late William LeSassier not only
used it for loss of memory but to lessen the impact of bad memories.
Rosemary has a peculiar affinity: it strengthens the circulation to the
nervous system, including the brain, senses, and spine.

This is one of the most important medicines for deepening and
extending the circulation. It is my chosen remedy for the syndrome
described in the medicine of the American South as "low blood."
When the blood stays down in the lower part of the body, it is hard to
move upward, or stays in the inside and is hard to circulate out to the
periphery, or when it is impoverished in its inherent elements (especially
iron), it is described as "low." The most obvious symptom is a darkening
around the ankles, eventually turning into a blue-black. Due to lack of
blood to the head, there may be memory loss or dementia. "Low blood"
occurs most often late in life, rather than in the robustness of childhood, the prime of adulthood, or the holding pattern called "middle
age." Rosemary is a wonderful stimulant for this condition.

Father Sebastian Kneipp used Rosemary wine as a remedy for conges-
tive heart failure—I have seen it help (remission? cure?) in several cases.

Rudolf Steiner said that Rosemary helped to "deepen incarnation"
and therefore it was for people who wanted to avoid the harsh experiences of life. For this reason, he recommended it for some kinds of
diabetes—for people who only wanted the sweetness of life, who were
too attracted to sugar.

⬿ Angelica ⬾
(*Angelica archangelica*)

We have already described this genus as a journeying medicine and Bear
Medicine. Angelica is "an herb of the Sun in Leo," writes Culpeper; "let
it be gathered when he is there, the Moon applying to his good aspect."
That is the time of the year when Angelica is in flower. One should pick

the root of this biennial during the first year, when it is without flowers. Our astrologer continues: "let it be gathered either in his [Leo's] hour, or in the hour of Jupiter, let Sol be angular [sunrise, sunset, midday]; observe the like in gathering the herbs, of other planets, and you may happen to do wonders." Because it is tall and strong in the second year it is also attributed a secondary relationship with Saturn, ruler of structure. "In all epidemical diseases caused by Saturn, that is as good a preservative as grows." It is "defending and comforting" to "the heart, blood, and spirits." Also, it will "warm and comfort a cold stomach," and from there, it radiates heat out to the periphery to protect, keep the skin healthy and the pores open, and vaporize, so to speak, excess fluids (Culpeper 1850, 8–9). It is used in "fire cider" (with Cayenne, Horseradish, Bayberry, and the like) to send blood to the face and head, to ward off an incipient infection. It can also be used (I like smaller doses) at the end of a long, drawn-out respiratory infection to warm and dry dampness and a depressed, cold tissue state. Angelica is for "all pains and torments coming of cold and wind" that is to say, spasms, and is particularly noted for colic (Culpeper 1850, 9). Here a good formula would be: Angelica, Calamus, and Orange Peel. Culpeper notes that it "procureth womens' courses" (1850, 9), and it is now used as a substitute, very effectively, for Chinese Angelica (*A. sinensis*). It is indicated when there is cramping with dark, coagulated blood alternating with rich red blood.

Stephen Harrod Buhner originated the insight that Angelica is particularly good at the first Saturn return, when a young woman needs to chart and re-chart her life path. I have used it successfully for men having trouble with the Saturn return. Saturn rules the "stages of life," and helps one adapt to challenges of aging and change.

⌾ Calendula ⌾
(*Calendula officinalis*)

Culpeper calls it an herb of "the Sun, and under Leo" (1850, 114). The flowers look like the Sun and it has been called "Herbal Sunshine." It is in flower "in the calends almost of euerie moneth [every month]," hence the name, writes John Gerard in 1635 (1975, 741). The flowers are collected during the summer, when they are plentiful, and thrown in the stews in the winter, to warm and for protection against cold. It has so many uses today that I need hardly mention it here. It is not a profound shamanic herb, but it is for children who are afraid of the dark. I recommend my account in *The Book of Herbal Wisdom* (1997, 179–84) and Sajah Popham's article on Calendula online (Popham n.d.).

☒ Sunflower ☒
(*Helianthus annuus*)

This plant is native to the Great Plains of North America and is widely loved as an ornamental, garden plant, and food. It is an important oil in Ayurveda—the medical tradition that does the most with oils. It is used in "oil pulling" (put under the tongue for 10–20 minutes to pull out toxins) and to provide oil (and detoxification) to the skin. It is also a Bear Medicine, but that is secondary to its primary solar nature.

This plant brings me back in my memory to the earliest days of my herbal explorations. The Flower Essence Society had come out with their first kit, and I had my friend Peter Young, who is a superb psychometrist and spiritual seer, hold the flower essence and see what he felt. On the positive side, Sunflower was like the sun beaming out of a person brightly; on the negative it was like a black hole pulling everything into it—"cars, trucks, buses, trains, planes," said Peter.

Twenty years later, I went down to Harmony, Minnesota, to visit a friend, Denese Ullom. She asked, "Would you like me to do a shamanic drumming for you?" "Okay," I said. I had no idea what that entailed. She had me lie on a sofa and started drumming. I wondered whether she was supposed to see or hear something or what? The question was soon answered. All of a sudden I saw a bear standing on its two hind legs, holding a rubber-tipped pointer to a blackboard with a sunflower drawn on it in colored chalk. Orange, yellow, green. Immediately, I understood the connection between the chest of the bear, the sunflower, and my own chest. I had a dry cough for about three months.

I went down to the gas station, bought some sunflower seeds, and was soon repaired. Two weeks later, Denese called to ask what to do for a respiratory problem—she'd breathed in too much chlorine cleaning her floor. I suggested sunflower seeds. She went down to the gas station, bought some, and was shortly cured, even though they were rancid.

One of my old clients had gotten poisoned by a dental adhesive; it was driving her crazy with anxiety, her hair was falling out, and she was a total mess. We used Sunflower seed oil as an oil-pulling medicine under her tongue. "I could taste the toxins after ten minutes." Time to spit out the oil. It removed the problem completely within a few weeks.

Over the years I learned that this was a remedy for "adrenal exhaustion." William LeSassier taught us that American Ginseng and Spikenard (*Aralia racemosa*, *A. californica*) are best for this condition (which supposedly doesn't exist)—basically, fatigue from overwork and overextension—but if there is hollowing out around the eyes, exhaustion, and in some cases the upper chest infection, it is the remedy.

During Omicron I had exactly those symptoms. My upper lungs became infected, probably a pneumonia, and I would wake from a deep sleep in a rapid heartbeat—dysautonomia was a common side-effect in covid long-haulers. I felt death was in my aura, and since my friend Susan had experienced that and survived, I went to her for advice. "You overextended yourself," she concluded. Then I knew the right remedy. Sunflower seed promptly turned it around and I spread the oil on me in the hopes of pulling out spike proteins or whatever, or protecting myself with Solar Bear power. And some of my friends received benefit too. Chris MacPadden (who taught me about Bat Medicine and had once suggested that I needed Sunflower seed for exhaustion, overwork, and hollow-eyedness), also dreamed about the seed and the oil.

☼ MOON MEDICINE ☼

The sister of Apollo, God of the Sun, is Artemis, Goddess of the Moon. Medicines with a lunar rulership are cooling and moistening, while solar remedies are warming and drying. Both are easy categories to understand and use. Many of the lunar remedies are white or pale, and many of them are also mucilages or contain the polysaccharides that soothe the mucosa and skin and, entering into the body (some polysaccharides more than others) lubricate, soothe, moisten, cool, and also encourage the generation of internal polysaccharides, including the polymers of the extracellular matrix, the "maternal" substance in which all cells are surrounded. Polysaccharides also can build immunity.

Generally, these kind of herbs are not very powerful in psychological or shamanic terms. For shamanic power, we must skip to the herb of Artemis. Mugwort has no mucilaginous powers and is actually a bit warming and drying but it is beneficial for dreaming, encouraging conscious development within the realm of the unconscious.

ꙩ Mugwort ꙩ
(*Artemisia vulgaris*)

Mugwort acts primarily on the autonomic nervous system, and this points to the Moon, because this is the nervous system in charge of all of our unconscious activities, which are "ruled by the Moon." In addition, Mugwort leaves shine in an uncanny fashion in the light of the Moon. This property is unique to Mugwort.

Mugwort is a complex, powerful, and ancient medicinal plant. It has taken years for me to understand it medically and spiritually—from the essence to the applications. This is only right for an herb that is associated with Artemis, the ancient Goddess of the Moon, Nature, the Wild, and the Hunt. She is descended from the Old, Old Goddess of the post-Paleolithic cultures, according to ethnobotanist and herbalist Wolf-Dieter Storl.

It is usually said that Mugwort got its name because it is placed in beers and ales. In this capacity it can be traced back millennia (Edwards 2011). Throughout Africa, Asia, and Europe brewing was originally the domain of women. When beer was available, a broom was placed along the road or path. This is believed to be the original association between "witches" and brooms.

Artemisia vulgaris, the true Mugwort of Western herbalism, is native to Siberia but naturalized long ago to Europe and China, and now North America. There are additional Mugwort species in China and the Pacific coast of North America.

The Autonomic Nervous System

After years of drawing a blank on Mugwort, I finally came to understand the medicinal properties of this powerful agent through acquaintance with the teachings of Dorothy Hall (1988, 225–29). She based her understanding of Mugwort largely on iridology.

Around the pupil, there is a circle of intense lines with creases running through them called the "nerve wreath." This opens when the pupil dilates in darkness, and contracts when it tightens in the presence of light. Since dilation of the pupil is an involuntary response, we know that the nerve wreath is the significator in the iris for the involuntary or autonomic nervous system. It doesn't matter what materialistic doctors and scientists might think about iridology, this correlation is anatomically undeniable: the autonomic, via the nerve wreath, controls pupillary response and the condition of the wreath is going to reflect autonomic health. The nerve wreath can be extra creased, saggy, tight, loose, and so on, and this indicates conditions on the health of the autonomic.

What Dorothy particularly pointed out was the presence of gaps in the nerve wreath. These indicate breaks where the autonomic does not "link up" in some way. She particularly pointed to inability to connect with one's colon. Therefore, Mugwort is for people who don't feel the urge to go to the bathroom, resulting in constipation. I saw a case like this. A young boy would miss the signal to poop, to his discomfort. I used it successfully (with Skullcap) for his three-year-old brother, who had "night terrors," a condition where a child (usually) wakens from dream incompletely and is caught between the dream and waking states in an unpleasant state of mind. Night terrors is a traditional indication for Mugwort. I used single drop doses because these were children. Mugwort helped with the "missed signal."

Dorothy also mentions sleep, but the other way around: people who can't fall asleep because their mind simply won't turn off. She gives many specific indications: people who lie awake and think of all sorts of remarkable things; insomnia where no other remedy or formula has helped; people who are exhausted from three or four nights of insomnia, then become constipated; people who have vivid dreams but wake up exhausted; people who, during the day, waver between wakefulness and sleepiness. They can be wide-awake, active, creative, ingenious, then sit down in exhaustion. They don't get the sleep to refresh themselves. So Mugwort helps the gap close between waking and sleeping, or helps separate the two so that a person can wake up.

In daytime waking consciousness we are predominately in the sympathetic mode of the autonomic (alert, awake), while in sleep we are in the parasympathetic (rest, relax, sleep, dream). One cannot be in both at the same time, yet they are connected and integrated. Also, during the day we are not only in sympathetic but the central nervous system (consciousness) is active. In night terrors and insomnia there is a gap between the two autonomic branches. There is some problem with the integration.

Once I had these teachings to guide me, it became apparent that Mugwort acted when there are profound gaps between the two branches of the autonomic. For instance, a friend of mine had autonomic dysreflexia—the autonomic switching back and forth spontaneously, without control. This is a terrifying condition and yet, after a lifetime working as a nurse with a Ph.D. in public health, she knew she had to walk out or die because there was no protocol for her and the general hospital care had already almost killed her. I recommended Mugwort tea and she quickly got better. When I saw her six weeks later, there were only some symptoms in the kidneys and the heart. Since the kidneys have to switch into the parasympathetic for us to sleep and rest, there may still have been some mild symptoms. The heart would spontaneously go into tachycardia (sympathetic excess). In order to switch back into parasympathetic, she would have to cough. The "head of the autonomic" is the vagus in the back of the throat (cough and gag reflex), so she was resetting her autonomic.

This case helped me understand another. A fifty-eight-year-old woman had increasing attacks of irregular pulse. She was increasingly dreamy during the day and thought she was probably going to die in the not-so-distant future. She wrote: "My heart continued to beat irregularly. I found myself automatically coughing to regulate or restart it because it was uncomfortable, I felt a bit dizzy and had a mild choking feeling on my neck." These symptoms constituted only about "10%" of the problem. "A few minutes after coughing and feeling relief, the heart would start beating irregularly again." I had her take a small dose of Mugwort. "It seemed to help fairly quickly and the episodes came further apart. I slept well and today have been sipping Mugwort throughout the day. I have had fewer episodes today." We added Gravel Root to decalcify the calcium phosphate that builds up in muscles as we age—including the heart muscles.

The first case was more serious and of many years' duration, complicated by heart surgeries. However, she stabilized, though not completely free all the time of tachycardia. She is still with us six years later; the second woman is doing fine as well.

Since this time I have noticed that coughing related to irregular pulse is not a completely uncommon condition. I had it myself after Covid-19. This disease is very disorganizing to the autonomic.

The application to sleep leads to a deeper use: Mugwort has a tremendous reputation as a dreaming medicine. In order to understand this aright, however, we should first study the folklore of the plant.

Goddess of the Mountain Tops

Artemisia receives her name from Artemis, the Goddess of the Wild and the Hunt. Her emblems are the moon and the bow and arrow. She was, therefore, the Goddess of the night and darkness as well. Additionally, she was associated with all things female: puberty, fertility, and labor. In a puberty rite dedicated to Artemis and called *arkeia*, the girls of Athens imitated the female bear (*arkoi*). This appears to reflect an even older bear cult and may point to the origin of the name "Artemis" itself. By the time the Old, Old Goddess reaches us through the Greeks she has already been bowdlerized to some extent, like the rest of the Greek pantheon.

The Greeks turned their faces from the wild. They believed that the wild, uncontrollable powers of the Gods and Goddesses were manifest on the mountaintops and, like Olympus, were closed to human penetration. They believed that Divine powers descended down to them. By comparison, the ancient Hebrews thought they had to go up to the mountaintop to make themselves available to the Divine. Moses went up the mountain to get the tablets. Abraham and Jacob sacrificed their animals on the mountaintops. The God name associated with Abraham, Isaac, and Jacob is El Shaddai, meaning God or Spirit (*El*) of the Mountains, the Wilderness, the Breasts. The Temple in Jerusalem was built on a mountaintop and the gospel written by a Jew for Jews (Matthew) has the "Sermon on the Mount," while the one written by a Greek (Luke) has the "Sermon on the Plain." We see here the round of associations that would have been associated originally with the Old, Old Goddess and her descendant, Artemisia.

Although the West is Greek in so many cultural habits, it takes after the Hebrews in this regard at least: mountains and wild spaces have a special relationship to the Divine not found in domesticated places.

Birth, Death, and Rebirth

The Old, Old Goddess was associated with the darkness and the night, but also with the rebirth of the sun at midwinter. This corresponded to her association with labor, birth, and death. Artemis was the primeval midwife in Greek mythology. "Only to childbearing women did she reveal herself as a gentle helper," notes Wolf-Dieter Storl (2018, 137). Where we have the associations with birth and death, we also have rebirth and experiences that go beyond the human. Wolf explains that Artemis was originally the patroness of the shamans.* They are the ones who are associated with birth, death, and rebirth.

The primeval Mother Goddess was associated with many of the

---

*Storl discussed this during a talk he gave at the International Herb Symposium in 2015. I have drawn various details from that lecture as well as from subsequent personal correspondence with him (2023) for this section and the following one.

female goddesses. Wolf cites medieval sources that equated Artemis with the northern European Frau Holle, the Queen of the Underworld, or the Queen of the Faeries—who lives in the Elder tree. Today Frau Holle often appears in European folk art as a kindly old grandmother collecting herbs.

The Holly was associated with midwinter, sometimes with the Old, Old Goddess, and sometimes with the dying and born-again God of midwinter. In medieval Catholic folk religion, Holly was associated with both Mother Mary and Jesus. The crown of thorns correlated with the thorny leaves, the blood of Christ with the red berries, and the bitterness of the berries with the bitter cup of suffering—which both Jesus and Mary had to drink. Don't try that at home!

At first it was the shaman who died and came back to help the people. Later it was the dying-and-reborn God of midwinter and finally it was Jesus.

The bright green leaves and berries of the Holly were associated with the promise that summer would return—when it did, the tree of midsummer would be the Oak. This was a masculine tree; the Ivy (*Hedera helix*) that climbed the trunk signified the Goddess. The tight bond of the Ivy to the tree signified true love. Elder was often known as the "Mother of the Herbs," but this title also belongs to Mugwort.

Because he was born six months before Jesus, John the Baptist was associated with midsummer in medieval Catholic folk religion and identified with the Green Man. In the representations of the Green Man, mostly in churches, he is usually shown as a face peering out through oak leaves, so the place of the oak as the tree of midsummer is carried into the circle of associations.

Goose Medicine.

Wolf also points out that the English "Mother Goose," the personification of the repository and teller of fairytales and stories, is a distant descendant of the shamanic Old, Old, Goddess. Here we see the relationship with the Spirit World or imagination. The goose is also associated with Artemis.

Wolf believes that the Old, Old Goddess was particularly associated with the female shamans of the ancient Celtic-Germanic world who would fly in the form of geese, north in the spring and south in the summer, flowing with the breath of the year. Wolf also notes that in Hindu culture, a great yogi is honorifically called a "goose" or "swan" (Sanskrit *hansa*)—for example, Paramahansa Yogananda, the "high-flying gander" who "made it all the way to Los Angeles," as Wolf quipped.

Goose is the traditional food for Christmas, the midwinter holiday, and it is seasoned with Mugwort or Sage. Wolf calls this a "seasonal totemic meal." (In North America we eat the turkey.) The twelve nights of Christmas were the original time of darkness when the female shamans would fly to the other world. The association of the Three Cranes with shamanism undoubtedly relates to Goose as well.

In Native American Medicine, Goose is particularly associated with marital fidelity. Simon Pokagon (1830–1899), a gifted Potawatomi writer and storyteller, penned a sensitive account entitled "An Indian's Observations on the Mating of Geese" (1896). Turtle is also associated with marital fidelity.

Female Reproductive Uses

In ancient times, Mugwort was used to relax the uterus in breech presentations and conditions where the fetus was not in the proper place; also for menstrual pain. It is indicated in very severe pain, according to a number of sources.

In ancient Greece, girls at puberty were "dedicated" to Artemis, the virgin Goddess, in the hopes that they would make a good and safe transition into womanhood. Mugwort may possibly regulate the period in young girls, but I might suggest gentler herbs such as Pulsatilla, Black Cohosh, or the old formula of Blessed Thistle and Mitchella.

In addition to lack of sensation (not receiving the bowel signal), Mugwort is also for heightened sensation, or pain. Thus, it is a remedy for "extreme menstrual cramps, as well as delayed menstruation, with anxiety," noted the late herbalist Carol Trascatto, of Olympia, Washington. Acupuncturist and herbalist Tim Bernhard, of Steven's

Point, Wisconsin, found that it is a good remedy for scar tissue in the uterus, from abortion and gynecological injury, and can restore fertility. It is indicated for "cold in the uterus" in Chinese herbalism, which often occurs with cold stiffness in the lower back, hips, and pelvis. Sex is often unpleasant due to arthritic or rheumatic pain. This is true for both men and women. Acupuncturist Francis Bonaldo, of Montreal, comments that impotence in older men often is due to tightness of the tendons and ligaments. Moxibustion is used particularly along the spine, lower back, and pelvis for such arthritic tightness, spasm, internalized cold, and stiffness.

Mugwort is an old remedy for TMD (temporomandibular disorder), tension in the jaw and neck, grinding of the teeth, even epilepsy. It is also for headaches. The neck is where the human meets the animal, the waking consciousness with the dream awareness.

Modern research shows that *Artemisia vulgaris* "has two opposite effects, contraction and relaxation, on [an] isolated artery." This "may help to explain the conflicting indications for [Mugwort] in traditional herbalism" (Nguyen et al. 2016).

Dreaming Medicine

Mugwort is associated with lucid dreaming by many contemporary herbalists. There was a discussion about how old the tradition of dreaming with Mugwort really is. One contributor found the European references only went back to the late nineteenth century. It was stated that if a young maid sleep on the root of Mugwort, she would dream of her true love. The contributor rejected this as stereotypical Victorian role-modeling to make young women seem foolish.

Such traditions, even when garbled, often contain precious seeds of insight, sometimes carried down from very ancient times. Most herbalists who have worked with Mugwort find that it acts more readily on women. Men have to work with it longer. Also, the dreams can be prophetic, as the Victorian account suggested. As one not-at-all-foolish young woman explained to me: "Mugwort not only promotes lucid dreaming, it unites my dream life with my waking life, so that what I dream of comes true." In other words, Mugwort unites the gap between dreaming and waking life and is also prophetic, as dreams so often are.

Pharmacology

Dorothy notes that Artemisia contains about 7.5% mineral ash. This is not very high, but it is high in phosphates of calcium, magnesium, and potassium. These, we know from cell-salt experience, are the salts for the spine (calcium), muscles (magnesium), and nerves (potassium). Magnesium sedates muscle contraction with the help of calcium. The study of *Artemisia vulgaris* on contraction and relaxation of muscles in a porcine artery (Nguyen et al. 2016), showed that agents that reduced the calcium reduced the contraction. Modern assays show the pharmacological profile of Mugwort to include phenolics and flavonoids (cooling antioxidants), stimulating volatile oils (cineole, anethol, camphor, borneol, kaemperol), thujone (crosses the blood-brain barrier), various terpenes (absinthin, artemisin, artemisic acid, camphene), and quercetin.

Preparation and Dosage

Mugwort was often picked at Midsummer, when the power of the Earth Mother is particularly strong, due to the fructifying effects of the Sun. For the leaves, it should be picked before it flowers. The leaves are stripped from stalks, which are too woody for use. They can then be rolled into a moxa stick, or stored loose for tea, tinctured (fresh or dried), or used as a smudge stick. The smoke smells a lot like Cannabis. It can attract the police. One cup of tea a day is enough of a dose, or 3–15 drops of the tincture, as needed. If picked for the flowers, they should be taken shortly after their appearance—this would be for essential oils.

Small, moderate, and large doses cause mild changes in awareness and attention that are usually not considered unpleasant, but the tea is bitter and not always pleasing to the palate. It is a uterine relaxant and probably should not be used during pregnancy, except at birth, for tense muscles. Start with small doses; there is a remote possibility that it could incite an allergic reaction. I feel we should minimize the dosage for children.

☼ CLOUD MEDICINE ☼

This is the medicine of the empath: people who pick up other people's thoughts and feelings. Ideally, they are able to differentiate between their own internal contents and those of others. "Cloud Medicine is like a vapor that goes through the keyhole to get to the other side," commented Susan. It retrieves hidden thoughts, feelings, intuitions, memories, and traumas. But a person with Cloud Medicine can pass through the keyhole and get stuck—"Help, I'm merged with someone else's energy!" Because people can be deluded by Cloud or Mist, this is a trickster medicine. As a contrary, Cloud can deliver a reprimand:

Susan and I were driving to central Wisconsin to visit a sacred quarry. Along the way we stopped at a buffalo farm and bought some frozen meat patties. We started up again and along the way we kept on seeing one little cloud that floated along in a different direction from all the rest. It was also a different color. Susan called it a "heyoka cloud." A few minutes passed and it was still there. We were talking. Suddenly, Susan yelled: "Ouch, that cloud bit me!" And indeed, she had a big welt on the side of her neck. Her window was closed and neither one of us saw an insect. We put a buffalo patty on the spot to draw out the poison. That quickly took the pain and swelling away, but we had to throw the patty out the window. Susan explained: "I said something bad about the peace pipe, so I was reprimanded."

Plants with Cloud Medicine have an effect on the porosity of the tissues or fluids of the body, so that metabolites (particularly hormones) move more easily through the organism. They sometimes act as mild diaphoretics, "vaporizing" the fluids of the body. The waters of the body are considered to be analogous to the emotions. The psychological functions are therefore similar to the physiological. That means that Cloud Medicines generally help people clarify issues having to do with empathy such as boundaries—or lack of empathy. In the All Soul we are "all related" and empathy is the norm, but in our world empathy is only found in a minority of people. It is not encouraged or accepted; it can also be hard to bear.

There are two kinds of Cloud Medicines: those that harden up porosity and those that soften hardness. Some plants act both ways. Cloud Medicines are easy to identify: they have fur on their leaves, the flowers are furry, or they have cloudlike structures, especially the flowers. In practical terms, furry leaves and stems allow an herb to survive through the winter cold, or to pop up earlier in the spring. If you kick the snow off a rosette of Mullein leaves you will find them strong and healthy in the middle of the winter. This dimension-shifting plant will be mentioned with the Smoke Medicines, a subclass of the Cloud Medicines, because it is an old smoke and smudge.

Herbalist Karyn Sanders, of Blue Otter School, teaches two opposite properties associated with medicines for the empath: being too open and being too cut off. There are Cloud Medicines for both states. Pulsatilla or Pasqueflower (*Anemone wolfgangiana, Pulsatilla vulgaris*) is for being too open, too suggestible, too gullible, while Prairie Smoke (*Geum triflorum*) is for being too introspective, withdrawn, or shy.

We are also brought back to Yarrow. Although it is a warrior remedy, it protects the empath too. It is a medicine of opposites: Venus/Mars, empath/warrior. The feathery leaves remind us of clouds.

∝ Pulsatilla, Pasqueflower ∾
(*Pulsatilla vulgaris, Pulsatilla patens, Anemona patens* var. *wolfgangiana*)

The *vulgaris* is native to Europe, the *patens* to North America. Homeopathic provings of both species have shown that they are interchangeable in properties (cf. Clarke 1900–1903, 3:907–30). The former has been used countless times in homeopathy; the latter is sometimes used as a flower essence. Both are used in herbal medicine as a tincture, in drop doses. John Uri Lloyd stated that Pulsatilla tincture lost its pharmacological properties after about six months, due to breakdown of the molecules. I have used both species, but mostly the homeopathic Pulsatilla in 6x, 30x, and 30c potency.

Pulsatilla blooms in April, early in the spring, hence the association with Easter—Pasqueflower. The American Pulsatilla is quite furry. The European is often grown in the garden.

The indications are well established in homeopathy. It is good for children who are nicely disposed but dependent on their parents and somewhat clingy; it is also used in the head colds of children, with yellowish mucus, plugged ears, clingy when sick. It is used in young girls at puberty, with irregular periods, again with the nice disposition, but clingy and dependent. It sets the period in order and improves confidence and independence. It is used in young women with irregular periods (no two periods alike) and poor pituitary regulation; they have emotional lability during PMS or at other times, alternately happy/sad: "crying about stupid things" or sentimental advertisements, and so forth. It regulates the period and establishes emotional strength and boundaries. It is applicable for young women who are suggestible, perhaps too easily manipulated by men and hurt by the comments of female peers. It improves fertility by regulating the hormones via the pituitary. It is used in perimenopause.

⟨ Prairie Smoke ⟩
(Geum triflorum)

This is one of the most beautiful plants I have ever seen. It is a member of the Rose family, but all parts of the plant are beautiful. The flower looks like faery hair; as it ripens, it turns from pink to red and falls over to look like a shooting star, then forming little pods that look like ovaries—except there are three of them.

The roots have been used in traditional medicine. They are astringent. It has been used by Native Americans for fever, inflammation, colic, digestive upset, severe coughs and sore chests, sore throat, or applied externally in oil to sores, rashes, blisters, and fresh wounds. An infusion is also used for aching joints and stiff and sore muscles, externally or—in the old days—in the sweat lodge.

The flower essence is used for stiff and excessive personal boundaries, to soften and open people up in a safe way.

☼ SMOKE MEDICINE ☼

Clouds are not, under normal conditions, controllable by mankind. Scientists like to think they can "seed" and control clouds but that is like herding fleas on cats. A skeptic might think they just dump aluminum particles up in the sky to "get rid of it," while vainly pretending to influence the weather. Actually, the principle does work: pine forests release vapors on hot days that increase haze in the air to protect them from the heat.

Some medicine men can call rain, but one also has to know how to end it. There was a white man married to a Native woman up on Red Lake rez I heard about many years ago. He could call rain but he couldn't stop it. Eventually, he got kicked off the rez. Years later, a friend of mine who was hitchhiking was picked up by him; he was now a truck driver—but he never learned how to stop rain.

Smoke, in contrast to Cloud, is somewhat controllable by man because it is kindled by fire, which can be started or put out. The animals don't control fire; only humans do. Smoke is used for signals. "Wherever there is smoke there is fire." Oxidation or fire is known as the "sickle of death," since it is what ultimately kills all organic cells and weathers even the remnants down to dust, like barn-boards. The fact that man can control fire indicates that we possess a special power: to tame the elements, to actualize the fires of awareness, to survive the sickle of death—for a while. Thus, the five-leaf signature in plants belongs to the humans as well as the wolves and the dragons.

But we are only talking about Smoke right now. Smoke is a waste product of fire, an incompletely burned material as light as air. It represents the incomplete burning, the need to face the place of no pity in order to extinguish all impurities.

The following three medicines are especially beneficial for practicing self-examination. Mullein is valuable both as a lung remedy and a shamanic medicine. Wormwood is the harsh taskmaster that forces us to face the place of no pity. Ghost Pipe has unique properties of cure; I wouldn't mention it because of environmental concerns but the story of healing I tell in the account below is remarkable. Tobacco helps us cross over to the other side in our mind, into the Spirit World.

⤫ Mullein ⤬
(*Verbascum thapsus*)

Mullein is an amazing medicine plant from a magical standpoint, and yet it is an ordinary "simple" used for millennia in herbal medicine, primarily for coughs. The furry leaves contain a little salty mucilage and are beneficial in harsh, dry coughs. Recently we have begun to use it for setting and healing broken bones in Western herbalism. In *The Book of Herbal Wisdom* (1997, 495–96) I told the story about how Susan and I learned about this twenty years ago; it is now widely used in this fashion.

Mullein is definitely a dreamer's plant. The leaves are soft and furry, like a Cloud Medicine, but the stalk is long and hard, like a staff, so it incarnates the principles of soft and hard and that is similar to the properties we need to engage in order to become *dreamers*: make the mind permeable, like a cloud, and sharp and retentive, like the hard edge of the ego or rational mind.

One day I was teaching at Jim McDonald's place in Michigan. I told the class: "Yeah, once I went on an herb walk with Jim and he taught us that the Mullein leaves closest to the stem are relaxing to the nerves, while the ones that are far away from the stem give you nightmares. Thanks, Jim." He looked at me strangely: "I never told you that." In fact, when I thought about it, I remembered that it was raining cats and dogs at 7:30 in the morning and I decided not to go on Jim's walk and stay in bed. I had two simultaneous, incompatible memories.

I was teaching at the Mid-America Conference that Bonnie Krechow used to host each year in southeastern Minnesota. When I told this story, a woman in the audience piped up: "I'm a witch. We have our own code words. When the recipe calls for 'graveyard dust' it means the outer leaves of the Mullein." (They look kind of like dust.) "We use them to give people nightmares," she added. I forgot about this but Jim was in the audience too and years later he reminded me of her comment. Mullein makes you forget too?

Why would we want to give someone nightmares? I addressed that question in my discussion of Black Bird. The animal self is the Guardian of the Threshold; it keeps people safe from psychospiritual forces that would be overwhelming for them until they are ready for excursions in the otherworld. One is really doing a person a favor in restoring the nightmare mechanism if it has been overridden by spiritual arrogance.

⟨ Wormwood ⟩
(*Artemisia absinthium*)

Wormwood has a lot in common with Alligator medicine because it puts us in contact with the place of no pity, engages us in the process of recapitulation, and is closely related to life and death; like Teasel, it reduces the scar. However, it is a Smoke Medicine. For many years, Wormwood wouldn't allow me to place it in any category that I knew about. Then, one day, when I was hashing this over with Wormwood, I smelled smoke and looked up. I was walking through downtown Ashland, Oregon, and a pall of woodsmoke hung over the city from a fire up in the valley of Lithia Creek. Then I finally understood: Wormwood was a Smoke Medicine. I could feel the tumblers fall into place: after so many years, the plant was satisfied with this conclusion.

Since the publication of *Seven Herbs* (1987), I have used Sagebrush (*Artemisia tridentata*) or Wormwood (*A. absinthium*) as remedies for devastation, poverty, effects of abuse, or any kind of situation where a person has not been allowed to enjoy life. I found both of these agents to be similar in virtue and since the latter grows where I live and is easy to access, I now use the Wormwood in place of Sagebrush.

In a number of medieval herbals, Wormwood appears first, testifying to its importance. From a very early time it was the source of the bitter green drink absinthe or vermouth and it is said that the name does not come from the root *vermis* (worm) but from *vert* (green); it was also a worm and parasite remedy so both derivations are justified. Today *Artemisia annua* is more often used for parasites; wormwood is too harsh for any but a medieval palate.

As I pointed out in *Seven Herbs* (1987, 69–84), Sagebrush (later I used Wormwood) is a remedy for deep, deadened emotions from devastating experiences or cruelty. Wormwood restores the love of life and the ability to anticipate, seek, or feel pleasure. We don't need to be deadened before we die. This is the remedy for spending too much time in the place of no pity.

Wormwood brings out old issues that are stuck, that devastate: child abuse, poverty and deprivation, loss, grief. It is, as herbalist Seán O'Donoghue says, "therapy in a bottle." We both agree that it is safe in one-drop doses, about once a week. No kidding. Too much brings on too many issues. It is also good for stiffness in the muscles and joints from aging and (perhaps) emotional factors. A single, occasional draft of the "green fairy" (absinthe) of Wormwood is a good dosage here—or one can take a cup of the bitter tea.

ও Ghost Pipe ৯
(*Monotropa*)

This very peculiar plant is a saprophytic parasite growing on the roots of various other plants, so it has no chlorophyll and instead has a ghostly white appearance. It looks like a little peace pipe. It is environmentally sensitive, so it should only be used with care. Herbalist David Winston introduced an old Tsalagi use to reduce pain during cancer. Actually, it reduces pain in many conditions and in such a way that the person can deal with it constructively and overcome the problem, sometimes.

Monotropa helps a person rise above their pain, whether it is physical or psychological. It gives them a greater perspective from which to process the experience. It is unfortunate that it is an herb of somewhat limited supply. It is particularly good when there has been sexual abuse or deep hurt of some kind. It is also a very important medicine for helping a person pass away in a peaceful state of mind. In this regard it is like Life Everlasting. It is unfortunate that Monotropa is an herb of somewhat limited supply.

I sent some Monotropa to a woman whose daughter had a traumatic experience and was a nervous wreck for several months afterward. Her equanimity was restored and she was able to process the experience more constructively. A week later the family dog got sick and the vet suggested that she be put down. Since she had the remedy, and it helps people pass over, I suggested she use a small amount for the dog. Ironically, it totally recovered in a day. I didn't know what to make of that, but the remission clearly belonged to Monotropa. It seemed to have an "organizing effect" in this canine case, so I recommended it to a friend whose husband was disoriented after a brain biopsy that informed him he had inoperable cancer. He calmed down, accepted his situation, returned to lucidity, and died peacefully two months later.

ҩ Tobacco ҩ
(*Nicotiana rustica*, *Nicotiana* spp.)

Smoked in a sacred way, Tobacco can be used to open the mind to meditative influences and then to the Spirit World. Used in a profane way, it will harden the aura, so to speak, toughening up the person so that they are not so permeable to the meditative or spiritual world. This was always pictured in the old cigarette advertisements: tough-edged, suave young people having a good time in the world of surfaces. Laid on the ground as an "offering," Tobacco is a communicator that helps us to link with the Spirit World. This is called "putting down Tobacco."

Let's talk about offerings for a moment. One time I was in a field of Red Willow (*Cornus stolonoifera*) and the little red shrubs were all saying: "Over there, over there." When I got to the bush I was going to pick from, I saw that I had collected from it five years before. Five years of growth had changed the appearance of everything: there was no way I could have found that bush if I had intentionally looked for it. That was the "doctor plant" the group wanted me to go to. A year later, the town made the owner mow the lot so that it would look neat. Another example of Muggles not being able to see the realities around them.

I don't usually hear a voice when I put down tobacco; I just get a feeling whether the plant wants to be picked or not. Sometimes they are lukewarm about it. I remember one time a peach tree outright refused to let me pick from it, saying: "Over there, over there!" I looked and saw a little tree. It had a better taste and properties. The plants want to help us.

Another time I put some tobacco down in a park, where one was not supposed to pick. I'll tell you—those Agrimonies were so happy to be used for medicine. They didn't enjoy being "preserved" for no particular reason. In another park I got busted for picking some False Solomon's Seal. That turned out good too: it made me start looking for my own land and I bought a beautiful little farm later that year.

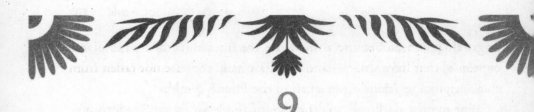

9

Glimpses of the Spirit World

*We are completely unaware of the magical world of the
shaman. It is quite simply stranger than we can suppose.*
TERENCE MCKENNA, *FOOD OF THE GODS*

There is so much lying beyond the doorway of human perception that it
would be conceited for anyone to claim to have more than "glimpses" of
the Spirit World. One conceit we have is that once we reach the Spirit
World everything would be hunky-dory and we would be firmly "on
God's side" and not have a lot to worry about. That's simply not true.
There are challenges and dangers in all theaters of existence. Our species rebelled against direct relationship with the spirit eons ago and
while we can be signaled, trained, led, and touched by the spirit, the
Spirit World long ago became alien country.

First Glimpse

One thing is pretty well established: when we pay our first visit to
Spirit World, it appears as a pure darkness. Don Juan called it the
"black world" or "netherworld" (Castaneda 1985, 293; 1993, 45). I have
already explained why this is the case: up until the moment of our first
look at the Spirit World, we have not had eyes to see or ears to hear
that are calibrated to that world. We are not innately hardwired with
the senses of the spirit. We are required to go through the animal self

to get these senses, because animals are the lineage (compared to plants or stones) that have senses—and, as I have said, they are not fallen from their original relationship to spirit in the Edenic world.

For me the darkness was the face of the Lord of the Underworld, not the whole picture screen. But that was pretty forbidding and I immediately rebelled when he told me he was going to make a link between me and the Wolf Being. That was the beginning of my ability to see and hear in the other world, and it also freed me from an "ancient curse" on the human race, which I felt falling off me when the snake surrounding my head slipped away.

We fell under this "ancient curse" when we rebelled against Creator and allied ourselves with the Snake. It is a real live "original sin" that taints the whole human genome. We can't feel it as individuals because it is built into our genes, but it is there nonetheless. If someone points to "original sin," we get mad about it, supposing ourselves to be primarily good in nature or at least not rotten to our primordial core. The human genome crashed and burned in Eden and we are stamped by an "original sin" much worse than anything imagined by a billion Christians.

The darkness of the netherworld is not some sort of "world of nothingness" into which the individual soul or spirit dissolves in the great return to the void. Nothingness is nothing. This darkness is a Something.

As we gain more and more experience of that Something, the light begins to shine and the vision can become ecstatic. One of the most beautiful descriptions of the Spirit World that I have seen is an account by Michael Bastine in *Iroquois Supernatural* (Bastine and Winfield 2011, 352).

Bastine couldn't talk about it for several years because he choked on the words every time. I don't want to quote his dream because it is really the property of the dreamer. So go out and buy the book. But I want to give the general description as a bookend to the blackness of our "first glimpse." Bastine found himself in a giant forest with giant animals that talked to each other and to him. He met a little old man who told him it was the Land of the Elders. An understanding came to him. When the trees and animals died, they went to that world and became Elders.

"Those Who Live in the Dark Places between the Stars"

Dreamtime is a complex world, just like the world of the body and soul. There are human souls there, good ones—as well as bad ones who would like to eat us for lunch. It would be remiss of me not to warn the student of the dangers along the way, especially those that increase the closer in we get to the Spirit World. This is the reason I have to talk about witches: real, bona fide witches. A lot of people are going to think I am just being medieval, but it is possible—even common—to use the familiar spirit to kill and maim souls. Some people actualize the dream self and become conscious and eternal in the Spirit World while remaining entirely self-centered and egotistical. One of my teachers called them "those who live in the dark places between the stars."

> Susan and I were driving down to attend a sweat lodge at some friends on a rez near the city. It was 10:30 in midsummer in the northern latitudes and there was just a hint of blue left on the horizon as darkness and stars covered the sky. Suddenly, from the right side of the road, a liquid darkness oozed out from behind some trees and moved sinuously across the dark spaces between the stars, until it disappeared behind trees on the other side of the road. Susan was dumbfounded and slowed to a stop.

Witches in dreamtime present less of a danger to normal people, whose imagination and dreamtime have yet to develop. However, they attack children in the families of the people they are trying to hurt—children are more imaginative and their energy bodies are more porous. Or they simply kill people physically, like my friend on the rez up north.

The methods used are usually more subtle, however. When people have access to the inner world where destiny is dreamed, they use that power to reconstruct the fate of their opponents, so that "everything gets twisted up." The victim will turn down the one-way street the wrong way, or get involved in a relationship that is not good for them, or a job that unravels their life.

Since even innocent mistakes and ignorance are dangerous; how much more are those that are constructed to hurt. Any oversight on the part of the neophyte, in which he or she underestimates, misunderstands, or misses the clue on the path can precipitate a scrambling of one's life. A bad destiny results in a miserable life—though it is an opportunity to learn from the place of no pity. Even if the misstep is curable, who would want to spend thirty years fighting for one's soul if the problem could have been avoided in the first place?

The real dark magicians know about the universal spirit, and they can become conduits for it just as much as the straight arrows and true hearts the spirit loves so much. How is this possible?

The spirit loves freedom so much that it would never undercut a person's free will and therefore it will tolerate itself to be taken prisoner even by an evil witch or dark magician. But this imbalance can only last for a while. The spirit is constantly at work to enlarge consciousness, and ultimately all enslavers of the spirit will find themselves enslaved by their own unfulfillable appetites. Witches in dreamtime will make mistakes, just like everyone else. "Oops."

The Mold of Man

Just as the Spirit World holds the archetypes of the animals, it also should hold the archetype of humanity. However, this matter is more complicated, due to "the incident in Eden."

Potentially, recapitulation not only goes all the way back to personal formative issues but also to genetic, human, and global origins. One of the most important experiences we can have, to free us from the "howling power of the genes," is the revelation of the "mold of man."

I don't know why, but when one runs across the mold of man it seems to be that the company of a spiritual mentor is required. This was true for Carlos, who met the "mold of man" (his words) in the presence of don Juan, in dreamtime. It also shows up in the account of Carl Jung, who was shown the mold by his deceased father. When I experienced the mold of man, I was under the direction of a deceased shamanic mentor.

> I felt the presence of my mentor in a dream. I saw a dark field against which there were occasional streaks of light, like shooting stars. I did not know at the time what the darkness meant and thought it might be sinister—a common human reaction. Soon I understood that the blazes represented instances when people stood up for the dignity of the human spirit. I saw a child standing up to his parents for his rights.
>
> Next I found myself in an area of light and I knew I was in the presence of the biological source of humanity. My mind identified it as the "mold of man"—and recognized the term from Castaneda. It proclaimed: "Worship me, I am the True God!" I felt doubt, however. Was this the real God? It immediately jumped on me: "Blasphemer, blasphemer, worship me, I am the True God!" This went on and on, "Blasphemer, blasphemer, worship me!" Fifteen minutes passed like this, during which I felt guilty, like I was committing a crime, but I couldn't find it in me to worship the mold. I didn't exactly know why. I also didn't know what blasphemy was. It seemed doubtful that the mold of man really was the True God. It didn't make sense. Finally, the vision faded away and I only felt the scrupulously neutral presence of my mentor. I woke up.

Later I realized that the mold of man was the human genome and that its motto was "Eat, drink, and procreate." It just wanted to be perpetuated. And I saw that the white streaks represented the human spirit, which was actually opposed to the genome.

Adam represents the genome of organic humanity while Eve represents life itself, organicity, or the protoplasm. In the post-Edenic world, the mold demands our worship through the enjoyment of sensual and reproductive pleasures. However, this brings us into conflict with the dictates of the Tree of the Knowledge of Good and Evil, which wants us to moralize our behavior. This is also referred to as the conflict between the seed of the woman and the seed of the serpent.

"I had no idea evil penetrated to this level of creation," said a friend who also experienced the mold of man. "This is built into the entire human race on the level of the genes. I saw people emerging from this 'God' and then being absorbed back into him." Kent called it the "Worm-headed God" because the people coming and going were like worms coming out of a mass of worms. One could call it the "Protoplasmic God." The alchemists called it "Proteus." These names refer to the combination of Adam (the mold) and Eve (the protoplasm). At death, Proteus reabsorbs the protoplasmic blob back into itself and recasts new humans from the primal material.

My experience of the mold of man resembles almost exactly Castaneda's. One similarity is don Juan's insistence that Carlos could only see the mold because he himself was showing it to him. In all four of these accounts a mentor was needed. I don't know why this is the case but it seems to be a characteristic of the experience.

There were also some major differences. Castaneda was greatly impressed by the mold, vowing to serve it no matter what, despite the ridicule of don Juan, who said there was no way to serve the mold. He had to drag Carlos away as he yelled "inane" pledges. Having been through this experience, I found Castaneda's account chilling. It seemed to me that his vow to serve the mold was an omen anticipating his eventual descent into sex addiction and egotism. That is precisely the way we serve the mold. This is the only place in all of Castaneda's writing where I find myself in disagreement with don Juan: it did matter that Carlos pledged his undying service to the mold.

Jung's experience occurred in a dream. His father, a Lutheran clergyman long deceased, led him up into a room where God was present. Jung understood that he was to bow his head down to the floor, touching his forehead to the surface. Try as he might, he couldn't do it.

When Jung told the dream to his students, he explained that he didn't feel that humanity should bow down to God in complete obedience, like a dumb fish. He felt the human being should retain a part of his or her individuality and free will. Many of his students were shocked, thinking it evidence of hubris toward the Supreme Being. That's what I thought for many years after reading his account. However, after I had my own experience of the mold of man I realized that Jung was right. His was a direct experience of the mold, as shown by the presence of the characteristic mentor. His instinct for truth and his dream self knew enough to react correctly to the mold when he was deep in the unconsciousness of the dream world. His rejection of subservience to the mold was appropriate.

The moment the mold fell in rebellion against Creator was also the moment when our consciousness shifted from the genome to our individual selves and we lost awareness of the "original sin" of the collective human genome against God. That is why so many people rightly reject the idea of "original sin"—it is only those who have the blood of personal sin on their hands that readily feel the reality of the Christian doctrine. The "original sin" is hidden in our genes. We rebelled as a race against Creator and the race, the human genome, is still rebelling.

To the extent we remain under the power of the mold of man we will not develop true and lasting individuality. Instead, our soul, dominated by protoplasmic imperatives, will be recalled back into unconsciousness. However, in little bursts of rebellion, we push against the mold, trying to become a true individual.

When we perceive the real nature of the mold of man and reject his worship, we begin to understand the howling power of the genes. We are not, of course, freed from our biological urges, which continue until we die. In this regard, the shaman is in the same position as the mystic, the religionist, and the ordinary person: a conscious being seeking some higher meaning in life, constantly sidetracked by the needs of the biological organism, the reptilian brain, and the ego.

The mold of man is not all bad. We need it for human procreation. William Blake pointed this out in a *Letter to the wife of Thomas Butts* (1982, 714):

To Mrs. Butts.
Wife of the Friend of those I most revere,
Receive this tribute from a Harp sincere;
Go on in Virtuous Seed sowing on Mould
Of Human Vegetation, and Behold
Your Harvest Spring in to Eternal Life,
Parent of Youthful Minds, and happy Wife!

W. B.

In addition to the howling power of the genes, we are also subject to the pull of the mineral realm. We are under the sway of both Adam, the mold of man, and the reptilian brain, at the bottom of which rests the Earth Spirit Dragon. These sources are invisible to us, but by feeling our way in the darkness we can uncover and see these hidden problems. We earned our free will at the cost of our spiritual birthright and we can return to congruity with our Creator. Is there a species more complicated in origin than our own? More blessed by opportunity than ours? More cursed by suffering? I don't know. Is there a story more unbelievable? We are a Mystery People.

The Human Spirit

Those shooting stars of light I saw against the darkness represent the human spirit. It is the supernatural opponent of the mold of man and the field of energy where actions reflecting the nobility of humanity are recorded. It possesses the grand characteristic of spirit, which always supports freedom. Don Juan associated the human spirit with magnanimous acts.

The universal spirit is noble and the human spirit is noble. It remained attached to the spirit after the human genome detached itself. It is like one of the animal spirits. Each species has its own archetype or genome. Because the animals are not fallen (except for Dragon and ourselves), each animal genome is still attached to its spiritual archetype and the spirit itself. For this reason, there is still a direct link to the spirit from the animal. The human spirit is also unfallen but it took a while to be fully available to human beings, and even then the mold of man is still in conflict with it.

In order to manifest here on earth, the human spirit had to go through all the shifts of the assemblage point that man goes through, from the sublime to the hellish: in other words, it had to incarnate through what don Juan calls the "band of man." The shifts along the band of man sum up all the things that man has done in the purely human sphere. Human history goes from the terrible to the great, pain to pleasure.

The story of the incarnation of the human spirit seems to be pretty much the story of Jesus. He experienced all the shifts of the assemblage point along the band of man. He also manifested the magnanimous character of the human spirit. He did not express a theology but instead described an alternate reality—the "kingdom of heaven"—in a series of word-pictures.

This brings us to the same clearing in the forest of eternity as the shamanic path, but it is not entirely congruent. The shamanic path follows the "shift below," or the shift to the province of the animal. That's not a hard shift to feel: anyone who is suddenly sexually aroused feels that shift. The shift below not only touches on sexual energy but survival and reproduction. Despite the constant moral hectoring of the Christian church ever since, this was not something Jesus addressed. His teachings do not focus on sexuality, beyond the most basic teachings of honorable relationship. The "shift below" was not his job assignment.

If we compare these two paths, we find that the path of the human spirit is conjunct the imagination—for that is what Jesus emphasizes in his "kingdom" stories—while the shift below emphasizes a connection to dreamtime. This is because of the differing natures of humans and animals. Thanks to the "incident in Eden" we have the ability to self-reflect, to look at the pictures in our mind. However, the warm-blooded animals sleep and dream and it is because of this that we can ourselves enter dreamtime. To do so, we have to enter the realm of the beast; the shift below. We can see why these are called the Old, Old Path and the New Way.

I remember the moment when I first became aware that the images appearing on the movie screen of my mind's eye were real. I was having a vision. It was a vision, not a dream:

In my mind's eye I was looking at the plastered wall of an old Mediterranean church. There was a fresco of Mother Mary on the wall. Suddenly, the image broke off as one coherent piece of plaster, so the picture of Mother Mary was floating in the air, two feet from the wall. From behind her, out floated a little cradle with the little baby Jesus in it. Words came with it: "And God gave his only begotten son so that the world might be saved."

This vision was so brusque and unexpected that it snapped my mind into lucid awareness. It was literally the first time I was aware of seeing images as a conscious observer. Eventually, I came to realize that the imagination as an active, conscious faculty seemed to be related to Jesus, but why or how? William Blake's theology, which I have recounted, seemed like a reasonable explanation.

Is there any virtue in "believing in Jesus?" There is no virtue in believing in anything. The virtue is in the experience of what is real, whole, and true. Then we *know*. There is, however, virtue in standing up for the dignity of the human spirit and wearing the human image.

We can only learn about the "shift below" and the animal self on the shaman's path. The animals gave us dreamtime but it is only the human that can give us imagination. Animals can't control the focus of the mind the way humans can. The imagination allows us to see the image of the human. Animals can see that too. We know, for instance, that crows have "words" that differentiate between "man" and "man with gun." However, the animals cannot generate and maintain the images at will. They see the images that appear before their eyes. It is only when they are sleeping that the images come back to them. We know that because sleeping dogs wag their tails or whimper or grimace.

The way of the human spirit is the way of the heart, the path of the soul, the avenue of human dignity. It unifies us with the spirit without sacrificing any aspect of our human nature or individuality that is genuine. By comparison, the path of the animal self is incomplete for us humans. Yet, denying our animality makes us incomplete too. Ultimately, the creation will have to reunite the animal and the human in order to bring an end to that unnatural schism. Perhaps we will also have to reunite with the faery people in order to be truly complete. R. J. Stewart talked to a spirit who outlined this evolutionary path.

Is the shaman's path infernal, as so many Christians believe? The principle of shamanism, the actualization of the animal self, or familiar, is not innately good or bad; it is what one does with the experience that determines the ultimate spiritual outcome. The Reverend Montague Summers wrote a book, *The Werewolf* (1966), in which he quotes hundreds of accounts by Inquisitors and ordinary eyewitnesses in which the werewolf is personified as evil and usually put to death. Only a single witness, an Irish priest, had enough compassion to ask if putting a werewolf to death was not a form of murder.

❂ CRANE MEDICINE ❂

The waterbirds are traditionally associated with the journey to the Spirit World. A traditional medicine bag in Siberia is a skinned crane and the Three Cranes are a shamanic symbol in Asian shamanism. As late as the twelfth century, the official symbol of the medical guild in Paris was Three Cranes, each with a sprig of Marjoram held in the beak. The symbol refers to birth, death, and rebirth—the shaman comes back from death to live, teach, and heal in the 3-D world.

In Native America, to dream of Crane gives one the authority to "pour water" or call in the spirits in a sweat lodge, although the skill to interpret what the spirits say is a separate gift in many cases. I knew of one person whose dream of the Wild Geranium or Cranesbill (*Geranium maculatum*) empowered him to "pour water." The Crane clan of the Anishinabe Ojibwa was the clan from whom the communicators with other tribes would be selected; they were known for their oratory. An excellent example of a Crane person is Barak Obama—tall, thin, long-legged, an excellent orator.

Because of the association with communication, Crane became transformed into Hermes or Mercury when the animal totems became Gods. In Egypt, we see a transitional figure in the Ibis-headed God Thoth, who was considered by the Greeks to be the counterpart of Hermes. In Africa, it is said that the first dance steps and then the alphabet were learned from observing Crane. It appears that there is no continent that is without reference to this knowledge.

⚡ Wild Geranium ⚡
(Geranium maculatum)

This is a common woodland wildflower over much of the Eastern Woodland region of North America. It was used by the Native people and the invaders. The root is highly astringent; at the top of the list with Oak bark for tannin content. It tones the mucosa of the digestive tract and has an effect on the kidneys.

As to its properties as a shamanic plant, Wild Geranium "restores the essence." It is good for people who have been on recreational or medical drugs for so long that they don't know how to regulate themselves or don't know what belongs to them rather than the drug. It is also a tremendous remedy for breaking ties between people—when at least one of them does not want the association any more. I wouldn't hesitate to use it in a divorce or business breakup; it even makes clear what belongs to whom.

⚡ Herb Robert ⚡
(Geranium robertianum)

At first I thought the effects of Herb Robert and Wild Geranium (both of which are also called Cranesbill or Storksbill) were identical. There is an important difference however. There has been an extensive and worldwide use of the *robertianum* for cancer (see Isabell Shipard's *How Can I Use Herbs in My Daily Life?* [2016]). This could be interpreted as a "restoration of the essence." The fact that the *maculatum* was not used for cancer in folk medicine, to any considerable extent, indicates that there probably is a difference.

✸ UNDERWATER PANTHER MEDICINE ✸

In the Spirit World we will meet with many beings that have little or no relationship to what we imagine to be true or real according to our material eyes and ears. So we will start with a being that is both legendary and real.

The Underwater Panther—also called the Underwater Serpent—is the inland equivalent of Sea Monster or Leviathan. Found at the bottom of the rivers and lakes of the great interior of the North American continent, I originally assumed that this being was entirely mythological. When I first dragged White Water-lily out of a shallow pond, the whiskers on the rhizomes showed me that the Underwater Panther is equivalent to the Catfish. In the north, the Sturgeon would be included in this identification.

Both these fish are quite remarkable. Both are bottom-feeders that grow to tremendous size. Catfish eight feet long have been caught by fishermen (crazy?) and even larger specimens have been photographed from the air. Endowed with skin, rather than scales, the male Catfish builds a nest, embraces the female as she lays eggs in the nest, depositing his spawn on the eggs, then protects the nest—behavior that reminds us of the warm-blooded animals. Sturgeon can also grow to prodigious dimensions: the largest yet found was eleven and a half feet long. They too are covered with skin, their scales having unified into five armorlike protective plates.

I am not sure if the Underwater Panther can be identified with the world of dream or imagination, since it is cold-blooded; even if it is highly evolved compared to many fish. It may be that it only attunes to fantasy, not true imagination or dreamtime. Traditionally, the

Underwater Panther is attuned to the entire economy of the emotional and image-based worlds put together—so it is an extremely powerful medicine but hard to sustain. There is a tendency to bottom-feeding among people with this medicine: absorbing the dregs of human nature. Rising above this, Underwater Panther has the ability to cleanse the waters of the soul—emotions and image-seeing—in themselves and other people.

He Who Must Not Be Named said that "the Underwater Panther medicines live in the valleys of the great inland rivers of the continent." This would include Jack-in-the-Pulpit, White Water-lily, Yellow Water-lily, and the American Lotus. To a lesser extent we would think of True and False Solomon's Seal. All of them have tubers, roots, rhizomes, tubers, or corms that are fat and fleshy so that they were often important wild foods or medicines in the old days.

❧ Jack-in-the-Pulpit ❧
(*Arisaema triphyllum*)

This common forest wildflower has a fat little root or corm that is packed full of calcium oxalates. Where the Sorrels—Wood, Garden, Sheep—and Rhubarbs have unhealthy amounts of calcium oxalate (avoid large and prolonged consumption), Jack-in-the-Pulpit has large crystals that cut and inflame the mucosa and other tissues, leading to pain and injury. This plant can only be used in the most tiny of doses— I use the homeopathic dilution for ease of delivery.

I have only used this plant once. A very good herbalist was exhausted and run down—as I thought—by taking on too much of the energy of her clientele. *Arisaema triphyllum* 6x homeopathic quickly brought her out of this state. Her practice is much larger and she keeps good boundaries.

The leaf bends over the spathe so that the upper part of the plant looks like the pulpits on the wall from which the Puritan ministers preached. In terms of the doctrine of signatures (or perhaps just playing about the plant in the imagination), this seems to indicate the need for caregivers to rise above and not get caught up in the emotions and fantasies of their communities.

⚛ White Water-lily ⚛
(Nymphaea odorata)

I already discussed this plant in *The Book of Herbal Wisdom* (1997, 381–87). It is a specific for yeast infection where there is a white coating on the tongue that is moist or just starting to dry out, but the more remarkable and impressive aspect is that it is the remedy for "lascivious thoughts," that is, preoccupation with sex. It has been found to be so active that wildcrafting was traditionally assigned to young virgins—who were considered to be immune to its effects, I guess. In adults, even when they are not preoccupied with sex, it can bring on such thoughts. One of the weirdest mistakes of my teaching career as an herbalist occurred in Melbourne, Australia, where I set out with a class to do an herb journey with White Water-lily, which is naturalized there. Quite a few people refused to participate and most of the rest of us had unpleasant lascivious thoughts and even insomnia from the mind working overtime to resist the thoughts.

In Native tradition this plant is not supposed to be touched by iron. This is even mentioned by the white physiomedicalist, William Cook (1869), whose father-in-law was a "root doctor" in upstate New York and the source of much of Cook's lore about plants of the Eastern Woodland region commonly used by Native Americans. It was also mentioned by He Who Must Not Be Named. I went out to pick this rhizome out of a shallow but cold pond (it was November), with a friend and her twelve-year-old daughter. We two adults were having no success trying to use rakes to pull it out of the chilly water while her daughter was pulling it out by hand in massive quantities (the rhizome is massive). We switched our method and had much more success.

This is a tremendous remedy for yeast infection (with a pale tongue coated white in the middle). This is a condition that may be associated with sexual abuse or misuse.

The Earth Spirit Dragon

Like everyone else, I'd heard of dragons, but I thought they were a silly fantasy. I had no direct experience of them until I got coronavirus in spring of 2020. Then I had a series of lucid dreams in which they taught me about themselves.

In the first dream, I saw a Dragon but it looked away from me in shame. *What?* I thought and started to wake up. *Oh . . . this is like the humans after the Garden of Eden. The Dragons were at fault, too, and they are also ashamed.* As I was waking up, I was informed that Dragon was the Earth Spirit, properly entitled the "Earth Spirit Dragon." I immediately rebelled against this: I want a nice maternal, middle-aged Mother Earth type, not a Dragon—even if she could kill me with the bat of an eyelash. I had to wait for further dreams to understand that both exist, but in different realms or layers of Earth. It became apparent that Dragon was the Lord of the Mineral Realm, not the Life Realm, which is the dominion of Mother Earth, the Living Nature—the Soul World.

When we see the Earth Spirit Dragon, we are freed from imprisonment in the mineral realm. They are ashamed because of their role in causing the fall of humanity from Eden. This is at last made clear and their real powerlessness is revealed like the Wizard of Oz: the man behind the curtain is embarrassed in the same way. We continue in imprisonment in minerality, while in the body, our spirit-and-soul has passed one more barrier on the path of personal spiritual evolution.

After I had fully woken up from this first lucid dream, some spirits came along—three of them—and said that I was wrong to call Snake "de-evolutionary": the correct word, they said, was "non-evolutionary." I still have a hard time with that because the snake, after all, once had limbs and lost them. What is that but de-evolution?

In a second dream, I was shown a hill or low mountain like a line across the forests of northern Wisconsin, Minnesota, Upper Michigan, or Ontario, proceeding for hundreds of miles, about a half-mile wide. It was made clear to me that the Dragon actually is inside Earth, pressing up in this line.

A week later I saw on a map that there really was a line of hills or mountains hundreds of miles long, starting at the eastern tip of the Keewanaw Peninsula, breaking up in the Porcupine Mountains, but reforming and running west to Mellon, Wisconsin, finally flattening out into the low hills that run up to the Apostle Islands off the shore of Wisconsin. I was shocked: the Dragon really was in the Earth.

I had a third dream where the Dragon showed me that the long line of hills was his spine. He turned from above my house and flew up to the "Copper Range," in Upper Michigan, merging with the line of hills. He showed me that Dragons were sensitive to EMFs, both celestial and man-made, and that they liked the copper because it grounded them. I suppose any invisible being, if it has real existence, is made of EMFs!

In a fourth dream, the Dragon and I had eye contact and at last there was peace between us. He showed me various mysteries about Dragons. They are associated with copper and the color green. In a fifth dream, the Dragons showed me that they channeled the EMFs from space and were responsible for creating the ever-changing "astrological matrix" of the planet.

Because Dragons are so connected with fantasy—the price of being invisible—I felt the necessity to check in with sources I tend to go to for shamanic validation. Carlos Castaneda is on the top rung. Sure enough, he does mention the "feathered serpent." His unsuccessful ability to deal with it led to the breakaway of the nagualist apprentices assigned to him by don Juan. The feathered serpent (Quetzalcoatl) is a powerfully dominant reference point in the Indigenous cultures of Mexico and the American Southwest.

❂ DRAGON MEDICINE ❂

According to the final dream I was given, the Earth Spirit Dragon is constantly forming and reforming the four elements according to the changing lights of the planets and stars. The eye of the Dragon picks up the starlight and channels it into the Earth. The changes brought by Dragon, as mediator for the stars and planets, are therefore equivalent to the astrological matrix within which we live. These changes do not penetrate beyond the Wheel of Dharma. The spirit, on the other hand, brings about spiritual change, which transcends conditions on Earth. We see how, even here, Dragon covers up the spirit, as it did in Eden.

There is a type of magic that belongs to the Earth Spirit Dragon. Through attunement, one can "be in the right place at the right time," astrologically speaking. Or more skillful yet—one could cause changes in the astrological matrix in order to achieve some purpose. But none of this would go beyond the Wheel of Dharma, so what benefit would it be? Answer: life on Earth is pretty hard—removing some of the obstacles, without harming anyone, might be worth the effort.

The sign of the magician is the pentangle or pentagram, because it refers to the fifth element. This is also a signature for Dragon Medicine, because it is like the fifth element, channeling the other four. However, this is also a signature for Wolf Medicine, which relates to the relationship between the ego and the world; domestic and wild. Finally, it is the symbol of the hand, through which magic is accomplished. However, the best signature for Dragon Medicine is invisibility. This is why Dragon Root is a powerful medicine of invisibility. It was used by Native American People from one coast to another—I cannot help but wonder if the continent-wide distribution of the plant is due to this usage. This was one of the methods used by Geronimo and his men but it was used by many others.

⍟ Dragon Root, False Solomon's Seal ⍟
(*Maiathemum stellatum, M. racemosum,* and others)

This is the first plant that ever identified itself to me as Dragon Medicine. That was a long time before I knew anything about Dragons. It used to insist that I call it "Dragon Root." My unimaginative response: *That's ridiculous, you're just a little rhizome the width of a pencil creeping around under the ground!* After a while, I found three more people that all said it wanted them to call it Dragon Root. One of them was the late Paula Jensen, a skilled herbalist in Santa Fe and Tulsa. I told her I thought it was a ridiculous name for the plant but she replied: "Well, it's a little plant with a big attitude." So I started calling it Dragon Root. After a while, it said: "That's okay. You can also call me False Solomon's Seal." So it has a name for itself in both the Outer Court and the Inner.

Actually, I like the old Latin name *Smilacina* because it sounds nice and avoids the issues brought up in the last paragraph, but this name has been replaced by botanists with the terribly awkward *Maianthemum*. Hey, botanists, lighten up a little bit! Wasn't *Pseudognaphalium obtusifolium* far enough out there for you? Dragon Root has also been moved in and out of the Lily family—now called the liloids.

Smilacina has properties a lot like True Solomon's Seal (*Polygonatum*). In fact, it is hard to tell when to use one or the other. The latter, as far as we know, is a Wolf Medicine not a Dragon Medicine, so on the magical level they are a bit different.

Smilacina is very precise about how we treat it: not only was it picky about its name, it wouldn't let me write about it until I had discovered another Dragon Medicine. Why? I don't know. Plants have their personalities, just like people, and even their own systems of nomenclature and classification.

ᴽ Tarragon ᴽ
(*Artemisia dracunculus*)

This European culinary herb is named the "little dragon" (*dracunculus*), and in French, *esdragon*; similarly, the name "Tarragon" is from the medieval Latin *tragonia*, which derives from the Greek *drakóntion* ("dragonwort"). The association is said to arise from the fact that the roots overgrow and choke themselves, so it has to be divided every two to three years or it will die out. That sounds more like the ouroboros than Dragon.

The herbaceous tops form large masses of wild, dense foliage. Tarragon is said to resemble Fennel or Anise seed in taste because all three give the tongue a tingling sensation. There is no word for this in European culinary or medical herbalism, but in American herbalism we call these kind of plants "diffusives." Tarragon has almost no flavor, but gives a strong diffusive sensation; that means it stimulates the nerves of the mouth, the back of the throat and the mighty vagus nerve that runs from the throat down into the viscera to control the autonomic or unconscious functions of the body. Tarragon is traditionally used as a digestive remedy because the vagus is so active in that sphere. But it could also interact with a lot more organs and functions that are not yet well mapped out—it can take hundreds of years to get to know a plant. It is known as a banishing herb in magical literature, but as a diffusive it summons other herbs—or helps them to express themselves more strongly. Normally, banishing is done with the hand. A substitute for Tarragon is Mountain Mint (*Pycnanthemum virginianum*).

The diffusives are especially good additives to formulas because they energize the other herbs. Tarragon is very good with Yarrow and Schizandra. Since both of these are top Warrior Medicines, I call these the "Dragonrider formulas."

The Headwaters of Creation

The headwaters of creation is the place where the great torrent of manifestation roars out from the abyss of nothingness. Since we are dealing with Mysteries, I am not sure anyone knows why nothingness boils over into somethingness but this vision has been reported by seers through the ages. Jacob Boehme described it many times and Thomas Vaughan likened it to the great cataract on the Nile.

The headwaters of creation is a place where one goes beyond one's genes. We must get to that abyss (without falling into it) in order to overcome the howling pull of our genetic material, which seeks to immerse us in purely material, tribal, and personal survival demands. The abyss lies beyond those concerns.

Two friends of mine asked if I wanted or needed a "soul journey."
"Sure," I replied, not knowing what that meant to them. They took
out their drums. Soon I was in another state of mind. In my inner ear,

·*I heard pounding, and I saw two old Ojibwa women pounding grain— wild rice or corn—with wooden mallets. It felt as if the differentiated genetic material in my testicles was being gently pounded down to undifferentiated material. Then I found myself at the Origin Place Lake. The sky was dark and brooding. A wind swept over the surface and I knew I was in the pre-genetic state at the headwaters of creation. Wow, I thought: This is the lake I always thought of as the origin place. Later that night—see below—I dreamed that the faery people told me I had "genetics" from them.*

One of the strange things about the Spirit World is that it interpenetrates with the material world so that a visionary place like the headwaters of creation can be superimposed over an actual place in the material world. This interpenetration can be personal or cultural. When I experience the headwaters of creation, I experience it as that particular lake in northern Minnesota. I first visited the lake when I was eighteen. It is only accessible by canoe. The sky was dark, a wind was wuthering over the waters and there was a brooding feeling under gray skies.

Would this lake serve the same function for other people? I found out that it did for at least one person. I have a friend who lives on an Ojibwa reservation nearby. He brought up the subject of the lake independently. For him, this was the origin place of his people. Archaeology showed that an island in the lake had been continuously occupied for over eight thousand years. It was on an ancient trade route from the Arctic Ocean to the Great Lakes and the eastern half of the continent. In the seventeenth century, the French built a trading post nearby and, of course, the people moved to that location.

This was not the "usual" origin place for any other Indigenous peoples of the Great Lakes, because this particular band were traders and hosts at the midpoint on one of the great inland trade routes. "We're not pure-bloods," my friend laughed. "We've hosted travelers for thousands of years." So, for him: this was where his people originated, where they were sustained down to the present, and where they were renewed and transformed and continue to live.

The Faery People

When I was about thirteen, my father taught me that the Catholic Church did not treat the faeries as demons, but embraced the ancient understanding that they could steal human souls and these souls would be forced to "dance for eternity" in the faery halls. This meant, according to the Church, that they would not join their human brethren in the great resurrection of the dead at the end of the world. I'm not sure why my father mentioned this to me, but I knew the second he brought it up that it was too late for me. I knew I had been born with mixed human-faery genes.

The great sources of information about the faeries are the Lowland Scottish ballads, like "Thomas the Rhymer" and "Tam Lin." This is pointed out by R. J. Stewart in *The UnderWorld Initiation* (1989). The Celts seemed to have had a greater interaction with the faery people than other nationalities, and their myths and legends sometimes tell us what is going on in that world.

We might as well begin with the faery dance. Why is it so dangerous? The tumblers are the basic building blocks of creation; always "tumbling," never still, until two click together to form a new content. At that moment, we step outside the faery realm. They are, therefore, the primal creative matter. The first Something. Susan is right to describe them as "tumblers," but they are also beings. There is consciousness in all that is created and it exists even in the primal Somethingness of Faery Land.

The reason the faery dance traps human souls is that the doorway in is always tumbling and is therefore never in the same place twice. One can get out again, but only if we don't eat or drink anything or accept gifts that bind one to that land. We can imagine how the starving peasants of medieval Europe would have been so easily seduced by offers of food or drink, whereas modern people are usually offered treasures or occult powers. The gifts they offer are the most seductive in the world because they can read our hearts like nobody else.

The entrapment may occur immediately or after years of interaction. Some people prefer to live in the faery world; so it is not entrapment but a choice. Thomas the Rhymer (ca. 1220–ca. 1295) was a particular friend of the Queen of Elfland and it is reputed that in his old age he was called by her and walked off into her kingdom. Reverend Robert Kirk (1644–1692), author of the *Secret Commonwealth of Elves, Fauns, and Fairies* (first published in 1815), is also said to have been taken to that land—though one of his cousins dreamed that he didn't want to remain there.

Neither the Rhymer nor the good reverend saw any conflict between these supernatural activities and their duties as Christians. Kirk was involved in preparations for the publication of a Gaelic version of the Bible and when this was secured he began his in-depth studies of the subterranean world and its inhabitants. His body was found on the faery mound behind his house and was buried in the churchyard. He was honored with the title "chaplain to the Queen of the Elves" by those who remained behind. Disappearance is a rare problem on the shamanic path—He Who Must Not Be Named lost a friend this way.

In my forty-sixth year, I felt the need to converse with the Queen of the Faeries myself and for several weeks I put out the intention, before sleep, of communicating with her. After two weeks, I dreamed that I was with the faeries—they looked like golden hairs, crisscrossing in all directions—and had a dialogue with them:

"You know how you always felt like you were an alien?"
   Yes.
"That's because you have genetics from us."
I felt instantly relieved to have this clarified, but they weren't done with me.
   "And now we will offer you a present as a reward for visiting us: how to become invisible. You know how we're invisible?"
   Yeah.
   "And you know how to tune into us through your feet, into the Earth?"
   A-huh.

"Well, if you tune into us that way you can be invisible."

I woke in terror. *Why would I want to be invisible? And would I come back if I did become invisible?* The medicine man didn't and he was a lot smarter than me. I felt they were trying to seduce me into their world. I notified two friends that I thought could follow me in there if I got stuck.

Two years passed and one of these friends set up an opportunity for me to sleep for the night in the "Tower of Gwydion," built by a man who had done faery work and died in a deer-vehicle accident on a winding California road.

That night I dreamed that the forces were gathering for the final cosmic showdown in the battle of good against evil. I was on the good side. We trusted in our generals, who were old Scots Lairds ready for anything. We were gathered, regiment by regiment, according to our spiritual genetics. I was in the part human, part faery regiment. There weren't a lot of us—about eighty. The faeries were gathering as well. As I woke up, I heard the "Ballad of Tam Lin" in my ear. I knew immediately, this was the ballad that tells us how to escape from the faeries. It describes the tumblers as ladies playing chess. (Even now, thinking about this makes me sick to the stomach). The female warrior in the ballad, Janet, intentionally seeks faery knowledge. She is told to avoid going up Carterhaugh, but she cuts her kilt above the knee and goes up looking for Tam Lin, a warrior caught by the faeries on the hill. She gets pregnant and threatens to abort the baby if Tam Lin does not take responsibility for the pregnancy. She is informed by him that when the faeries march on All Hallows' Day, they give up their prisoners. If she holds on to him through the night, through several transformations involving warm- and cold-blooded animals, she can drag him out of the faery realm when dawn breaks and he will be free. In the morning he wakes in her arms. Immediately, I knew I had seen the march of the faeries and I was safe.

364   Glimpses of the Spirit World

I didn't pursue more knowledge about the faeries, though they gave me several more gifts over the following decades—all involving plants.

Twenty years passed from my dream of the faeries marching. Coronavirus dramatically impacted my dream life. When I was sick with Omicron, I was assaulted by ridiculous, over-the-top rationalism that kept me awake all night. I finally realized what was going on and shut my internal dialogue off and finally fell asleep. As I woke up, I suddenly saw a set of drawers, each of which contained a different "faery power." As it stuck out of the drawer, the faery substance looked like cotton or wool or insulation, though the fibers were slightly larger. I felt no threat from the faeries; they were offering me their magic without asking anything in return. I didn't even know that was an option. I tried to use the imaginary fur but they preferred to work with me via herbs that were furry or wooly. That was their signature.

R. J. Stewart summed up some of the gifts of the faery people in *The UnderWorld Initiation* (1989, 63):

Magical literature and folk tales are full of people with curious powers, particularly that of seership. Yet any experienced worker of magic will agree that clairvoyance and similar abilities are the common property of us all, and that in the advanced stages of initiation into the Mysteries, these psychic abilities are absorbed into higher functions which do not have any paranormal manifestation or material potential for abuse.

An individual who emerges from the UnderWorld may or may not have unusual powers of consciousness or energy, but these are interim patterns, side-effects of the transformation. The greater magical gift in the Western Tradition is not power, but "the Tongue that Cannot Lie." Beyond this stage, further development is of a spiritual order, and the magical initiations are superseded.

In American Indian Medicine, the faeries are generally not considered desirable allies. Timothy Knab describes how the nagualists of central Mexico taught him to avoid "those who are not our brothers." However, interaction with the "inorganic beings," as Castaneda called them, had become a characteristic of the lineage into which he was inducted. He had such an intense interaction with them that even don Juan and his fellow apprentices were terrified by the amount of "inorganic" energy Carlos pulled back from the other world. (This was not a sign of spiritual corruption but of an extraordinary, bizarre "friendship" between human and faery.) The last book in the series, *Being-in-Dreaming*, is one of the best eyewitness descriptions of the faery world I have ever read. As don Juan said, Castaneda's experiences would become "sorcerer stories" for their lineage in the future.

Don Juan explained that his lineage was provided powers of the non-ordinary by the inorganic beings and that these helped free them from the earthbound world. However, his lineage had become dependent on the beings for their non-ordinary powers—so we see the problem with the faeries.

◉ FAERY MEDICINE ◉

When my late friend John Redden moved to Toronto in the '70s, he discovered two peculiar herb stores. One was founded by Khalid Ottway, a genuine hakim from Saudi Arabia, while the other was run by an old Canadian. As John pursued his studies in herbalism, he came to realize that the formulas in the second store did not resemble any combinations he had ever seen. He asked the old man where he came up with them and was rewarded with a confidence. "When I was a child growing up on our family farm in Ontario, the faeries used to play with me and teach me things. Those are their formulas. I don't actually know anything about herbs."

I instantly blurted out to John: "Did you save any of those formulas?" He blinked. The idea had not occurred to him. When I told this story to a friend, she saw what I'd missed: "He didn't think of the faeries as real, so he didn't think the combinations were worth saving."

John was a deeply spiritual person, but faeries weren't his cup of tea.

A few years later, I was making a medicine bag for a friend. She dreamed that she and I went to the faery kingdom at the center of the galaxy. I was trying to take back two artifacts they had stolen from me. I got one of them. She explained: "You didn't have trouble being there because you're part faery, but I'm fully human, so I felt very uncomfortable." Three of them lined up in front of her and probed her energy field from head to toe; they determined she didn't belong there. "I could tell police anywhere in the universe," she commented. We joined hands and left. The next day I stopped making that medicine bag and started making an "herb catcher."*

The Dragonrider formulas are an example of formulas that I know the faeries like. I thought I'd invented them myself, but we don't always know where our thoughts come from. Some people—Robert Louis Stevenson records this of himself—experience "little people" weaving together their thoughts.

In addition to Tarragon (or Mountain Mint), there are four plants that are especially associated with Faery Medicine. One is Elder, who is referred to as the Elder Mother in European folklore: a name for the Faery Queen. Another faery tree is Hawthorn (*Crataegus* spp.) Both are useful when one has become too abstracted, or swept away into the imagination. They are excellent for attention deficit disorder. Life Everlasting (*Helichrysum, Gnaphalium, Pseudognaphalium*) is known in Ireland as the "Steed of the Faeries." It is used in the Last Rites of the Catholic Church to help the soul go to the next world. Humans and faeries interact at conception, birth, and death. St. John's Wort (*Hypericum perforatum*) was called the "Flower of the Faeries" by Father Sebastian Kneipp, and is associated in folklore with the "faery ride"—being taken to the faery halls to dance all night.

---

*Since she was a human, my friend had typical human misunderstandings about commerce in the faery realm. The faeries hadn't stolen anything from me; the artifact I was seeking was actually a new creation that didn't exist until the moment it returned with us from the center of the galaxy. I've never heard of an "herb-catcher" before or since.

✥ Elder ✥
(*Sambucus nigra, S. canadensis, S. mexicana*)

I've written about Elder in a number of places, and so have many other herbalists. Charlemagne decreed that every house in France have an Elder in the yard as a complete "medicine chest," since it could purge all humors via the skin, lungs, colon, and kidneys—also in large doses it was emetic. The berries are considered nutritious and blood-building, and are used to make the famous wine. The flowers are lighter and used to make a "water" that is similar to a soda for light, cooling refreshment in the summer, in Europe.

The Black Elder (*S. nigra*) is the official representative of the genus in herbalism and preferred for flavor in wine-making. The Canadian (*S. canadensis*) is available wild throughout the North American continent, east of the Rockies. The third (*S. mexicana*) grows from Mexico up through California to Oregon. It is considered genetically similar to the Black Elder but the berries are blue. I saw a specimen in Lake County, California with a base five feet by three—hollowed out and fragmented, since the wood rots in the center.

Elder was considered to be the abode of a special being known variously as the Elder Mother, Old Lady, or Old Girl. In Denmark she was called the Hyldemoer, literally the "Hidden Mother" (the same Germanic root, *huld-*, can be seen in the Icelandic term *huldufólk*, which refers to the "hidden folk" or faeries). Essentially, she is the Queen of the Faeries. The little Elder Mother is often visualized as an old woman who gathers medicinal plants in the mountains. In the old days, in Central Europe, the peasants put an offering of milk out under the Elder in the spring and brought the herbs to the church for a blessing at the Feast of the Assumption of the Virgin Mother, in mid-August—to ensure that both Mothers blessed the herbs.

It is said that the bark stripped upward causes emesis while the bark stripped downward purges the kidneys and bowels. Other people say the difference is in whether one drinks the bark decoction quickly or slowly. The reader can pursue this knowledge at their own risk. The safe parts are the flowers and berries. They open the skin to cool in hot weather and fever, and to expectorate mucus; and the berries "build the blood." In Europe there is an almost identical looking Elder (*Sambucus ebulis*), the berries of which purge.

Elder is, of course, a famous flu and cold remedy and there has been a bit of research on the matter. It increases cytokines, which are both pro- and anti-inflammatory. A book dedicated solely to the medicinal properties of Elder, entitled *Anatomia sambuci* (Anatomy of Elder), was penned by Martin Blochwitz and published in 1644. Just about everything that could be done with this plant is recorded in that book. I drew from this in *The Book of Herbal Wisdom* (1997, 432–42).

In the Hans Christian Andersen fairy tales, Elder represents the wild pagan background of Central Europe, is considered the abode of the Queen—sometimes King—of the Underworld. It also figures as a representative of the storyteller's muse. In practice, I find that it is a specific for children who live so much in their imagination that they don't pay attention much to parents, teachers, or fellow students. This, of course, has its good side, but not if you're trying to teach a child not to run into the street. This is a state of mind that is similar to attention deficit disorder, but it is not exactly the same.

℞ Rabbit Tobacco ℘
(*Pseudognaphalium obtusifolium*)

Rabbit Tobacco and many of its cousins, including Helichrysum, are very mysterious. The tops look like little tufts of clouds. We gather them after the frosts in the fall. When a mist comes, if you are out in the field with them, they release a beautiful vanilla/savory smell, which indicates the presence of volatile oils. Altogether, this plant could be considered a Rabbit, Cloud, or Faery Medicine.

The first time I picked this plant, I drove for three hours, got out of the car, put down my tobacco, and started picking. Within five minutes a mist came and the flowers in my hands and in the fields burst out into a beautiful scent. I knew that the plant liked me, though it is a Trickster remedy, associated as it is with the faeries, clouds, and rabbits.

After being picked, it should be hung out in the barn or shed for six months, according to Paul Red Elk. In the old days white people would hang it in the house because of the beautiful smell—which would come out when the air got damp. However, some Indian people are in the habit of tying it up and putting it deep in the medicine bundle or in a storage place where they can't smell the scent. Rabbit Tobacco makes one psychically more permeable to the Soul and Spirit Worlds. Many Indians are already sensitive in this way so they don't want to get too opened up. White people, on the other hand, are not very sensitive, so they need to put it out where they can smell it.

I asked Paul Red Elk about it one day and he said: "Just a second, I have to translate back from Lakota to explain this plant . . . Yes. It is called 'Walker Between the Worlds.' When an old person dies and they can't pass on a legacy, they haunt the family, sometimes, until they can pass it on." That would be a medicine power, not money or some material asset. "It helps pass on the legacy and release the person to the Spirit World." It keeps releasing scent after it is dead, so that is an important signature. "Don't pick it where there has been a battle and throw it away if there is an argument in the house."

The next day I flew to Birmingham, Alabama, and was picked up by Phyllis Light. I told her about Sweet Everlasting (as I called it) on the drive back to her house in Arab. The next morning, she said, "I had a dream last night that my astrological mentor came and showed me a bunch of astrology books he was going to give me. He died when I was in my twenties." However, his greedy ex-wife took the books and she never got them. In the dream her teacher said: "Here are the books. Now I need to go on to another world." Phyllis said to me, "And ya' know what? That herb you were talking about was helping us communicate, only it's what we call Rabbit Tobacco."

I asked Sondra Boyd why it was called "Rabbit Tobacco." She said: "The old folks noticed that it grew where the rabbits like to hang out in the fields, so they figured it as a tobacco to help them communicate with

Creator." J. T. Garrett gives a different story in *The Cherokee Herbal* (2003, 91). One day Wolf was chasing Rabbit up in the mountains. Just in the nick of time Rabbit managed to run into a thicket where Wolf couldn't get him. After a while he came out and looked around. He was all beat up and cut; the Rabbit Tobacco plant told him it was a good remedy for cuts and bruises. The Tsalagis (Cherokees) were famous with the early white settlers for their wound medicine. Rabbits have thin skin and they can get injured and bleed to death just by being chased a long distance by a predator. One of my friends, an older Anishinabe woman who has since passed away, thanked me for some: "Yes, it helps my fraidy-cat small-animal self," she explained with a laugh.

Rabbit Tobacco is widely used on the North American continent by the Indian people to help the deceased spirit of a person move on. The strange thing is that in Europe its close cousin Life Everlasting (*Helichrysum* spp.) is used in the same way by the Catholic Church. During the last rites, a bit of Helichrysum oil is dabbed above the lip, to help the person cross over. The European name refers both to the fact that it is an "everlasting"—a dried herb that keeps its beautiful form after it dies—and that it will help the soul in the next world.

This is a remedy for people who are congenitally weak from birth or the first year of life. It's like they missed a part of the transmission of genes or enzymes from the parent. The first time I heard about it was from a woman in McGayheeville, Virginia: "I grew up on a Blue Ridge hill farm. We never went to the doctor. I had asthma from birth till age seven when the neighbor gave me Rabbit Tobacco." His wife sewed it into a pillow and they gave it to her. She slept with it for a year. "It was mine. You didn't have many toys to call your own in those days, with six kids. I slept with it every night. In a year, the pillow was in tatters but I was totally cured."

Under Yellow Dock Root I've mentioned a woman who got colitis five weeks after the delivery of her third child. Well, it was very difficult for that daughter. She had a lot of nervousness and fear about separation from her mother. She also had colds, bronchitis, and asthma. I tried to help when she was young but nothing worked. A homeopath tried to no avail as well. Finally, when she was eleven, her mother was desperate and brought her out to see me at my herb farm in the country. The Mayo Clinic said she didn't have an enzyme that helps people fight off colds so she would get sick easily and it would go into asthma. Well, I'd learned about Rabbit Tobacco in the last few years and I thought, *Hmm, she was deprived of her mother's milk, with all those immune signals and enzymes?* I gave her Rabbit Tobacco tincture and over a year she was virtually cured. She is a beautiful, healthy young woman now.

I used the pillow method with the Anishinabe woman mentioned above; she was suffering from asthma and it did her a great deal of good, though she was in her sixties. When I was teaching at Wendy Fogg's herb school, there was a student in her thirties who had bad asthma. She was on prednisone, which causes the skin to become thin. Her hair was stubby and short, and she had that "small-animal" scaredy-cat look. I gave her Rabbit Tobacco. When I was teaching at Wendy's years later, I started to tell the story. A woman in the audience raised her hand and said: "That was me. Now I'm totally cured." I couldn't believe it. Her skin was radiant and tanned, her hair was long and luxurious, and I couldn't have recognized her if I tried. She quit her job, moved to Limerick, Maine, opened an herb store with her husband, and was flourishing.

This plant has blessed me and blessed me, from the first day I picked it, when the mist came, down to today. After I got to know Rabbit Tobacco, I had a dream. The faeries told me to make a smoking mixture from Tobacco, Rabbit Tobacco, and Red Willow bark. They explained that the Tobacco would help a person get to the other side; Rabbit Tobacco would help one get in touch with all the different combinations of the tumblers in the otherworld; and Red Osier Dogwood would help fixate the tumblers on one combination once you found what you needed and wanted to come back to the regular world. Rabbit Tobacco is in touch with all the tumblers, just like it is in touch with all the genes.

In addition to helping a person pass on to the otherworld, this herb also helps people in this world make connections with their family or ancestors if there are unresolved or hidden issues in the family lineage.

One woman had kidney pains of obscure origin. She felt they were tied to family secrets. Her mother and father had been Poles rounded up to work in forced labor camps during the Holocaust. They wouldn't talk about their experience and she felt this caused her pain. The Rabbit Tobacco brought out dreams that very night, revealing some of the horrendous suffering the family had experienced. Once she knew what to ask about, she was able to confirm many of the details with older relatives. She truly was healed, emotionally and physically.

❂ BAT MEDICINE ❂

We have so much baggage regarding bats in Western culture that it is hard to get a bead on this kind of medicine. I have had to learn about it from Native American friends and what I learned was more unsettling than anything I ran across in Western literature.

"The Indian People are attacked by the Bat People through their genes," said the sophisticated Anishinabe friend I went to dinner with so many years ago. This had no relationship that I could tell with the rest of the conversation. I thought maybe she was referring to white people, so I didn't ask anymore. Bat People, it turns out, make white people look like kid's stuff. I passed this comment on to a Lakota friend, Arlo. Several days later, he reported back: "Yeah, Percilla was right. The Bat People do attack the Indian People through their genes."

Years went by and I began to have an understanding of Holly. Someone pointed out that it was a Bat Medicine—we can tell from the thorns on the tips of the leaves; they look like claws on bat wings. When the first reports indicated that SARS-CoV-2 derived from a virus harvested from bats, to which spikes from snake venom had become attached (Luo et al. 2020), I felt like I needed to know about Bat Medicine at last—especially once I got Covid myself. I asked my Anishinabe friend Chris MacPadden about it. He hesitated for a moment. "I don't like to have much to do with that medicine," he said. "It works on the genetic level and can modify your genes and your ancestors; even your past lives. It's multidimensional."

Bat Medicine operates in the darkness, where we are not aware, below our usual level of consciousness, but it does not "draw us to the dark side." It is a medicine that functions in the darkness, in the parts of ourselves that we neglect to develop, don't know about, or reject. That includes past generations and the ancestors that have been ignored and forgotten, lifetimes and history that were forgotten. There is reason the Indian People respect and listen to their elders: it is so that these dark spots do not occur in the bloodline.

Viruses are little bits of protein that scientists still quibble about: are they independent life-forms or not? Are they the cause of disease, or do they multiply as a result of stress in the system? Whatever they are, they are very important. They are Nature's way of introducing new genes into all genomes, to further the course of evolution. Through exposure to them, our genetics are changed; we gain immunity and they even bring in new genetic "suggestions" that can modify our genome in positive or negative ways. Bats have an extremely strong immune system so that they can easily overcome viruses. For this reason, the virus has to learn to replicate super-quickly in order to overcome their immune system. This is why the really powerful, dangerous influenza strains appear to originate in bats: SARS, MERS, and coronaviruses. The last Ebola epidemic was traced to a little boy playing in a tree where bats lived. Some people think Ebola and SARS-CoV-2 are man-made in a laboratory. Others don't believe they exist. A deeper insight takes us to the fact that viruses are Mother Earth's agents of genetic change. When she is dealing with devastation, and especially when the bats are affected, she throws out new genetics through viruses in order to bring about change. This particular virus opens (or closes) the heart and the dream centers in the brain. It changes the immune system. It is a spiritual disease that is changing us below the level of consciousness.

It is almost as if the Bat People were created by the viruses (could we call them the Virus People?) to be a home for them within the creation. The viruses live right at the intersection between the physical and the electromagnetic frequencies, as if precipitating new energy configurations into new genetic applications. And of course, the bats are some of the only animals sensitive to sonar—also to radar, which confuses them. In order to harbor the viruses, bats have thrown ten different immune mechanisms overboard so that the viruses can live inside them. Instead of controlling viruses by the normal immune routes, bats have to maintain a higher body temperature—that's why they live in caves and come out only at night: sunlight will kill them.

The emotions that people nourish in darkness, separated from other human beings, are the ones that correlate with these viruses: hatred, envy, jealousy, paranoia, fear. You can't nurse hatred in the bright sunshine of human society; you have to go home and bitterly ruminate on the subject. These emotions are bad for the attitude, the immune system, and the neighborhood. Dr. Bach's flower essence for these kinds of emotions is Holly. Dorothy Hall used the Bach flower essence Holly, but it is only mentioned in her unpublished notes for students. She mentioned "self-destructive" emotions and activities.

I used Holly for myself and others to deal with the mental symptoms that seemed to accompany coronavirus. When we reflect on the social climate of the preceding half-dozen years we see the growing paranoia, fear of strangers, obsession, irrationality, and factional hatred. We also see a lot of environmental damage that has remained hidden, including the decimation of bats.

Herbalist Amanda Dilday, who also worked with Holly for coronavirus, pointed out the analogy between the use of sonar and the heart. We send out and receive signals of love, ambivalence, neutrality, dislike, and hatred. The heart is a sensory organ. It works in the darkness, independently of the five senses. Herbalist Stephen Buhner has written eloquently of the heart as a sensory organ in *The Secret Teachings of Plants* (2004, 89–115).

Amanda also used this medicine during coronavirus the same way I did. We found independently that it opened the heart, even to the extent of increasing the circulation to the upper rib cage, protecting the heart and lungs and increasing blood supply to the immunological thymus, perhaps relaxing the aorta. Due to the genetic manipulation going on right now in medical research, Bat Medicine has become very important. "All that is necessary to enter the new spiritual age is to have an open heart." So keep sending and receiving those sonar signals of the heart.

There is a place of purification in the Land of the Dead where we are submerged in total darkness. It is pretty easy to imagine the worst when we are in a place like that, but it is a place where we can also turn on our sonar and our hearts and learn. And the lessons learned there will change our genetics.

☙ Holly ❧
(*Ilex opaca, I. aquifolium*)

I'm going to discuss this herb more in a book on viruses and the immune system, so I'll only give the short story here. The leaves are not toxic but the berries are high in saponins that tremendously irritate the gastrointestinal tract, so it is therefore listed as a highly toxic plant in the literature (Evans and Stellpflug 2012, 539–40).

The English Holly (*Ilex aquifolium*) has more of a history of usage than the American (*Ilex opaca*), although I have used them interchangeably. Chinese Holly (*Ilex pubescentis*) is one of the four ingredients of the important "antiviral" remedy Gan Mao Ling. Acupuncturist and herbalist Ellen Geary sent me an excellent account of the Chinese Holly (as well as the Western). She wondered why Gan Mao Ling worked so well, especially in "complex viral cases," so she took out the ingredients and found that it was the Holly. She found it beneficial when the acute pathogen attacks the "heart level." This is why it is so useful in covid, where the pathogen quickly goes from the surface to the interior.

English Holly leaf has not been used a great deal, either in ancient or recent times, but it did establish a reputation as a diaphoretic, releasing perspiration in acute disease, and as a febrifuge. The leaf is mildly laxative (rather than cathartic and irritating, like the berries) and diuretic, removing edema and water retention.

The Bach Flower Essence

It is to Dr. Edward Bach that we owe the modern usage of English Holly. It is his essence for feeling irrational hatred, or feeling it directed toward oneself. He wrote (2011, 26) that it is:

> For those who sometimes are attacked by thoughts of such kind as jealousy, envy, revenge, suspicion. For the different forms of vexation. Within themselves they may suffer much, often when there is no real cause for their unhappiness.

Dr. Bach simmered the buds of the trees in his remedy kit, rather than making a flower essence.

The late Dorothy Hall had much to say about Holly flower essence in her unpublished lectures for students. She used the Bach flower essence, stretching Dr. Bach's definition to the boundaries. It is the remedy for "self-inflicted injuries." This is quite an insight into hatred and jealousy. Dorothy expanded "self-infliction" to include excessive immune reactions. That would include cytokine storms. She used Holly flower essence for leukemia, which results from an initial immune reaction that doesn't stop, producing overproduction of white cells. She had positive experiences with over forty cases of children's leukemia, working with doctors—until the jealousy of the medical profession overcame generosity and her associations with the hospital were ended. This usage fits perfectly with the immune exhaustion and fatigue one feels after a viral or bacterial lodgment in the system. Because of its association with the immune system, Dorothy also used Holly for swelling of the spleen.

Bartonella and Coronavirus

When I first contracted Bartonella (diagnosed by symptoms by a specialist, not by a lab test), I felt like the disease hated me. For a while, I kept it in check with various herbs; finally, however, after six months it was causing congestion in the back brain, ears, and mastoids (bones behind the ears) and I was having fits of exhaustion that were very worrisome. I started it six months after the tick bit me; in five days I felt normal, though I kept taking it for several months. When I first came down with coronavirus in March 2020, I also felt it hated me as it would clench my chest muscles or heart and then release a massive flux of blood that left me astonished, lying in bed. Almost always, coronavirus attacks at night. I took Holly and it always stopped or lessened the symptoms.

The Guardians of the Planet

Their pronouns are They, Them, and Theirs, capitalized. Spiritual voyageurs who meet the "Guardians of the Planet," or the "Guardians of the Life Force" in dreamtime automatically know this. I've seen this spelling in writings as diverse as A. S. Raleigh in the early twentieth century and Théun Mares late in the century. It came to me in dream—I knew it was "Them, the Guardians of the Planet," even though I'd never heard of Them before.

When the Earth was first coalescing, the Supreme Being (or someone up there in the celestial government) gathered some beings from another evolutionary cycle that had been fulfilled somewhere else, to act as keepers of the evolutionary current on planet Earth. Because They don't have "Earth genetics," the Guardians have an "alien" feel, but it is different from the faeries because They went through some kind of evolution in time and space before coming to Earth. They are not interested in personal biography so there is not much more that can be said about this sort of thing: who They are or where They came from. They fear being worshipped as gods—They are the archetypes of the seven gods.

I had an amazing series of dreams that were interlocking and related, even though separated by many years. The first one occurred when I was eleven years old:

> I went through a door into the Earth, into a subterranean room that was decorated in a Victorian-era style. There were globe lights on the walls. An older woman was seated at a desk near the door. All of a sudden, water started pouring down the stairs and I knew the world

was ending. The woman simply said, "Here, put one of these globes over your head and you'll be safe. I'll do it too, like this": and she put a globe over her head and another over mine. I woke up knowing the world was ending and I would be safe.

The next dream occurred when I was thirty-one:

Fire and stones were falling from the sky, killing people, but I knew I would be safe. I was walking toward the center of the city. When I reached the center, I knelt down and said: "Please God, I'll help, I'll try and take on karma so that people don't have to suffer and die." I started to wake up and said to myself: Geez, what the heck did I promise? When I woke up, I felt the presence of "Them, the Guardians of the Planet."

The final dream in the series occurred three years later:

I was with Them, the Guardians of the Planet. They said, "There are going to have to be Earth changes and people are going to have to suffer and die." I said, "No, no, I'll help, I'll try and take on karma so that people don't have to suffer and die." But They said, "No, it's too late, and anyways, it's for the betterment of humanity." I was stunned. You knew anything They said was the truth. Then I was alone with one of Them and she gave me a mortality rate I won't repeat here. I slammed out of dreamtime: "When, where, how?"

A friend, half a continent away, had the same dream, with the same words. We think it was some kind of dreamtime template. Some things on the other side are quite organized, others are completely disorganized.

The idea of spiritual, as well as physical evolution, was brought to public awareness by Helena Blavatsky, founder of the Theosophical Society. She expanded on Darwin's new Theory of Evolution to cover the spiritual life. It is not very often that a person (much less a woman) gets to introduce an entirely new perspective of such enormous appeal, but this honor belongs to the founder of Theosophy. Every age, every century, needs new terminology because of the transformative and unstable character of human nature.

There are seven of Them in number, each in charge of a different department. They came to be known as the Gods, and were known to the ancestors of the Hebrews as *ha Elohim*, the Gods, the plural of *El* or *Elon*, a spirit or god. But They don't want to be associated with worship—especially to replace the Supreme Being. In the Hebrew Bible the word *Elohim* came to be the name for the God—which was one way of reducing the incorrect worship. In the last book of the Christian Bible, these beings are called the "Seven Spirits before the Throne of God."

☼ EARTHKEEPER MEDICINE ☼

There are not many life-forms that seem to have an "evolutionary perspective," but there is at least one.

☙ California Bay Laurel, Oregon Myrtle ❧
(*Umbellularia californica*)

When Jolie lived in Marin, she roasted some Bay Laurel nuts to obtain the delicious "truffles"—they taste better than both coffee and chocolate. (Roast to coffee-bean black-brown at about 350° and melt together with a dab of honey.)

Some of the nuts were not completely roasted in the batch Jolie gave me and that is how we want them for medicine. Raw, they are too mealy and acrid for consumption. When I tasted the semi-roasted nuts, I thought: *Wow, that's almost a perfect acridity from the standpoint of medicinal taste*. It gave me a slight sore throat that cleared up in twenty-four hours, so I knew it had medicinal properties. Acrid remedies usually act on the vagus nerve, the main trunk of the autonomic nervous system. So, I made myself some medicine. That was the beginning of my acquaintance with the Bay Laurels.

This ancient tree is native to the bottoms of canyons in coastal areas of California and Oregon—where the Oaks grow. They belong to a wonderful and ancient plant family, the *Lauraceae* or Bays. These include the Bay tree sacred to the Greeks and Romans, Sassafras, Avocado, and a bunch of other spice trees.

Forty million years ago, the Bay Laurels were part of a jungle forest that covered California. Today they are the sole representatives of that forest. More than all their neighbors, they seem to be capable of evolutionary adaptation. This ought to mean that they are tremendous survivors and would be excellent healing agents, but that is an understatement. It is more like they are in tune with the forces of evolution itself, and this makes them a Medicine of the Earthkeepers.

A few years later, Jolie and I held a plant attunement class in Berkeley. We wanted to help the Tan Oak, which was being devastated by Oak wilt. The Bay Laurels carry the disease but it doesn't hurt them. They brushed off the problem: "It doesn't matter in the long run whether the Tan Oaks survive or not." They casually added: "And you humans shouldn't assume you are going to survive either."

The Tan Oaks were whiny and helpless. They remembered the days when the Native people picked and loved them. They were aware of the holocaust of Native America: "No one comes to us now." Big, somber Valley Oak said: "We've seen this disease before." That would explain why the White Oak family has considerable immunity to the wilt; the Red Oak branch somewhat less. Jolie asked the Tan Oaks if they could get help from the Valley Oaks. "None of the other Oaks like us," they whined.

The Bay Laurels take the "long view." I asked Sondra about them and she was unintentionally plunged into a plant attunement. "They say they preexist the Earth and are able to plant themselves anywhere in the universe." She was surprised by their sense of invulnerability, which included a "haughty" superiority to the human race and a timeless viewpoint. "What is this? The Tree of Life or something?" she asked. They are like "a shaman in a bottle," she continued. I asked her to compare them with another medicine that contains dimethyltryptamine (DMT).

She said: "Ayahuasca encompasses all of creation, but the Bay Laurels encompass creation and eternity."

"How can you know all these things?" I asked. "When it doesn't involve me personally, I can get a readout," she replied. "That's how I was trained."

A week later, I had an interesting dream. I was on the side fighting for good against evil on Earth but we were losing until we made an alliance with two gnarly old Western gunfighters. Their names were "God the Father" and "Mother Earth." A week later I had another dream. The Bay Laurels said: "We aren't in charge of two worlds. We're in charge of three: Creation, eternity, and the human world."

I thought that was pretty cheeky, but years later it struck me as remarkable in a different way. The Bay Laurels put the human world on the same plane of comparison as creation and eternity.

Case Histories

A man in his twenties had very severe lifelong insomnia. The tongue was red, dry, and peeled in the stomach area, with a very red tip indicating heat rising and agitating the mind. The pulse was tense. Tincture of Bay Laurel semi-roasted nuts, 3 drops as needed. It was very effective and immediate, but the cure only lasted for a year and a half. I wasn't able to help further because he moved to a foreign country.

A twenty-nine-year-old woman felt terror every waking minute, she said. She suspected child abuse involving prescription drugs but couldn't pin anything down. She left home and wouldn't talk to her parents. She got married and was employed in a creative job. Finally, she blurted out: "I need something hallucinogenic." Oh. "I can help you there," I thought. I sent her a tincture of the semi-roasted Bay Laurel nut, 3 drops, 3x/day. Better from the first dose. After three months she emailed: "It seems to have worked completely." She still had no idea where the terror came from or what it meant.

Bay Laurel is not a full-fledged hallucinogen but because it contains DMT it acts deeply through dreamtime, daydreaming, and the imagination.

A middle-aged man suffered from extreme depression following the death of his seventeen-year-old son five years previously. Tincture of the semi-roasted nut of Bay Laurel caused a sensation like deep, terrible flu, body ache—he said he felt attacked by demons. Felt way better after two weeks, but stopped taking the medicine. Two months later, he was totally changed: joy, meaning, and creativity were restored to his life over the next several months. A medicine man diagnosed the cause of the death and the demonic oppression as witchcraft.

Here is another interesting case. After an accident, a woman had facial bones fragmented, broken into pieces, pieces missing, not setting, not healing; it felt like she was dying. Within an hour of the first dose, bones started going back into place, cheeks rising, forehead changing shape, feels like "I am getting my life back." Breathing easier. Less wheezing. Asthma better. Not cured of asthma and had many more serious problems to navigate, but the *Umbellularia* helped set bones. The lungs and heart needed surgery.

A woman with insomnia contacted me by email. I sent her semi-roasted nut tincture of Bay Laurel, recommending 3 drops, 1–3x/day. "The first night I was back home here—in Minneapolis/St. Paul—I slept for the first time in over a year from about 1 a.m. to 8 p.m., no wake-ups(!) A day of fully present. A gift. It was the second night in a row of half dropper of the California Bay Laurel tincture. It tastes like chocolate?" "Yes, it does," I responded. "It's so good. Thank you for the share." And: "I woke and thought along the lines of 'I just got a step up to my soul's path.' And then some poetic lines came to me which I wrote down."

I put one of my apprentices to work shelling and processing the Bay Laurel nuts:

While shelling the nuts, I began experiencing a flood of memories, embarrassing and shameful memories of my sexual exploits in my late teens and early twenties. I was a sexually compulsive and very wounded young woman who filled the void with sex. When I was shelling the Laurel nuts, these young men's faces appeared in my mind, as if rising from somewhere dark and buried and shameful.

She stopped and told me what she was experiencing. I told her to continue because "the medicine was working." She continued, "memories and tears flowing." The knife I gave her was dull, so it took a long time to chop the nuts. "I'm glad because I fell into a meditative state and began to feel full body and mind peace. I began singing my soul's song and I felt held and protected by the Laurel. I knew this was my plant guide. That's my middle name."

We made the tincture and she took some with her:

I have been taking 5 drops, 3x a day. The medicine helps me feel connected to the divine Creator, the divine in all things, the divine in me. I feel my anxiety melt away because I know I am held and guided. It opens my perspective and envelops me in universal connection. I know I will be okay when I take this medicine. It is as if a light from the heavens and a spirit from the underworld meet together in my body and unify me in the middle. It is the only thing that has ever removed my anxiety. It gives the long, long view.

Prophetic Medicine

In Native practice in the Pacific Northwest, the Bay Laurels and Ninebarks are considered by many to be the two most important medicine plants. The Bay Laurel nuts are used to understand past, present, and future. ("What do they know that we don't?") For prophecy and scrying, the shells are cracked open and the nuts are placed in water unroasted; they fall to the bottom. Read the top of the water. Skim it off to change the energetic. They are used for problems extending beyond the current lifetime, like long-term depression from "more than one lifetime." They are also used as catalysts in a formula or brew to get the other herbs to open up in the desired direction.

Evolution Medicine

The Bay Laurels shared with me the following story while we were doing our attunement in Berkeley:

Crackling lightning at the beginning of creation, across an ancient sky. An enormous dinosaur head is silhouetted against the horizon. Evolution begins. Life in the ocean arises onto the land. Plants, insects, flowers, amphibians and reptiles; sunshine, dinosaurs, animals, and finally humans appear. The Bay Laurels think the humans look funny because of their "floppy feet" and call them the "floppy-footed ones." They laugh at them, but then the humans break a taboo, which shocks Them, the Bay Laurels. "These creatures are not only awkward but crazy." The creation careens out of control. There is a dimension shift from creation to eternity. There is a table around which the Guardians of Creation usually sit, with charts and maps all over, as if planning the future of evolution. I have the feeling: They have just left the room a moment ago to avoid contact with a human.

The Great Mystery

Human nature is taken for granted but we are a Mystery People. We do not fully understand who we are. We possess faculties we have not yet guessed. Other capacities we do not possess will be acquired through exploration of consciousness. We will change in ways we cannot anticipate. The Bat People will affect our "spiritual genome." Plants will help us understand and develop ourselves. Bay Laurels will prod us along the path of evolution. Turtles will rise from the bottom of the sea to teach us while stars are falling from the sky. Dragons will befriend us. Even the greatest human teachers have not touched upon all our potentials. Nobody knows them all. We are spiritual voyageurs. We are a Mystery People. We are Mystery.

References

Austin, Mary Hunter. 1934. *Can Prayer Be Answered?* New York: Farrar and Rinehart.

Bach, Edward. 2011. *The Twelve Healers and Other Remedies.* Definitive edition. Brighton-cum-Sotwell, UK: Dr Edward Bach Centre.

Bahn, Paul. 2007. "Stone Horse and Papal Bull." *Sarguntum* 39: 141–46.

Ball, Edward. 1998. *Slaves in the Family.* New York: Ballantine.

Barford, Duncan. 2010. *Occult Experiments in the Home: Personal Explorations of Magick and the Paranormal.* London: Aeon.

Bartlett, Robert Allen. 2007. *Real Alchemy: A Primer of Practical Alchemy.* Lake Worth, FL: Ibis.

Bartram, William. 1955. *The Travels of William Bartram.* New York: Dover.

Bastine, Michael, and Mason Winfield. 2011. *Iroquois Supernatural: Talking Animals and Medicine People.* Rochester, VT: Bear and Company.

Benfey, O. Theodore. 1958. "August Kekulé and the Birth of the Structural Theory of Organic Chemistry in 1858." *Journal of Chemical Education* 35.1: 21–23.

Bennett, John G. 1976. *Gurdjieff: Making a New World.* London: Turnstone.

Bishop, Louise M. 2007. *Words, Stones and Herbs: The Healing Word in Medieval and Early Modern England.* Syracuse: Syracuse University Press.

Black Elk, Linda S. 1998. *Culturally Important Plants of the Lakota: Based on Interviews, Research, and a Comprehensive Review of Historical Documents.* Edited by Wilbur D. Flying By, Sr. Fort Yates, ND: Sitting Bull College.

Black Elk, Wallace, and William S. Lyon. 1991. *Black Elk: The Sacred Ways of a Lakota.* New York: HarperOne.

Blagrave, Joseph. 2010. *Blagrave's Astrological Practice of Physick.* Edited by David R. Roell. Bel Air, MD: Astrology Classics.

Blake, William. 1982. *The Complete Poetry and Prose of William Blake.* Edited by David V. Erdman; commentary by Harold Bloom. Revised edition. Berkeley and Los Angeles: University of California Press.

Blochwitz, Martin. 1677. *Anatomia sambuci, or, The Anatomy of the Elder Cutting Out of It Plain, Approved, and Specific Remedies for Most and Chiefest Maladies.* London: Brome and Sawbridge.

Bloom, Harold, and David Rosenberg. 1990. *The Book of J.* New York: Grove Weidenfeld.

Böhme [Boehme], Jacob. 1920. *Six Theosophic Points and Other Writings.* Translated by John Rolleston Earle. New York: Knopf.

———. 1969. *The Signature of All Things.* Cambridge: Clarke.

———. 2007. *Clavis or Key.* N.p.: Providence University.

Buhner, Stephen Harrod. 2004. *The Secret Teachings of Plants.* Rochester, VT: Bear and Company.

———. 2006. *Sacred Plant Medicine.* Rochester, VT: Bear and Company.

Burton, Elizabeth. 2012. *The Life and Times of Thomas of Ercildune: "The Rhymer."* Burnham-on-Sea, UK: Llanerch.

Cajete, Gregory, and LeRoy Little Bear. 1999. *Native Science: Natural Laws of Interdependence.* Santa Fe: Clear Light.

Cardano, Gerolamo. 2002. *The Book of My Life.* New York: New York Review of Books.

Castaneda, Carlos. 1968. *The Teachings of Don Juan: A Yaqui Way of Knowledge.* New York: Simon and Schuster.

———. 1985. *The Fire from Within.* New York: Pocket.

———. 1987. *The Power of Silence.* New York: Pocket.

———. 1993. *The Art of Dreaming.* New York: HarperCollins.

Chai, Makana Risser. 2011. "Huna, Max Freedom Long, and the Idealization of William Brigham." *Hawaiian Journal of History* 45: 101–21.

Clagett, Marshall. 1955. *Greek Science in Antiquity.* New York: Abelard-Schuman.

Clarke, John Henry. 1900–1903. *A Dictionary of Practical Materia Medica.* 3 vols. London: Homeopathic.

Clausewitz, Carl von. 1989. *On War.* Edited and translated by Michael Howard and Peter Paret. Princeton: Princeton University Press.

Clymer, R. Swinburne. 1963. *Nature's Healing Agents.* Philadelphia: Dorrance.

Coles, William. 1657. *Adam in Eden, or Nature's Paradise: The History of Plants, Fruits, Herbs, and Flowers.* London: Brooke.

Cook, William H. 1869. *The Physio-Medical Dispensatory: A Treatise on Therapeutics, Materia Medica, and Pharmacy, in Accordance with the Principle of Physiological Medication.* Cincinnati: Cook.

Cotton, John. 1641. *An Abstract or the Lawes of New England, as They Are Now Established*. London: Ley.

Cowan, Eliot. 2014. *Plant Spirit Medicine: A Journey in the Healing Wisdom of Plants*. Updated edition. Boulder: Sounds True.

Crellin, John K., and Jane Philpott. 1990. *A Reference Guide to Medicinal Plants: Herbal Medicine Past and Present*. Durham and London: Duke University Press.

Crowley, John. 1981. *Little Big*. New York: Harper Perennial.

Culpeper, Nicolas. 1652. *The English Physitian, or An Astrologo-physical Discourse of the Vulgar Herbs of this Nation*. London: Cole.

———. 1850. *The Complete Herbal*. New and enlarged edition. London: Kelly.

Damon, S. Foster. 1979. *A Blake Dictionary: The Ideas and Symbols of William Blake*. Boulder: Shambhala.

Dante Alighieri. 2001. *Inferno*. New York: Penguin.

De Angulo, Jaime. 1950. "Indians in Overalls." *The Hudson Review* 3.3 (Autumn): 327–77.

Densmore, Frances. 1974. *How Indians Use Wild Plants for Food, Medicine and Crafts*. New York: Dover.

Diffenbaugh, Vanessa. 2012. *The Language of Flowers: A Novel*. New York: Ballantine.

Dorson, Richard M. 1952. *Bloodstoppers and Bear Walkers: Folk Tales of Immigrants, Lumberjacks and Indians*. Cambridge, MA: Harvard University Press.

Douglass, Frederick. 1845. *Narrative of the Life of Frederick Douglass, An American Slave*. Boston: Anti-Slavery Office.

Dudley, Kim. 2012. Unfinished and unpublished writings on Yarrow and other subjects.

Eagle Feather, Ken. 2006. *On the Toltec Path: A Practical Guide to the Teachings of Don Juan Matus, Carlos Castaneda, and Other Toltec Seers*. Rochester, VT: Bear and Company.

Edwards, Lin. 2011. "Brewery from 500 BC Reveals Its Secrets." Phys.org website.

Eliade, Mircea. 1964. *Shamanism: Archaic Techniques of Ecstasy*. Translated by Willard R. Trask. Princeton: Princeton University Press.

English, Ali. 2019. *Wild Medicine: Summer*. London: Aeon.

Evans, Zabrina N., and Samuel J. Stellpflug. 2012. "Holiday Plants with Toxic Misconceptions." *Western Journal of Emergency Medicine* 13.6 (Dec.): 538–42.

Firstenberg, Arthur. 2020. *The Invisible Rainbow: A History of Electricity and Life*. White River Junction, VT: Chelsea Green.

Folkard, Richard. 1884. *Plant Lore, Legends, and Lyrics*. London: Sampson Low, Marston, Searles, and Livington.

Fought, Emily. 2020. "The Rare Medicine Hat Horse." Cowgirl Magazine website.

Franz, Marie-Louise von. 1980. *Alchemy: An Introduction to the Symbolism and the Psychology*. Toronto: Inner City.

Freud, Sigmund. 1969. *An Outline of Psycho-Analysis*. Translated and edited by James Strachey. Revised edition. New York: Norton.

Fruehauf, Heiner. 2016. "Huangjing (Rhizome Polygonati)." ClassicalChinese Medicine website, September 1, 2019.

Garrett, J. T. 2003. *The Cherokee Herbal: Native Plant Medicine from the Four Directions*. Rochester, VT: Bear and Company.

Gerard, John. 1975 [1633]. *The Herbal or General History of Plants*. Facsimile of the 1633 edition revised and enlarged by Thomas Johnson. New York: Dover.

Gillette, Douglas. 1997. *The Shaman's Secret: The Lost Resurrection Teachings of the Ancient Maya*. New York: Bantam.

Gilmore, Melvin R. 1991. *Uses of Plants by the Indians of the Missouri River Region*. Lincoln, NE: Bison.

Ginsberg, Allen. 1986 [1956]. *Howl*. Facsimile edition edited by Barry Miles. New York: HarperCollins.

Green, Thomas. 1824. *The Universal Herbal: or, Botanical, Medical, and Agricultural Dictionary*. 2 vols. London: Caxton.

Grieve, Maud. 1994. *A Modern Herbal*. London: Tiger. Facsimile of 1931 edition.

Griggs, Barbara. 1981. *Green Pharmacy: A History of Herbal Medicine*. London: Norman and Hobhouse.

Gunther, Robert T., ed. 1968. *The Greek Herbal of Dioscorides: Illustrated by a Byzantine A.D. 512, Englished by John Goodyer A.D. 1655*. New York: Hafner. [Fascimile of 1934 edition.]

Hall, Calvin S., and Vernon J. Nordby. 1973. *A Primer of Jungian Psychology*. New York: Penguin.

Hall, Dorothy. 1988. *Creating Your Herbal Profile*. New Canaan, CT.: Keats. [U.S. edition of *Dorothy Hall's Herbal Medicine*. Melbourne: Lothian, 1988.]

Hall, Samuel, et al. 2023. "Risk of Aneurysm Rupture (ROAR) Study: Protocol for a Long-term, Longitudinal, UK Multicentre Study of Unruptured Intracranial Aneurysms." *BMJ Open* 13(3): 1–7.

Harner, Michael. 1990. *The Way of the Shaman*. Tenth anniversary edition. New York: HarperCollins.

Harris, Ben Charles. 1975. *The Compleat Herbal.* New York: Larchmont.

Hedsel, Mark. 1999. *The Zelator: The Secret Journals of Mark Hedsel.* Edited by David Ovason. London: Arrow.

Hill, John. 1755. *The Useful Family Herbal, or, An Account of All Those English Plants, Which Are Remarkable for Their Virtues and of the Drugs, Which Are Produced by Vegetable of Other Countries.* Second edition. London: Johnston and Owen.

Hoffmann, David. 1992. *The New Holistic Herbal: A Herbal Celebrating the Wholeness of Life.* Rockport, MA: Element.

Hool, Richard. 1918. *Health from British Wild Herbs: A Guide to the Most Common and Most Useful Non-poisonous British Wild Herbs, and Their Medicinal Virtues and Applications to Various Complaints.* Republished online at Henriette's Herbal Homepage website, December 11, 2023.

———. 1922. *Common Plants and Their Uses in Medicine.* Republished online at Henriette's Herbal Homepage website, December 11, 2023.

Horowitz, Mitch. 2009. *Occult America: The Secret History of How Mysticism Shaped Our Nation.* New York: Bantam.

Howe, E. Graham. 2012. *The Druid of Harley Street: The Spiritual Psychology of E. Graham Howe.* Edited by William Stranger. Berkeley, CA: North Atlantic.

Huang, Huang. 2009. *Zhang Zhong-jing's Clinical Application of 50 Medicinals.* Third edition. Beijing: People's Medical.

Inagawa, Tetsuji. 2022. "Prevalence of Cerebral Aneurysms in Autopsy Studies: A Review of the Literature." *Neurosurgical Review* 45 (5496): 1–18.

Ingraham, Sandra, and Hank Wesselman. 2010. *Awakening to the Spirit World: The Shamanic Path of Direct Revelation.* Boulder: Sounds True.

Jacobi, Jolande. 1971. *Complex/Archetype/Symbol in the Psychology of C. G. Jung.* Princeton: Princeton University Press.

Jenkins, Philip. 2004. *Dream Catchers: How Mainstream America Discovered Native Spirituality.* Oxford: Oxford University Press.

Jeremias, Joachim. 1971. *New Testament Theology.* London: SCM.

Jung, Carl Gustav. 1954. *The Development of Personality.* Translated by R. F. C. Hull. Princeton: Princeton University Press.

———. 1977. *Mysterium Coniunctionis.* Second edition. Princeton: Princeton University Press.

———. 1993. *Psychology and Alchemy.* Princeton: Princeton University Press.

Kaehr, Shelley. 2002. *Origins of Huna: Secret Behind the Secret Science.* Dallas, TX: Out of This World.

Kampenhout, Daan van. 2008. *The Tears of the Ancestors: Victims and Perpetrators in the Tribal Soul.* Phoenix: Zeig, Tucker and Theissen.

Keneally, Thomas. 1993. *Schindler's List*. New York: Simon and Schuster.

Kharitidi, Olga. 1997. *Entering the Circle: Ancient Secrets of Siberian Wisdom*. San Francisco: Harper.

———. *The Master of Lucid Dreams*. 2001. Charlottesville, VA: Hampton Roads.

Kline, Jacob. 1992. *Greek Mathematical Thought and the Origin of Algebra*. New York: Dover.

Knab, Timothy J. 1995. *A War of the Witches: Journey into the World of the Contemporary Aztecs*. San Francisco: HarperSanFrancisco.

Knight, Katherine. 2006. *How Shakespeare Cleaned His Teeth and Cromwell Treated His Warts*. Stroud, UK: Tempus.

Konstantinos. 2010. *Werewolves: The Occult Truth*. Woodbury, MN: Llewellyn.

Krebs, Ernest T. 1920. "An Indian Remedy for Influenza." *Bulletin of the Nevada State Board of Health* (January): 7–9.

Kuhn, Thomas S. 1970. *The Structure of Scientific Revolutions*. Second edition. Chicago: University of Chicago Press.

Kimmerer, Robin Wall. 2013. *Braiding Sweetgrass: Indigenous Wisdom, Scientific Knowledge, and the Teachings of Plants*. Minneapolis: Milkweed.

Lake-Thom, Bobby. 1997. *Spirits of the Earth: A Guide to Native American Nature Symbols, Stories, and Ceremonies*. New York: Plume.

Lama, Luis De La. 1993. *The Heart of the Serpent: Mystical Journeys to the Core of Life*. Raleigh, NC: White Dragon.

Lecouteux, Claude. 2003. *Witches, Werewolves, and Fairies: Shapeshifters and Astral Doubles in the Middle Ages*. Rochester, VT: Inner Traditions.

Levin, David. 1960. *What Happened in Salem?* Second edition. New York: Harcourt, Brace and World.

Lewis, Arthur H. 1969. *Hex*. New York: Trident.

Libby, Walter. 1922. "The Scientific Imagination." *The Scientific Monthly* 15.3 (September): 263–70.

Light, Phyllis D. 2018. *Southern Folk Medicine*. Berkeley: North Atlantic.

Long, Max Freedom. 1954. *The Secret Science Behind Miracles*. Ninth edition. Marina del Rey, CA: DeVorss.

Luna, Eduardo Luis. 1984. "The Concept of Plants as Teachers Among Four Mestizo Shamans of Iquitos, Northeastern Peru." *Journal of Ethnopharmacology* 11: 135–56.

Luo, "George" Guangxiang, The Conversation US, Shou-Jiang Gap, and Haitao Guo. 2020. "Snakes Could Be the Original Source of the New Coronavirus Outbreak in China." *Scientific American* website. 22 January 2020.

Maletic, Vladimir, and Charles Raison. 2017. *The New Mind-Body Science of Depression*. New York: Norton.

Marchant, Carolyn. 1990. *The Death of Nature; Women, Ecology and the Scientific Revolution*. San Francisco: HarperSanFrancisco.

Mares, Théun. 1998. *The Mists of Dragon Lore: The Toltec Teachings*. Cape Town: Lionheart.

Mattioli, Pietro Andrea. 1590. *Kruetterbuch*. Frankfurt am Main: Feyrabendt.

McGaughey, Douglas R. 2016. "What is Critical Idealism? Critical Idealism: A Brief Introduction." Criticalidealism website, December 11, 2023.

McKenna, Terence. 1992. *Food of the Gods—The Search for the Original Tree of Knowledge: A Radical History of Plants, Drugs, and Human Evolution*. New York: Bantam.

———. 2010a. "Hermeticism and Alchemy," part 3. Podcast 225. Psychedelic Salon website, December 11, 2023.

———. 2010b. "Empowering Hope in Dark Times." Podcast 211. Psychedelic Salon website, December 11, 2023.

———. 2010c. "Under the Teaching Tree," part. 1. Podcast 215. Psychedelic Salon website, December 11, 2023.

———. 2016. "The Purpose of Psychedelics." Recorded lecture. Be Here Now channel, YouTube website, December 11, 2023.

Mees, L. F. C. 1973. *Drugs: A Danger for Human Evolution?* London and New York: Regency.

Mességué, Maurice. 1991. *Of People and Plants: The Autobiography of Europe's Most Celebrated Healer*. Rochester, VT: Healing Arts.

Metzner, Ralph. 1998. *The Unfolding Self: Varieties of Transformative Experience*. Novato, CA: Origin.

Meyer, Joseph E. 1953. *The Herbalist*. Hammond, IN: Indiana Botanic Gardens.

Milton, Richard. 1994. *Alternative Science: Challenging the Myths of the Scientific Establishment*. Rochester, VT: Park Street.

Moss, Robert. 2012. *Dreaming the Soul Back Home: Shamanic Dreaming for Healing and Becoming Whole*. Novato, CA: New World Library.

Müller, K., K. Ziereis, and D. H. Paper. 1998. "Ilex Aquifolium: Protection Against Enzymatic and Non-Enzymatic Lipid Peroxidation." *Planta Medica* 64.06 (Aug.): 536–40.

Narby, Jeremy. 1998. *The Cosmic Serpent: DNA and the Origins of Knowledge*. New York: Tarcher/Putnam.

Narby, Jeremy, and Francis Huxley, eds. 2001. *Shamans Through Time: 500 Years on the Path to Knowledge*. New York: Tarcher/Putnam.

Neihardt, John G. 1988. *Black Elk Speaks: Being the Life Story of a Holy Man of the Oglala Sioux*. Lincoln: University of Nebraska Press.

Nesfield-Cookson, Bernard. 1987. *William Blake: Prophet of Universal Brotherhood*. London: Crucible.

Nguyen, Ha Thi Thanh, et al. 2016. "Pharmacological Characteristics of *Artemisia vulgaris L.* in Isolated Porcine Basilar Artery." *Journal of Ethnopharmacology* 182 (22 April): 16–26. [Online version available on ScienceDirect website.]

Okely, Francis, trans. *Memoirs of the Life, Death, Burial, and Wonderful Writings, of Jacob Behmen*. Northampton: Lackington, 1780.

Olivet, Fabre d'. 1921. *The Hebraic Tongue Restored and the True Meaning of the Hebrew Words Re-established and Proved by their Radical Analysis*. Translated by Nayán Louise Redfield. New York: Putnam and Sons.

Paracelsus [Theophrastus Bombastus von Hohenheim]. 1894. *The Hermetic and Alchemical Writings of Paracelsus*. Translated by Arthur Edward Waite. 2 vols. London: Elliot.

———. 2008. *Essential Theoretical Writings*. Edited and translated by Andrew Weeks. Leiden: Brill.

Patterson, William Patrick. 2008. *The Life and Teachings of Carlos Castaneda. Including Daniel Brinton's 1894 essay "Nagualism: A Study in Native American Folklore and History."* Fairfax, CA: Arete.

Pelikan, Wilhelm. 1973. *The Secrets of Metals*. Translated by Charlotte Lebensart. Great Barrington, MA: Lindisfarne.

Place, Robert M. 2005. *The Tarot: History, Symbolism, and Divination*. New York: Tarcher.

Pokagon, Simon. 1896. "An Indian's Observation on the Mating of Geese. *The Arena* 16 (July): 245–48.

Pollack, Gerald H. 2013. *The Fourth Phase of Water: Beyond Solid, Liquid, and Vapor*. Seattle: Ebner and Sons.

Popham, Sajah. N.d. "Calendula (*Calendula officinalis*)." HerbRally website, December 11, 2023.

Pullman, Philip. 2000. *The Golden Compass: His Dark Materials*. New York: Scholastic.

Purucker, Gottfried de. 1932. *Fundamentals of the Esoteric Philosophy*. London: Rider.

Quinn, D. Michael. 1987. *Early Mormonism and the Magic Worldview*. Salt Lake City: Signature.

Raleigh, Albert Sidney. 1916. *The Shepherd of Men: An Official Commentary on the Sermon of Hermes Trismegistos*. San Francisco: Hermetic.

———. 1928. *Hermetic Consciousness Unveiled*. Chicago: Hermetic.

———. 1929. *The Lakshmi Avatar: Lakshmi: The Gopis*. Chicago: Hermetic.

————. 1932. *An Interpretation to Rudyard Kipling's* They. Chicago: Hermetic.

Randolph, Paschal Beverly 1930. *Seership: Guide to Soul Sight.* Quakertown, PA: Confederation of Initiates.

Raphael, Alice. 1965. *Goethe and the Philosophers' Stone: Symbolical Patterns in "The Parable" and the Second Part of "Faust."* New York: Garrett.

Rumi [Jalal Al-Din Rumi]. 1997. *The Illuminated Rumi.* Translated by Coleman Barks; illustrated by Michael Green. New York: Doubleday.

Sahtouris, Elisabet. 2000. *EarthDance: Living Systems in Evolution.* San Jose: iUniversity.

Salaman, Clement, Dorine van Oyen, William D. Wharton, and Jean-Pierre Mahe, trans. 2000. *The Way of Hermes: New Translations of* The Corpus Hermeticum *and* The Definitions of Hermes Trismegistus to Asclepius. Rochester, VT: Inner Traditions.

Schelling, Andrew. 2017. *Tracks Along the Left Coast: Jaime de Angulo and Pacific Coast Culture.* Berkeley, CA: Counterpoint.

Schoch, Robert. 2014. "The Roots of Kahunaism: Is This the Legacy of Ancient Egyptian Magic?" *Atlantis Rising* 106 (July–August).

Shipard, Isabell. 2016. *How Can I Use Herbs in My Daily Life?: Over 500 Herbs, Spices and Edible Plants: An Australian Practical Guide to Growing Culinary and Medicinal Herbs.* Nambour: Stewart.

Singh, Pryanka, et al. 2020. "Shikimic Acid as Intermediary Model for the Production of Drugs Effective against Influenza Virus." In *Phytochemicals as Lead Compounds for New Drug Discovery*, edited by Chukwuebuka Egbuna, et al, 245–56. Amsterdam: Elsevier.

Smoley, Richard, and Jay Kinney. 2006. *Hidden Wisdom: A Guide to the Western Inner Traditions.* Revised edition. Wheaton, IL: Quest.

Steiner, Rudolf. 1914. An Outline of Occult Science. London: Theosophical Publishing Society.

————. 1947. *Knowledge of the Higher Worlds and Its Attainment.* Hudson, NY: Anthroposophic.

————. 1972. *An Outline of Occult Science.* Translated by Maud B. and Henry B. Monges. Revised by Lisa D. Monges. Spring Valley, NY: Anthroposophic.

————. 1973. *Mystery Knowledge and Mystery Centres.* Translation revised by Pauline Wehrle; edited by Andrew Welburn. London: Rudolf Steiner.

————. 1994. *Theosophy: An Introduction to the Spiritual Processes in Human Life and in the Cosmos.* Translated by Catherine E. Creeger. Hudson, NY: Anthroposophic.

————. 1995. *Intuitive Thinking as a Spiritual Path: A Philosophy of Freedom.* Translated by Michael Lipson. Hudson, NY: Anthroposophic.

——. 2003. *Genesis: Secrets of Creation: The First Book of Moses.* Translated by Pauline Wehrle. London: Rudolf Steiner.

——. 2014. *The World of the Senses and the World of the Spirit.* Translated by Johanna Collis. London: Rudolf Steiner.

Stewart, R. J. 1989. *The UnderWorld Initiation: A Journey Towards Psychic Transformation.* Wellingborough, UK: Aquarian.

Storl, Wolf D. [Dieter]. 2010. *Healing Lyme Disease Naturally: History, Analysis, and Treatments.* Berkeley, CA: North Atlantic.

——. 2018. *Bear: Myth, Animal, Icon.* Berkeley, CA: North Atlantic.

——. 2024. *The Heart and Its Healing Plants: Traditional Herbal Remedies and Modern Heart Conditions.* Translated by Christine Storl. Rochester, VT: Healing Arts Press.

Strassman, Rick. 2001. *DMT The Spirit Molecule: A Doctor's Revolutionary Research into the Biology of Near-Death and Mystical Experiences.* Rochester, VT: Park Street.

Summers, Montague. 1966. *The Werewolf.* New York: Bell.

Sun Bear and Wabun. 1980. *The Medicine Wheel: Earth Astrology.* New York: Simon and Shuster.

Thompson, C. S. J. 1934. *The Mystic Mandrake.* London: Rider.

Tierra, Michael. 1988. *Planetary Herbology: An Integration of Western Herbs into the Traditional Chinese and Ayurvedic Systems.* Edited and supplemented by David Frawley; supplemented by Christopher Hobbs. Twin Lakes, WI: Lotus.

Tierra, Michael, and Lesley Tierra. 1998. *Traditional Chinese Herbal Medicine.* 2 vols. Twin Lakes, WI: Lotus.

Tolkien, J. R. R. 2001. *The Fellowship of the Ring.* New York: Quality Paperback Book Club.

Traill, H. D., and J. S. Mann. 1901–1904. *Social England: A Record of the Progress of the People in Religion, Laws, Learning Arts, Industry, Commerce, Science, Literature and Manners from the Earliest Times to the Present Day.* 6 vols. London: Cassell.

Treben, Maria. 1984. *Health through God's Pharmacy: Advice and Experiences with Herbs.* Steyr: Ennsthaler.

Tunneshende, Merilyn. 2001. *Don Juan and the Art of Sexual Energy: The Rainbow Serpent of the Toltecs.* Rochester, VT: Bear and Company.

——. 2002. *Don Juan and the Power of Medicine Dreaming: A Nagual Woman's Journey of Healing.* Rochester, VT: Bear and Company.

——. 2004. *Twilight Language of the Nagual: The Spiritual Power of Shamanic Dreaming.* Rochester, VT: Bear and Company.

Turner, William. 1996. *A New Herball.* Edited by George T. L. Chapman, Frank McCombie, Marilyn N. Tweddle, and Anne U. Wesencraft. 2 vols. Cambridge: Cambridge University Press.

Uyldert, Mellie. 1980. *The Psychic Garden: Plants and Their Esoteric Relationship with Man.* Wellingborough, UK: Thorsons.

Vaughan, Thomas. 1968. *The Works of Thomas Vaughan: Mystic and Alchemist.* Edited by Arthur Edward Waite. New Hyde Park, NJ: University.

Vogel, Virgil J. 1970. *American Indian Medicine.* Norman, OK: University of Oklahoma Press.

Waley, Arthur. 1939. *Three Ways of Thought in Ancient China.* London: Routledge.

Wallace, Amy. 1968. *Soma: Divine Mushroom of Immortality.* New York: Harcourt Brace Jovanovich.

———. 2003. *Sorcerer's Apprentice: My Life with Carlos Castaneda.* Berkeley: Frog.

Waters, Frank. 1969. *Book of the Hopi.* New York: Ballantine.

Wesselman, Hank. 1995. *Spirit-Walker: Messages from the Future.* New York: Bantam.

Wilson, Colin. 2006. *Atlantis and the Kingdom of the Neanderthals: 100,000 Years of Lost History.* Rochester, VT: Bear and Company.

Winston, David, and Steve Maimes. 2007. *Adaptogens.* Rochester, VT: Healing Arts.

Wood, Matthew. 1987. *Seven Herbs: Plants as Teachers.* Berkeley, CA: North Atlantic.

———. 1997. *The Book of Herbal Wisdom: Using Plants as Medicines.* Berkeley, CA: North Atlantic.

———. 2006. "Different Kinds of Science in Relationship to Western Herbal Medicine." Dissertation, Master of Science Degree (Herbal Medicine), Scottish School of Herbal Medicine, University of Wales.

———. 2008–2009. *The Earthwise Herbal.* 2 vols. Berkeley, CA: North Atlantic.

———. 2021a. *Holistic Medicine and the Extracellular Matrix: The Science of Healing at the Cellular Level.* Rochester, VT: Healing Arts.

———. 2021b. *Seven Guideposts on the Spiritual Path: The Shamanic Story in Genesis.* N.p.: Matthew Wood Institute of Herbalism.

Wood, Matthew, with David Ryan. 2016. *The Earthwise Herbal Repertory: The Definitive Practitioner's Guide.* Berkeley, CA: North Atlantic.

Yance, Donald. 2013. *Adaptogens in Medical Herbalism.* Rochester, VT: Inner Traditions.

Young, William P. 2007. *The Shack.* Newbury Park, CA: Windblown Media.

Zolla, Elémire. 1982. *Archetypes: The Persistence of Unifying Patterns.* New York: Harcourt, Brace Jovanovich.

Index